Lecture Notes

Endocrinology and Diabetes

Amir Sam

BSc (Hons), MB BS (Hons), MRCP
Wellcome Trust Clinical Research Fellow and SpR in Endocrinology and
  Diabetes, Hammersmith Hospital, Imperial College, London, UK

Karim Meeran

MD, FRCP, FRCPath
Professor of Endocrinology, Imperial College Healthcare NHS Trust,
  London, UK

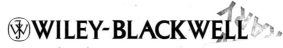

WILEY-BLACKWELL

A John Wiley & Sons, Inc., Publication

D0549757

Library of Congress Cataloging-in-Publication Data

Sam, Amir H.
  Lecture notes. Endocrinology and diabetes / Amir Sam, Karim Meeran.
    p. ; cm.
  Includes index.
  ISBN 978-1-4051-5345-4 (pbk. : alk. paper)
  1. Endocrinology–Outlines, syllabi, etc. 2. Diabetes–Outlines, syllabi, etc. 3. Endocrine glands–Diseases–Outlines, syllabi, etc. I. Meeran, Karim. II. Title. III. Title: Endocrinology and diabetes.

  [DNLM: 1. Endocrine System Diseases. 2. Diabetes Mellitus. WK 140 S187L 2009]
  RC649.S26 2009
  616.4–dc22
                        2009002846

ISBN: 9781405153454

A catalogue record for this book is available from the British Library.

Set in 8 on 12 pt Stone Serif by SNP Best-set Typesetter Ltd., Hong Kong
Printed and bound in Singapore by Ho Printing Singapore Pte Ltd

1 2009

Contents

Preface

In the conception of this book, we used our teaching experience to cover the main topics in endocrinology and diabetes in a simple and easy-to-understand style.

We have tried to discuss the basic anatomy and physiology of the endocrine system, which is fundamental to the understanding of pathophysiology and presentation of the endocrine diseases. *Lecture Notes: Endocrinology and Diabetes* also contains detailed sections on the practical management of diabetes and endocrine disorders. Therefore we believe that this book is suitable for medical students and doctors training in endocrinology, and can be used for exam revision as well as rapid consultation in the clinic.

Amir Sam
Karim Meeran

Acknowledgements

We are grateful to Mr Fausto Palazzo, Dr Roberto Dina, Professor Pierre-Marc Bouloux, Dr John Frank and Dr Owais Chaudhri for kindly providing some of the illustrations used in this book. Additionally, we would like to express our thanks to Dr Kevin Shotliff and John Wiley & Sons for the diabetic retinopathy images used in Chapter 37, which were taken from *Practical Diabetes International*, Volume 23, pages 418–20. We are also grateful to Dr Waljit Dhillo, Dr Victoria Salem and Dr Sufyan Hussain for their useful advice.

Abbreviations

5-HIAA 5-hydroxyindoleacetic acid
ABPI ankle–brachial pressure index
ACCORD Action to Control Cardiovascular Risk in Diabetes trial
ACE angiotensin-converting enzyme
ACR albumin-to-creatinine ratio
ACTH adrenocorticotrophic hormone
ADH antidiuretic hormone
ADVANCE Action in Diabetes and Vascular Disease: Preterax and Diamicron MR Controlled Evaluation trial
AGB adjustable gastric banding
AGE advanced glycosylation end-product
AHO Albright's hereditary osteodystrophy
AIDS acquired immune deficiency syndrome
ALT alanine transaminase
AMPK adenosine monophosphate-activated protein kinase
APS autoimmune polyglandular syndrome
ARB angiotensin receptor blocker
AVP arginine vasopressin
BFGF basic fibroblast growth factor
BMD bone mineral density
BMI body mass index
BMP-7 bone morphogenic protein-7
CAH congenital adrenal hyperplasia
CARDS Collaborative AtoRvastatin Diabetes Study
CARE Cholesterol and Recurrent Events trial
CDGP constitutional delay of growth and puberty
CEA carcinoembryonic antigen
CNS central nervous system
CPT I carnitine palmitoyltransferase-I
CRH corticotrophin-releasing hormone
CSW cerebral salt wasting
CT computed tomography
CTLA-4 cytotoxic T-lymphocyte antigen 4
CVD cardiovascular disease
DAFNE Dose Adjustment for Normal Eating

DCCT Diabetes Control and Complications Trial
DEXA dual-energy X-ray absorptiometry
DHEA dehydroepiandrosterone
DHEA-S dehydroepiandrosterone sulphate
DIEP Diabetes in Early Pregnancy study
DKA diabetic ketoacidosis
DMSA dimercaptosuccinic acid
DPP-IV dipeptidyl peptidase-IV
ECG electrocardiogram
EDIC Epidemiology of Diabetes Interventions and Complications study
eGFR estimated glomerular filtration rate
ESR erythrocyte sedimentation rate
ESRD end-stage renal disease
FIELD Fenofibrate Intervention and Event Lowering in Diabetes study
FNA fine needle aspiration
FSH follicle-stimulating hormone
GAD glutamic acid decarboxylase
GEMINI Glycemic Effects in Diabetes Mellitus: Carvedilol-Metoprolol Comparison in Hypertensives
GFR glomerular filtration rate
GH growth hormone
GHRH growth hormone-releasing hormone
GLP-1 glucagon-like peptide-1
GSH glucocorticoid-suppressible hyperaldosteronism
HbA$_{1c}$ glycated haemoglobin
hCG human chorionic gonadotrophin
HDL high-density lipoprotein
HHS hyperosmolar hyperglycaemic state
HIF hypoxia-inducible factor
HIV human immunodeficiency virus
HPA hypothalamic–pituitary–adrenal
HRT hormone replacement therapy
ICSI intracytoplasmic sperm injection
IGF-I insulin-like growth factor-I
IGFBP-3 insulin-like growth factor-binding protein-3

IRMA intraretinal microvascular abnormality
IRS insulin receptor substrate
ITT insulin tolerance test
IVF in vitro fertilization
JNK c-Jun amino-terminal kinase
LADA latent autoimmune diabetes in adults
LDL low-density lipoprotein
LH luteinizing hormone
MAPK mitogen-activated protein kinase
MC4R melanocortin-4 receptor
MDRD Modification of Diet in Renal Disease study
MEN multiple endocrine neoplasia
MI myocardial infarction
MODY maturity-onset diabetes of the young
MRI magnetic resonance imaging
MSH melanocyte-stimulating hormone
MTC medullary thyroid carcinoma
NET neuroendocrine tumour
NF neurofibromatosis
NPH neutral protamine Hagedorn
NSAID non-steroidal anti-inflammatory drug
NSC National Screening Committee
NVD new vessels on disc
NVE new vessels elsewhere
OGTT oral glucose tolerance test
PAC plasma aldosterone concentration
PCOS polycystic ovary syndrome
POMC proopiomelanocortin
POPADAD Prevention of Progression of Arterial Disease and Diabetes study
PPAR peroxisome proliferator-activated receptor
PPNAD primary pigmented nodular adrenocortical disease

PRA plasma renin activity
PSA prostate-specific antigen
PTH parathyroid hormone
PTTG pituitary tumour transforming gene
PTU propylthiouracil
PYY peptide YY
RANK receptor activator of nuclear factor kappa B
RANKL RANK ligand
RYGB roux-en-Y gastric bypass
SD standard deviation
SDHB succinate dehydrogenase subunit B
SG specific gravity
SHBG sex hormone-binding globulin
SIADH syndrome of inappropriate antidiuretic hormone
SOS Swedish Obese Subjects study
SRS somatostatin receptor scintigraphy
StAR steroidogenic acute regulatory protein
STAT signal transduction and activators of transcription
T$_3$ triiodothyronine
T$_4$ thyroxine
TGF transforming growth factor
TNF tumour necrosis factor
TRAb thyroid-stimulating hormone receptor antibody
TRH thyrotrophin-releasing hormone
TSH thyroid-stimulating hormone
UKPDS United Kingdom Prospective Diabetes Study
VEGF vascular endothelial growth factor
WHI Women's Health Initiative trials
WHO World Health Organization

Chapter 1

Thyroid anatomy and physiology

Anatomy

The thyroid gland consists of left and right *lobes* connected by a midline isthmus (Fig. 1.1). The isthmus lies below the cricoid cartilage, and the lobes extend upward over the lower half of the thyroid cartilage. The thyroid is covered by the strap muscles of the neck and overlapped by the sterno-cleidomastoids. The pretracheal fascia encloses the thyroid gland and attaches it to the larynx and the trachea. This accounts for the upward movement of the thyroid gland on swallowing.

The thyroid gland develops from the floor of the pharynx in the position of the foramen caecum of the adult tongue as a downgrowth that descends into the neck. During this descent, the thyroid gland remains connected to the tongue by the thyroglossal duct, which later disappears. However, aberrant thyroid tissue or thyroglossal cysts (cystic remnants of the thyroglossal duct) may occur anywhere along the course of the duct (Fig. 1.2). Such thyroid remnants move upward when the tongue is protruded.

The thyroid gland is composed of epithelial spheres called *follicles* (Fig 1.3), whose lumens are filled with a proteinaceous colloid containing *thyroglobulin*. Two basic cell types are present in the

follicles. The follicular cells secrete thyroxine (T_4) and triiodothyronine (T_3) and originate from a downward growth of the endoderm of the floor of the pharynx (see above). The parafollicular or C cells secrete calcitonin and arise from neural crest cells that migrate into the developing thyroid gland. The follicles are surrounded by an extensive capillary network.

Physiology

Thyroid hormones act on many tissues. They regulate:
- organogenesis, growth and development (central nervous system, bone)
- energy expenditure
- protein, carbohydrate and fat metabolism
- gut motility
- bone turnover
- heart rate and contractility, and peripheral vascular resistance
- beta-adrenergic receptor expression
- muscle contraction and relaxation
- the menstrual cycle
- erythropoiesis.

Iodine is essential for normal thyroid function. It is obtained by the ingestion of foods such as seafood, seaweed, kelp, dairy products, some vegetables and iodized salt. The recommended iodine intake for adults is 150 µg per day (250 µg per day for pregnant and lactating women). Dietary iodine

Lecture Notes: Endocrinology and Diabetes. By A. Sam and K. Meeran. Published 2009 by Blackwell Publishing. ISBN 978-1-4051-5345-4.

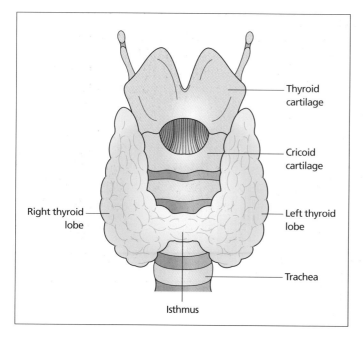

Figure 1.1 Thyroid gland.

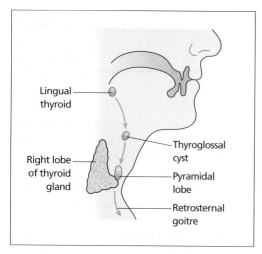

Figure 1.2 Possible sites of remnants of the thyroglossal duct.

is absorbed as iodide. Iodide is excreted in the urine.

Thyroid hormone synthesis

Figure 1.4 illustrates different steps in thyroid hormone synthesis:

- *Thyroglobulin* is synthesized in the rough endoplasmic reticulum and is transported into the follicular lumen by exocytosis.
- Iodide is transported into the thyroid follicular cells via a sodium–iodide symporter on the basolateral membrane of the follicular cells. Iodide transport requires oxidative metabolism.
- Inside the follicular cells, iodide diffuses to the apical surface and is transported by pendrin (a membrane iodide–chloride transporter) into the follicular lumen.
- *Thyroid peroxidase* (TPO) enzyme catalyzes the process of oxidation of the iodide to iodine and its binding (organification) to the tyrosine residues of thyroglobulin to form monoiodotyrosine (MIT) and diiodotyrosine (DIT).
- DIT and MIT molecules are linked by TPO to form *thyroxine* (T_4) and *triiodothyronine* (T_3) in a process known as coupling.
- Thyroglobulin containing T_4 and T_3 is resorbed into the follicular cells by endocytosis and is cleaved by lysosomal enzymes (proteases and peptidases) to release T_4 and T_3. T_4 and T_3 are then secreted into the circulation.
- Uncoupled MIT and DIT are deiodinated, and the free tyrosine and iodide are recycled.

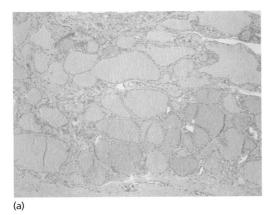

(a)

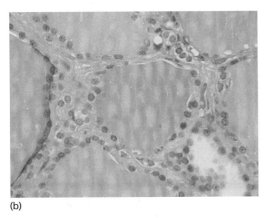

(b)

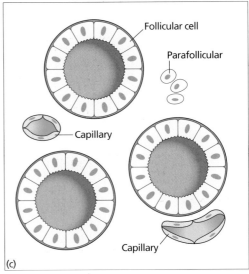

(c)

Figure 1.3 (a) A low-power histological image of thyroid tissue showing numerous follicles filled with colloid and lined by cuboidal epithelium. (b) A high-power view of follicles lined by cuboidal epithelium. (c) Thyroid follicles (lined by follicular cells), surrounding capillaries and parafollicular cells.

The thyroid gland stores T_4 and T_3 incorporated in thyroglobulin, and can therefore secrete T_4 and T_3 more quickly than if they had to be synthesized.

Extra-thyroidal T₃ production

T_4 is produced entirely by the thyroid gland. The production rate of T_4 is about 100 μg per day. However, only 20% of T_3 is produced directly by the thyroid gland (by coupling of MIT and DIT). Around 80% of T_3 is produced by the deiodination of T_4 in peripheral extra-thyroidal tissues (mainly liver and kidney). The total daily production rate of T_3 is about 35 μg.

T_4 is converted to T_3 (the biologically active metabolite) by *5'-deiodination* (outer-ring deiodination). 5'-Deiodination is mediated by deiodinases type 1 (D1) and type 2 (D2). D1 is the predominant deiodinating enzyme in the liver, kidney and thyroid. D2 is the predominant deiodinating enzyme in muscle, brain, pituitary, skin and placenta. Type 3 deiodinase (D3) catalyzes the conversion of T_3 to reverse T_3 (the inactive metabolite) by 5-deiodination (inner ring deiodination), as shown in Fig. 1.5.

Changes in T_3 concentration may indicate a change in the rate of peripheral conversion and may not be an accurate measure of the change in thyroid hormone production. For example, the rate of T_3 production (by 5'-deiodination of T_4) is reduced in acute illness and starvation.

Total and free T₄ and T₃

Approximately 99.97% of circulating T_4 and 99.7% of circulating T_3 are bound to plasma proteins: *thyroid-binding globulin* (TBG), *transthyretin* (also

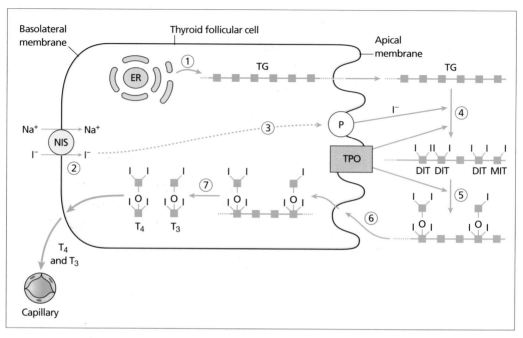

Figure 1.4 Steps in thyroid hormone synthesis. (1) Thyroglobulin (TG) is synthesized in the endoplasmic reticulum (ER) in the thyroid follicular cells and is transported into the follicular lumen. The small blue squares represent the amino acid residues comprising TG. (2) Iodide is transported into the follicular cell by the sodium–iodide (Na^+/I^-) symporter (NIS). (3) Iodide diffuses to the apical surface and is transported into the follicular lumen by pendrin (P). (4) Iodide is oxidized and linked to tyrosine residues in TG to form diiodotyrosine (DIT) and monoiodotyrosine (MIT) molecules. (5) Within the TG, T_4 is formed from two DIT molecules, and T_3 is formed from one DIT and one MIT molecule. (6) TG containing T_4 and T_3 is resorbed into the follicular cell by endocytosis. (7) TG is degraded by lysosomal enzymes to release T_4 and T_3 molecules, which move across the basolateral membrane of the follicular cell into the adjacent capillaries. TPO, thyroid peroxidase.

known as thyroid-binding pre-albumin), albumin and lipoproteins.

Only the unbound thyroid hormone is available to the tissues. T_3 is less strongly bound and therefore has a more rapid onset and offset of action. The binding proteins have both storage and buffer functions. They help to maintain the serum free T_4 and T_3 levels within narrow limits, and also ensure continuous and rapid availability of the hormones to the tissues.

Free thyroid hormone concentrations are easier to interpret than total thyroid hormone levels. This is because the level of bound hormone alters with changes in the levels of thyroid-binding proteins, even though free T_4 (and T_3) concentrations do not change and the patient remains euthyroid (Fig. 1.6). Box 1.1 summarizes factors that may alter TBG levels.

> **Box 1.1 Factors that may alter thyroid-binding globulin (TBG) levels**
>
> **↑ TBG**
> Hereditary TBG excess (X-linked dominant)
> Pregnancy
> Drugs, e.g. oestrogen, tamoxifen, opiates, phenothiazines, 5-fluorouracil, clofibrate
> Hepatitis
> Acute intermittent porphyria
>
> **↓ TBG**
> Genetically determined
> Malnutrition
> Chronic liver disease
> Nephrotic syndrome
> Drugs, e.g. androgens, corticosteroids, phenytoin
> Cushing's syndrome
> Acromegaly

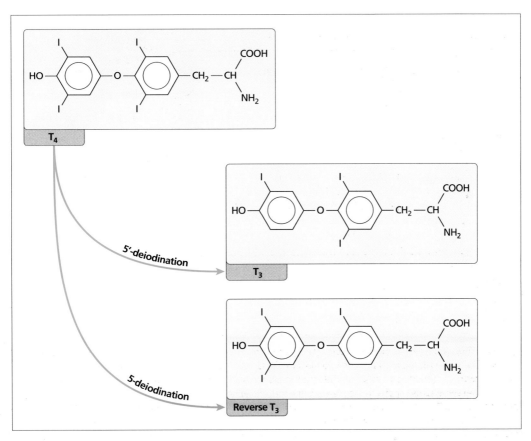

Figure 1.5 The conversion of T₄ to T₃ by 5'-deiodination and to reverse T₃ by 5-deiodination.

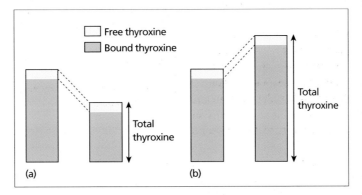

Figure 1.6 (a) If serum thyroid-binding globulin (TBG) levels are decreased, the level of thyroid hormone bound to TBG also decreases (the dark blue part of the bar). However, homeostatic mechanisms will maintain the free thyroid hormone levels (the light blue part of the bar). Note that although free hormone levels are unchanged, the 'total' hormone levels measured will be lower. (b) If TBG levels are increased, the level of thyroid hormone bound to TBG also increases (the dark blue part of the bar). However, homeostatic mechanisms will maintain the free hormone levels (the light blue part of the bar). Note that although free hormone levels are unchanged, the 'total' hormone levels measured will be higher.

Other causes of increased serum total T_4 and T_3 levels include familial dysalbuminaemic hyperthyroxinaemia (due to the presence of an abnormal albumin with a higher affinity for T_4) and the presence of anti-T_4 antibodies. Patients with these conditions are euthyroid, have normal serum thyroid-stimulating hormone (TSH) levels, and usually have normal serum free T_4 and T_3 levels when measured by appropriate methods.

Thyroid hormone metabolism

T_4 is degraded at a rate of 10% per day. Around 40% of the T_4 is deiodinated to T_3 and 40% to reverse T_3. The remaining T_4 is conjugated with glucuronide and sulphate, deaminated and decarboxylated, or cleaved between the two rings.

T_3 is degraded (mostly by deiodination) at a rate of 75% per day. Reverse T_3 is degraded even more rapidly than T_3, mostly by deiodination.

Regulation of thyroid hormone production and release

T_3 and T_4 synthesis and secretion is stimulated by the *thyroid-stimulating hormone* (TSH) released from the anterior pituitary gland (Fig. 1.7). TSH production and release is increased by hypothalamic *thyrotrophin-releasing hormone* (TRH).

Thyrotrophin-releasing hormone

TRH is a tripeptide synthesized and released by the hypothalamus. TRH content is highest in the median eminence and paraventricular nuclei of the hypothalamus. TRH stimulates TSH secretion by activating a G-protein-coupled receptor and the phospholipase C-phosphoinositide pathway, resulting in mobilization of calcium from intracellular storage sites.

Chronic TRH stimulation also increases the synthesis and glycosylation of TSH, which increases its biological activity.

Thyroid-stimulating hormone

TSH is a glycoprotein secreted by the thyrotroph cells of the anterior pituitary. TSH is composed of

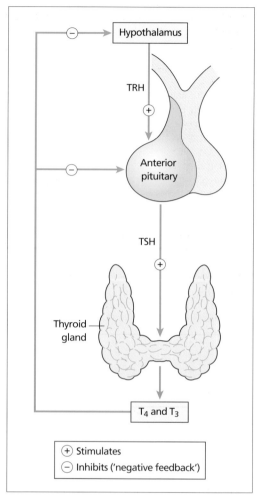

Figure 1.7 Hypothalamic–pituitary–thyroid axis. TRH, thyrotrophin-releasing hormone; TSH, thyroid-stimulating hormone.

alpha and beta subunits that are non-covalently bound. The alpha subunit is the same as that of luteinizing hormone, follicle-stimulating hormone and human chorionic gonadotrophin. However, the beta subunit is unique to TSH. TSH binds to specific plasma membrane receptors and activates adenylyl cyclase. TSH also stimulates phospholipase C activity.

TSH stimulates every step in thyroid hormone synthesis and secretion. It also stimulates the expression of many genes in thyroid tissue and causes thyroid hyperplasia and hypertrophy.

T_3 formed from the deiodination of T_4 and T_3 that enters the cells from the serum is transferred to the nucleus. The thyroid hormone receptors (TRs) heterodimerize with the retinoid X receptor and act as nuclear transcription factors. TRs bind thyroid hormone response elements in the promoter region of thyroid hormone-responsive genes. In the absence of T_3, TRs bind co-repressor proteins that repress transcription. On T_3 binding, co-repressors are displaced and co-activator proteins bind the TRs, resulting in histone acetylation, generation of a permissive chromatin structure and induction of gene transcription.

There are two T_3 nuclear receptors—alpha and beta—encoded by separate genes located on chromosomes 17 and 3. Two forms of each TR are generated by alternative splicing. Only the beta-1, beta-2 and alpha-1 receptors bind T_3. Liver predominantly expresses beta receptors, whereas heart and bone express alpha receptors. The hypothalamus and pituitary express beta-2 receptors which mediate the negative feedback regulation.

T_4 and T_3 inhibit TSH synthesis and release both directly (by inhibiting transcription of the TSH subunit genes) and indirectly (by inhibiting TRH release). T_4 and T_3 also decrease the glycosylation and hence bioactivity of TSH.

TSH secretion is regulated by very small changes in serum T_4 and T_3 concentrations. However, an important exception is that the reduced T_3 levels in patients with non-thyroidal illness have little effect on TSH secretion. This may be due to a greater contribution of serum T_4 to the nuclear T_3 content of the pituitary than other tissues.

Box 1.2 shows a list of the causes of increased and decreased TSH concentration.

Mechanism of action of thyroid hormones

Thyroid hormones enter cells via active membrane transporter proteins (e.g. MCT8). Inside the cells,

Chapter 2

Hypothyroidism

Hypothyroidism results from insufficient secretion of thyroid hormones.

- *Primary* hypothyroidism is characterized by low serum free thyroxine (T_4) and high serum thyroid-stimulating hormone (TSH) levels (due to a reduced negative feedback effect of T_4 on TSH synthesis/secretion).
- *Subclinical* hypothyroidism is defined as normal serum free T_4 and T_3 levels and a high serum TSH. This reflects the sensitivity of TSH secretion to very small decreases in thyroid hormone secretion.
- *Central* hypothyroidism is much less common and results from reduced TSH secretion from the anterior pituitary (secondary hypothyroidism) or reduced thyrotrophin-releasing hormone (TRH) secretion from the hypothalamus (tertiary hypothyroidism).

Epidemiology

The prevalence of congenital hypothyroidism in the UK is about 1 in 4000 of the population. The frequency of hypothyroidism varies from 0.1% to 2% of adults. Hypothyroidism is 5–8 times more common in females. Primary hypothyroidism accounts for more than 95% of cases of hypothyroidism. Around 5% of adults and 15% of women over the age of 60 have subclinical hypothyroidism.

Aetiology

Box 2.1 summarizes the causes of hypothyroidism.

Subclinical hypothyroidism (see above) may result from the same causes as primary hypothyroidism or from inadequate T_4 replacement in a patient with overt hypothyroidism.

Congenital hypothyroidism may be secondary to thyroid agenesis, dysgenesis or inherited defects in thyroid hormone biosynthesis.

Box 2.1 Causes of hypothyroidism

Congenital
Thyroid agenesis, dysgenesis or inherited defects in thyroid hormone biosynthesis

Acquired
Primary
Chronic autoimmune (Hashimoto's) thyroiditis
Iatrogenic (drugs, thyroidectomy, radioiodine, neck radiotherapy)
Iodine deficiency/excess
Thyroiditis

Central
Pituitary/hypothalamic damage (e.g. due to tumours, trauma, radiotherapy, hypophysitis, infarction, infiltration)

Lecture Notes: Endocrinology and Diabetes. By A. Sam and K. Meeran. Published 2009 by Blackwell Publishing. ISBN 978-1-4051-5345-4.

Acquired hypothyroidism may be primary or central as mentioned above. Primary hypothyroidism may be due to chronic autoimmune (Hashimoto's) thyroiditis, iatrogenic causes (e.g. drugs, thyroidectomy, radioiodine), iodine deficiency/excess or thyroiditis.

Chronic autoimmune (Hashimoto's) thyroiditis is caused by cellular and antibody-mediated injury to the thyroid tissue. There are two forms, goitrous and atrophic, which have similar pathophysiology but are different in the extent of thyroid follicular cell hyperplasia, lymphocytic infiltration and fibrosis. Chronic autoimmune thyroiditis is usually but not always permanent. These patients are more likely to have a personal or family history of other autoimmune conditions, such as Addison's disease and type 1 diabetes mellitus, vitiligo (Fig. 2.1), pernicious anaemia and premature ovarian failure. An increased incidence of Hashimoto's thyroiditis is also found in those with Down's or Turner's syndrome.

Drugs such as the antithyroid drugs carbimazole and propylthiouracil (used to treat hyperthyroidism) may cause hypothyroidism. Amiodarone is an iodine-containing drug and may cause both hypothyroidism (see below) and thyrotoxicosis (see Chapter 3). Other drugs that may cause hypothyroidism include lithium, alpha-interferon and interleukin-2. Patients on these drugs should have their serum TSH checked every 6–12 months.

T_4 has a half-life of 7 days, and hypothyroidism occurs about 2–4 weeks following total *thyroidec-tomy*. After subtotal thyroidectomy for the treatment of Graves' disease, hypothyroidism occurs within the first year in the majority of patients. The annual risk of hypothyroidism in those who are euthyroid at 1 year is 0.5–1%. Some patients become transiently hypothyroid after 4–8 weeks but recover several weeks or months later.

Following *radioiodine therapy* for the treatment of Graves' disease, the majority of patients become hypothyroid within the first year. The rest have a 0.5–2% annual risk of hypothyroidism. Some patients with toxic multinodular goitre or thyroid adenomas who receive radioiodine therapy also become hypothyroid.

External irradiation of the neck may result in hypothyroidism with a gradual onset. Many patients develop overt hypothyroidism after several years of subclinical hypothyroidism.

Iodine deficiency and excess can both cause hypothyroidism. Iodine deficiency is the most common worldwide cause of hypothyroidism and is more prevalent in mountainous areas. Iodine excess can also result in hypothyroidism by inhibiting iodine organification and T_4 and T_3 synthesis (Wolff–Chaikoff effect).

In *postpartum* and *subacute thyroiditis*, transient hypothyroidism (lasting weeks to a few months) may follow transient thyrotoxicosis.

Rarer causes include infiltrative diseases, for example fibrous (Reidel's) thyroiditis, haemochromatosis, sarcoidosis, amyloidosis, leukaemia, and consumptive hypothyroidism due to an ectopic production of the type 3 deiodinase in vascular and fibrotic tumours, which metabolizes T_4 to reverse T_3.

Clinical presentations

Hypothyroidism often has an insidious and non-specific onset. Patients may present with fatigue, lethargy and cold intolerance. Clinical presentations of thyroid hormone deficiency result from a generalized slowing of metabolic processes and an accumulation of hydrophilic glycosaminoglycans in the interstitial spaces of the tissues (*myxoedema*). Box 2.2 summarizes the clinical presentations of hypothyroidism in adults and possible explanations for these manifestations.

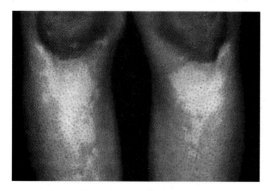

Figure 2.1 Vitiligo in a patient with Hashimoto's thyroiditis.

Box 2.2 Clinical presentations of hypothyroidism

General
Tiredness, cold intolerance, depression, goitre

Skin and hair
Skin: dry and coarse (decreased acinar gland secretion), pale (reduced blood flow), yellowish tinge (carotenaemia), oedematous (accumulation of glycosaminoglycans in the dermis with associated water retention)
Coarse hair, hair loss and brittle nails

Cardiovascular
Bradycardia, exertional breathlessness and reduced exercise tolerance (reduced heart rate and contractility as thyroid hormone regulates genes involved in myocardial contractility and relaxation), exacerbation of heart failure or angina, diastolic hypertension (increased systemic vascular resistance), pericardial effusion, hypercholesterolaemia and hypertri-glyceridaemia (decreased lipid metabolism)

Respiratory
Exertional breathlessness, hypoventilation (respiratory muscle weakness and reduced ventilatory responses to hypoxia and hypercapnia), obstructive sleep apnoea (macroglossia), pleural effusion

Gastrointestinal
Constipation (decreased gut motility), weight gain (reduced metabolic rate and accumulation of glycosaminoglycan-rich fluid), ascites (rare)

Reproductive
Hyperprolactinaemia (high thyrotrophin-releasing hormone in primary hypothyroidism stimulates prolactin production)
Women: oligomenorrhoea/amenorrhea or menorrhagia, early abortion
Men: reduced libido, erectile dysfunction, delayed ejaculation, reduced serum total testosterone due to low sex hormone-binding globulin levels

Neurological
Slowing of intellectual activities, movement and speech, impaired memory, delayed relaxation of deep tendon reflexes, carpal tunnel syndrome, peripheral neuropathy, cerebellar ataxia, encephalopathy, muscle abnormalities (asymptomatic rise in serum creatine kinase, muscle cramps, proximal muscle weakness, rarely rhabdomyolysis)

Myxoedema coma
May present with coma, hypothermia, hypercapnia and hyponatraemia. Precipitating factors include infection, cold exposure, trauma and drugs (hypnotics or opiates) in patients with severe hypothyroidism

Anaemia
Normocytic anaemia, macrocytic anaemia (in those with pernicious anaemia associated with autoimmune thyroiditis), microcytic anaemia (in female patients with menorrhagia)

Metabolic
Hyperlipidaemia, hyponatraemia (reduced cardiac output sensed by the carotid sinus baroreceptors can result in increased antidiuretic hormone release; also decreased glomerular filtration results in reduced free water excretion), hyperhomocysteinaemia

In secondary hypothyroidism due to hypothalamic/pituitary disease, the symptoms are usually milder than in primary hypothyroidism and may be masked by symptoms of other hormone deficiencies (see Chapter 12). For example, hot flushes secondary to hypogonadism may make the cold intolerance caused by hypothyroidism less obvious.

Investigations

The diagnosis of hypothyroidism is made by measuring serum TSH and free T_4. In many developed countries, congenital hypothyroidism is diagnosed during the routine screening of all infants by measuring TSH or T_4 in blood obtained from a heel prick in the first week of life.

Table 2.1 shows the results of thyroid function tests in primary, subclinical and secondary hypothyroidism. In general, younger patients presenting with primary hypothyroidism have much higher TSH levels than older patients.

Other laboratory test abnormalities in hypothyroid patients include *hyperlipidaemia* and *hyponatraemia*.

Patients with central hypothyroidism should have pituitary function tests and a magnetic resonance imaging scan of the hypothalamus and pituitary. A TRH test may occasionally be done to differentiate between pituitary and hypothalamic causes of TSH deficiency. A dose of 200 µg of TRH is given intravenously over 2 minutes. Blood samples are taken at 30 and 60 minutes. The 60-minute value exceeds the 30-minute value in hypothalamic hypothyroidism.

Pituitary enlargement may occasionally be seen in severe primary hypothyroidism owing to hypertrophy and hyperplasia of the thyrotroph cells. It is important to distinguish this entity, which is reversible with T_4 replacement, from a pituitary adenoma.

Treatment

Hypothyroidism usually requires lifelong treatment with synthetic levothyroxine. Exceptions include cases of transient hypothyroidism following subacute or postpartum thyroiditis, or reversible hypothyroidism due to a drug that can be stopped.

Treatment objectives are the resolution of symptoms, a normalization of TSH and a reduction in the size of the goitre in patients with Hashimoto's thyroiditis.

There is no proven benefit in using a combined T_3/T_4 replacement.

Dose and administration of levothyroxine

Younger patients (under 50 years) can be started on levothyroxine 50 µg daily. Thyroid function tests are repeated after 6 weeks and the dose is increased by 25 µg until the TSH is in the normal range and ideally as close to 1.0 mU/L as possible.

Older patients should be started on a lower dose (25 µg daily) as they may have ischaemic heart disease, and levothyroxine increases myocardial oxygen demand. The dose may be gradually increased; however, a suboptimal replacement may have to be accepted if an optimal dose causes cardiac symptoms.

The average dose of levothyroxine in hypothyroid adults is about 100 µg per day, but the range varies from 50 to 200 µg daily. It is important to advise patients on the potential adverse effects of levothyroxine over-replacement, such as arrhythmias and osteoporosis.

Table 2.1 Thyroid function tests in various forms of hypothyroidism

	Thyroid-stimulating hormone	Free thyroxine	Free triiodothyronine
Primary hypothyroidism	↑	↓	↓ or N
Subclinical hypothyroidism	↑	N	N
Central hypothyroidism	↓ or inappropriately N	↓	↓ or N

N, normal.

Levothyroxine should be taken on an empty stomach, and medications that interfere with its absorption (e.g. ferrous salts, cholestyramine) should be taken several hours after the levothyroxine dose. Some drugs (e.g. phenytoin, carbamazepine) may increase levothyroxine metabolism.

Patients with poor compliance with levothyroxine replacement may occasionally receive their total weekly dose of levothyroxine once per week. This should probably be avoided in coronary heart disease.

Follow-up and monitoring

Levothyroxine has a half-life of 1 week and it takes about 6 weeks (six half-lives) to reach a steady-state concentration. Serum T_4 increases first, and then TSH secretion starts to fall. Follow-up appointments for clinical assessment, measurements of thyroid function and adjustment of the dose should be arranged every 6 weeks. After stabilization of TSH levels and establishment of the proper maintenance dose, clinical assessment and serum TSH measurements should be carried out annually.

When levothyroxine is commenced, TSH occasionally rises further initially before it starts to fall. This may be because the pituitary itself has begun to suffer from the profound hypothyroidism and has failed to make TSH. On commencement of the levothyroxine, the pituitary starts to recover.

It is worth noting that hair loss may initially be made worse by commencing levothyroxine. This is because new hair follicles start growing and push up the old hair follicles. It may take about 9 months before this stabilizes.

Special circumstances

Myxoedema coma

Myxoedema coma should be treated aggressively as it has a high mortality of up to 80%. Patients should be monitored closely in an intensive care unit. Mechanical ventilation should be instituted for respiratory failure. Blood should be taken for culture, free T_4, T_3, TSH and cortisol before starting treatment. Treatment must be started before diagnosis is established.

- No consensus has yet been reached about the optimal replacement regimen of *thyroid hormone* replacement. An accepted regimen includes the administration of intravenous levothyroxine 300–500 μg (depending on the patient's age, weight and risk of myocardial ischaemia or arrhythmia) followed by daily intravenous doses of 50–100 μg until the patient can take oral levothyroxine. If there is no improvement within 24–48 hours, intravenous T_3 (10 μg, 8-hourly) is added.
- Intravenous *hydrocortisone* (100 mg 6–8-hourly) must be given until coexisting adrenal insufficiency can be excluded.
- Treat possible *precipitating factors* such as infection with broad-spectrum antibiotics.
- Replace intravenous *fluids* (and glucose) appropriately.
- Correct *hypothermia* using a heating blanket. Aim for an hourly rise of 0.5°C in core temperature. Rapid external warming can cause inappropriate vasodilatation and cardiovascular collapse.

Suspected adrenal insufficiency

Levothyroxine replacement in patients with untreated adrenal insufficiency can precipitate an Addisonian crisis (see Chapter 6). A short Synacthen test should always be done prior to levothyroxine replacement if adrenal insufficiency or secondary hypothyroidism is suspected. Hydrocortisone must be given with the levothyroxine if adrenal insufficiency is confirmed.

Subclinical hypothyroidism

Indications for levothyroxine replacement in subclinical hypothyroidism include pregnancy, a serum TSH above 10 mU/L, goitre, symptoms of hypothyroidism such as fatigue, constipation or depression, or high serum antithyroid peroxidase (microsomal) antibody. Patients who are not treated should have periodic thyroid function tests to detect progression to overt hypothyroidism.

Oestrogen therapy

Oestrogens may increase the need for levothyroxine. In women receiving levothyroxine replacement, serum TSH should be measured about 12 weeks after starting oestrogen therapy to determine whether an increase in levothyroxine dose is needed.

Surgery

Patients on thyroxine replacement who are unable to eat or drink following surgery should receive intravenous levothyroxine (80% of oral dose) *only* if they have not resumed oral intake after 5–7 days.

Transient hypothyroidism

Transient hypothyroidism, for example following thyroiditis, can last from a few weeks to as long as 6 months. Patients with minimal symptoms may not require therapy. Symptomatic patients should receive levothyroxine for several months. A normal serum TSH level 6 weeks after stopping levothyroxine indicates a recovery of thyroid function.

Pregnancy

See Chapter 31.

Key points:

- Primary hypothyroidism (low serum free T_4 and high serum TSH) may be due to chronic autoimmune (Hashimoto's) thyroiditis, iatrogenic causes (antithyroid drugs, thyroidectomy, radioiodine), iodine deficiency/excess or thyroiditis.
- Clinical presentations of thyroid hormone deficiency result from a generalized slowing of metabolic processes and an accumulation of hydrophilic glycosaminoglycans in the interstitial spaces of the tissues (myxoedema).
- Hypothyroidism usually requires lifelong treatment with synthetic thyroxine. Hypothyroid patients with a history of ischaemic heart disease should be started on a lower dose of levothyroxine.
- Levothyroxine replacement in patients with untreated adrenal insufficiency can precipitate an Addisonian crisis.

Chapter 3

Thyrotoxicosis

Thyrotoxicosis is the syndrome resulting from an excess of circulating free thyroxine (T_4) and/or free triiodothyronine (T_3). Thyrotoxicosis may be due to either increased thyroid hormone synthesis (*hyperthyroidism*) or increased release of stored thyroid hormone from an inflamed thyroid gland (e.g. in subacute thyroiditis).

- *Primary* hyperthyroidism is characterized by raised free T_4 and/or T_3 and low thyroid-stimulating hormone (TSH). TSH is suppressed due to the negative feedback effect of thyroid hormones on TSH synthesis/secretion.
- *Secondary* hyperthyroidism is characterized by raised T_4 and T_3 due to increased TSH secretion from a pituitary tumour ('thyrotroph adenoma').

T_3 toxicosis (high free T_3, normal free T_4, low TSH) tends to occur early in the course of hyperthyroidism, when patients have relatively few symptoms. T_4 toxicosis (high free T_4, normal free T_3, low TSH) may be seen in hyperthyroid patients in whom a concurrent non-thyroidal illness reduces the conversion of T_4 to T_3.

Subclinical hyperthyroidism is defined as suppressed TSH in the presence of normal free T_4 and T_3. These patients may have few or no symptoms or signs of hyperthyroidism.

Lecture Notes: Endocrinology and Diabetes. By A. Sam and K. Meeran. Published 2009 by Blackwell Publishing. ISBN 978-1-4051-5345-4.

Epidemiology

Thyrotoxicosis affects 1% of females and 0.1% of males. Graves' disease accounts for 70–80% of all cases of hyperthyroidism. Toxic multinodular goitre is the most common cause of hyperthyroidism in the elderly. Secondary hyperthyroidism is very rare.

Aetiology

Box 3.1 summarizes the causes of thyrotoxicosis.

Box 3.1 Causes of thyrotoxicosis

Graves' disease
Toxic multinodular goitre
Toxic adenoma
Thyroiditis (de Quervain's and postpartum)
Secondary hyperthyroidism (due to a TSH-secreting pituitary adenoma)
Drugs: excessive exogenous thyroxine, amiodarone

Rarer causes
Metastatic thyroid cancer
McCune–Albright syndrome
Ectopic thyroid tissue (e.g. struma ovarii)
Gestational thyrotoxicosis
Human chorionic gonadotrophin-secreting trophoblastic tumours

---

Graves' disease

Graves' disease is caused by autoantibodies that stimulate the TSH receptor and hence thyroid hormone synthesis and secretion, and thyroid growth (causing a diffuse goitre). Possible precipitating and predisposing factors include genetic susceptibility (suggested by an association with certain alleles of CTLA-4 and HLA) and environmental factors such as infection.

The mechanisms that may be involved in the pathogenesis of Graves' hyperthyroidism include molecular mimicry (similarity between some infectious/exogenous antigens and human proteins) and thyroid cell expression of HLA class II molecules (which may act as antigen-presenting cells to initiate an autoimmune response).

Patients with Graves' disease may have a personal or family history of other autoimmune disorders such as vitiligo, alopecia areata, pernicious anaemia, type 1 diabetes mellitus, myasthenia gravis or coeliac disease.

Toxic multinodular goitre and toxic adenoma

These are the result of focal and/or diffuse hyperplasia of thyroid follicular cells whose function is independent of regulation by TSH. Between 20% and 80% of toxic adenomas and some nodules of toxic multinodular goitres have somatic mutations of the TSH receptor gene that confer autonomous hyperactivity.

Thyroiditis

Thyroiditis (e.g. subacute viral, postpartum) can result in thyrotoxicosis by the release of preformed thyroid hormones from a damaged thyroid gland into the circulation.

Subacute (de Quervain's) viral thyroiditis presents initially with thyrotoxicosis followed by hypothyroidism several weeks later. Recovery of normal thyroid function occurs 3–6 months later, but 10% of patients may have late relapses. A similar but painless thyroiditis may occur 3–6 months after delivery (postpartum thyroiditis)

possibly due to the exacerbation of a previously subclinical autoimmune thyroiditis. The thyrotoxic phase lasts for about 1–4 weeks.

Secondary hyperthyroidism

Secondary hyperthyroidism due to a TSH-secreting pituitary tumour is very rare. A similar biochemical picture (high free T_4/T_3 and normal or high TSH) may be seen in the uncommon 'thyroid hormone resistance syndrome' (see below).

Amiodarone

Amiodarone (an iodine-containing antiarrhythmic drug) may affect thyroid function in several ways. Amiodarone inhibits the conversion of T_4 to T_3 and results in a high or high-normal free T_4, low-normal free T_3 and initially high TSH that normalizes within 2–3 months. In addition, amiodarone may cause both hypothyroidism (see Chapter 2) and thyrotoxicosis.

In amiodarone-induced thyrotoxicosis, clinical manifestations are often masked by the drug's beta-blocking activity. Patients may present with atrial arrhythmias, exacerbation of ischaemic heart disease or heart failure, unexplained weight loss, restlessness or low-grade fever. There are two types of amiodarone-induced thyrotoxicosis. However, some patients may have a mixture of both types:
- *Type 1* thyrotoxicosis is caused by amiodarone's high iodine content, which provides the substrate for excessive thyroid hormone synthesis in patients with a previously silent multinodular goitre.
- *Type 2* thyrotoxicosis is due to a direct toxic effect of the drug on the thyroid gland, resulting in a destructive thyroiditis and the release of preformed T_4 and T_3.

Subclinical hyperthyroidism

This condition may be endogenous (due to the same conditions that cause overt hyperthyroidism) or due to excess exogenous T_4.

Clinical presentations

Clinical presentations of thyrotoxicosis are summarized in Box 3.2.

Box 3.2 Clinical presentations of thyrotoxicosis

General

Heat intolerance, anxiety, irritability, hyperactivity, fatigue, insomnia

Skin, nails and hair

Increased sweating, warm moist skin (increased blood flow), palmar erythema, pruritus
Onycholysis (loosening of the nails from the nail bed)
Hair loss
Graves' disease: pretibial myxoedema, acropachy
Alopecia areata and vitiligo (associated with autoimmune disorders)

Ocular

Lid retraction and lid lag
Graves' ophthalmopathy: periorbital oedema, grittiness, increased tear production, chemosis, proptosis (unilateral in 5–10%), ophthalmoplegia, optic nerve compression

Cardiovascular

Palpitations (sinus tachycardia, atrial fibrillation)
Widened pulse pressure (a combination of systolic hypertension and reduced peripheral vascular resistance), congestive heart failure, mitral valve prolapse/regurgitation

Respiratory

Exertional breathlessness (due to increased oxygen consumption and carbon dioxide production, and respiratory muscle weakness), tracheal obstruction secondary to large goitre

Gastrointestinal

Diarrhoea, increased appetite, weight loss, weight gain (10% of younger patients), dysphagia (due to a large goitre)

Neurological

Tremor, proximal muscle weakness, brisk tendon reflexes, inability to concentrate, chorea
Hypokalaemic (thyrotoxic) periodic paralysis: seen particularly in Asian men, characterized by intermittent weakness, usually after exercise or a high-carbohydrate meal

Psychiatric

Depression, apathetic thyrotoxicosis in the elderly, psychosis (rare)

Genitourinary

Females: oligomenorrhoea/amenorrhoea
Males: gynaecomastia, reduced libido, erectile dysfunction, abnormal or decreased spermatogenesis, polyuria (possibly due to primary polydipsia or hypercalciuria)

Musculoskeletal

Osteoporosis (thyroid hormone stimulates bone resorption), raised serum alkaline phosphatase (increased bone turnover), hypercalcaemia

---

Examination of the neck may reveal a diffusely enlarged goitre (90% of patients with Graves' disease), a multinodular goitre or a solitary nodule. A diffuse goitre may also be seen in painless thyroiditis and TSH-secreting pituitary tumours. Sub-acute (de Quervain's) thyroiditis presents with a small tender goitre, and patients may have had a preceding flu-like illness.

Clinical signs specific to Graves' disease include *ophthalmopathy, pretibial myxoedema* and *thyroid acropachy*. These are mediated by different autoantibodies that may co-exist in Graves' disease.

Graves' ophthalmopathy

Graves' ophthalmopathy (Fig. 3.1) may be clinically obvious in 20–25% of patients with Graves' hyperthyroidism at the time of diagnosis of the hyperthyroidism. It is more common in females. Many more (>90%) may have evidence of ophthalmopathy on computed tomography/magnetic resonance imaging (CT/MRI) of the orbits. Around 10% of patients with Graves' ophthalmopathy do not have Graves' disease; they may have autoimmune hypothyroidism or thyroid autoantibodies.

Graves' ophthalmopathy may present with periorbital oedema, conjunctival oedema (chemosis) and injection, grittiness, corneal ulceration, proptosis (60%), ophthalmoplegia and diplopia (40%), retrobulbar pain or pain on eye movement, and optic nerve compression (6%), which may result in impaired visual acuity or visual field defects. Graves' ophthalmopathy may be unilateral in 15% of patients.

Pathogenesis involves activated T cell cytokines and TSH receptor antibodies that activate TSH receptors on fibroblasts and adipocytes. This sets off an inflammatory process and causes the secretion of hydrophilic glycosaminoglycans, resulting in an increased retro-orbital volume.

Patients with thyrotoxicosis due to any cause may have *lid retraction* and *lid lag* (sclera visible above the iris as the patient looks downward) caused by sympathetic overactivity, possibly mediated by increased beta-adrenergic receptors.

Pretibial myxoedema

Pretibial myxoedema (Fig. 3.2) is specific to Graves' disease. It is seen in up to 2% of patients and results from an accumulation of hydrophilic glycosaminoglycans secreted by fibroblasts in the dermis. Pretibial myxoedema is characterized by raised, pigmented, orange-peel textured nodules or plaques on the anterior aspect of the leg or the dorsum of the foot. They are usually asymptomatic, but may be pruritic or painful.

Thyroid acropachy

Thyroid acropachy (Fig. 3.3) is seen in fewer than 1% of the patients with Graves' disease and resembles clubbing. It is due to periosteal new bone formation in the phalanges.

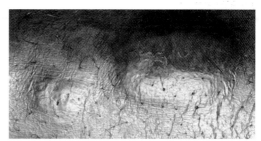

Figure 3.2 Pretibial myxoedema.

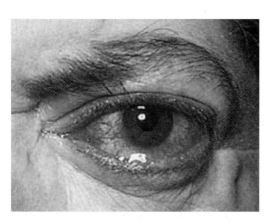

Figure 3.1 Graves' ophthalmopathy.

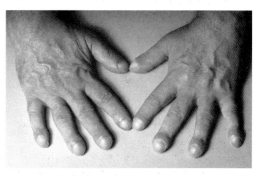

Figure 3.3 Thyroid acropachy.

Thyroid storm

A thyroid storm ('thyrotoxic crisis') may present with:
- fever, sweating
- cardiovascular symptoms: tachyarrhythmias, cardiac failure
- neurological symptoms: agitation, delirium, seizure, coma
- gastrointestinal symptoms: diarrhoea, vomiting, jaundice.

It has an untreated mortality of 50%. It may be precipitated by thyroid surgery, radio-iodine, iodinated contrast agents, withdrawal of thionamides (antithyroid drugs) and acute illnesses such as infection, stroke, diabetic ketoacidosis or trauma.

Investigations

Thyroid function tests

- In *primary hyperthyroidism*, thyroid function tests show suppressed serum TSH and high free T_4 and or free T_3.
- In *secondary hyperthyroidism*, TSH is either high or inappropriately normal in the presence of a raised free T_4/T_3. The differential diagnosis of this state includes thyroid hormone resistance (see below).
- In *subclinical hyperthyroidism*, TSH is low, but free T_4 and free T_3 levels are normal. Therefore free T_3 levels should always be measured when TSH is low in the presence of a normal T_4 to differentiate between subclinical hyperthyroidism and T_3 thyrotoxicosis.

Patients on amiodarone therapy should have their thyroid function checked before starting therapy, every 3–4 months during treatment and for at least 1 year after the drug has been stopped.

Radioisotope uptake scan

A radioisotope (intravenous [i.v.] ^{99}technetium pertechnetate or oral ^{123}iodine) uptake scan is helpful in differentiating between different causes of thyrotoxicosis (Fig. 3.4):

- Graves' disease is characterized by a diffuse increased uptake of the radioisotope. (Normal uptake is up to 3% of the administered dose.)
- Toxic multinodular goitre is characterized by multiple areas of increased radioisotope uptake ('hot' nodules) with suppression of uptake in the rest of the gland.
- A solitary toxic adenoma is seen as a single area of increased radioisotope uptake ('hot nodule') with suppression of uptake in the rest of the gland.
- A low or absent radioisotope uptake indicates either thyroiditis (inflammation and destruction of thyroid tissue) or an extra-thyroidal (e.g. exogenous) source of excess thyroid hormone.

The scanning time is earlier with ^{99}technetium pertechnetate (maximum thyroid uptake occurring within 30 minutes of i.v. injection), and there is no need to stop antithyroid drugs before the scan (technetium is transported into the thyroid follicular cells, but it is not organified).

Patients must not have any iodine-containing medications, supplements or radiocontrast dyes before the radioisotope scan as they block radioisotope uptake. It is essential to make sure that the patient is not pregnant prior to the radioisotope scan.

TSH receptor-stimulating antibodies

TSH receptor-stimulating antibodies are positive in Graves' disease. However, this test is expensive, and the aetiology of thyrotoxicosis can often be determined with a combination of thyroid function tests and a radioisotope uptake scan.

Some laboratories measure 'TBII' (TSH-binding inhibitor immunoglobulin). This test shows that there is an antibody that competes with TSH for the TSH receptor, but it does not differentiate between stimulating and blocking antibodies (some patients with Graves' disease have a mixture of stimulating and blocking TSH receptor antibodies).

Antithyroglobulin and antithyroid peroxidase (microsomal) antibodies are present in up to 87% of patients with Graves' disease. However, these have low specificity and are present in 15% of healthy females and 5% of males.

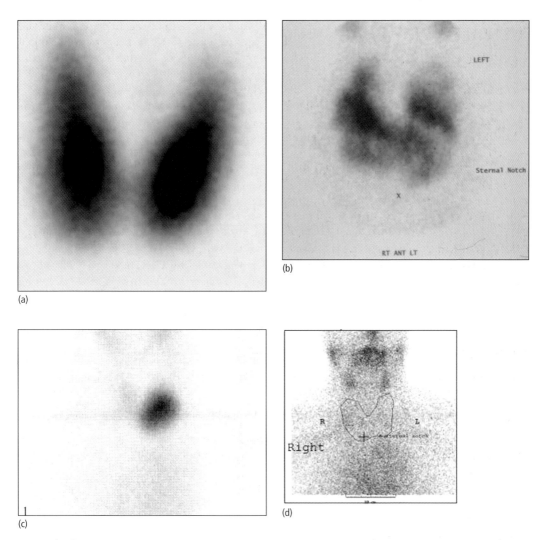

(a)

(b)

(c)

(d)

Figure 3.4 [99]Technetium pertechnetate uptake scan: (a) Graves' disease, (b) toxic multinodular goitre, (c) solitary toxic adenoma, and (d) thyroiditis.

Other investigations

Thyroiditis

Erythrocyte sedimentation rate (ESR) is elevated in patients with subacute viral de Quervain's thyroiditis.

Graves' ophthalmopathy

CT or MRI (STIR sequence) of the orbits may be used in the assessment and follow-up of patients with Graves' ophthalmopathy.

Secondary hyperthyroidism

A pituitary MRI should be requested in cases of secondary hyperthyroidism. A differential diagnosis of secondary hyperthyroidism is thyroid hormone resistance (see below).

Amiodarone-induced thyrotoxicosis

A detectable uptake on a radioisotope uptake scan suggests type 1 amiodarone-induced thyrotoxicosis (see above). Low or absent uptake may be due to either type 2 amiodarone-induced thyrotoxicosis (i.e. thyroiditis) or the iodine content of amiodarone itself in those who have recently been taking the drug. Therefore a radioisotope uptake scan is only useful in those who have not recently been on amiodarone, and even then it may be difficult to interpret given its very long half-life. Colour-flow Doppler ultrasonography may distinguish type 1 (increased vascularity) from type 2 (reduced vascularity) amiodarone-induced thyrotoxicosis. However, this test requires an experienced sonographer.

Treatment

All patients with primary hyperthyroidism should be told about the three options available for treatment (Box 3.3). For the treatment of secondary hyperthyroidism, see Chapter 12.

In patients with severe thyrotoxic symptoms, *beta-blockers* such as propranolol (20–80 mg three

> **Box 3.3 Treatment options in thyrotoxicosis**
>
> Antithyroid drugs (thionamides)
> Radio-iodine
> Surgery (thyroidectomy)

times a day) may be used temporarily (initially, for 4–8 weeks). Atenolol (100 mg daily) is an alternative.

Graves' disease

In Europe, most patients with Graves' disease below the age of 50 years receive antithyroid drugs as initial treatment (see below). Radio-iodine is more commonly used in North America. However, if thyrotoxicosis relapses, a second course of antithyroid drugs is unlikely to result in remission, and definitive treatment (radio-iodine or surgery) is preferred. An alternative is the indefinite use of low-dose antithyroid drugs, with the risk of recurrence if drugs are inadvertently stopped.

In patients with Graves' disease who are over 50 years of age, radio-iodine or surgery should be encouraged as recurrent thyrotoxicosis may be dangerous in the presence of coincidental heart disease. A 12–18-month course of thionamides has a 50% relapse rate in women and a 95% relapse rate in men. Thus men tend to be offered radio-iodine as primary treatment.

Pre-treatment with antithyroid drugs prior to radio-iodine or surgery may be required in those who do not tolerate the symptoms of hyperthyroidism. Symptoms are usually controlled in 4–8 weeks with antithyroid drugs. Pre-treatment with antithyroid drugs may reduce the risk of thyroid storm and transient thyroiditis. However, pre-treatment with antithyroid drugs is associated with a higher rate of failure, and a larger dose of radio-iodine may be necessary.

Toxic multinodular goitre and toxic adenoma

Patients with multinodular goitre and toxic adenoma are ideally treated with radio-iodine or surgery depending on the patient's preference. Surgery is preferred in those with retrosternal extension or large goitres. However, long-term antithyroid drugs may be used in those who refuse or cannot have radio-iodine or surgery.

Antithyroid drugs

The antithyroid drugs *carbimazole, methimazole* and *propylthiouracil* (PTU) reduce T_4 and T_3 production by inhibiting thyroid peroxidase. PTU also inhibits the peripheral conversion of T_4 to T_3. Carbimazole has the advantage of once-daily dosing. Up to 50% of female patients with Graves' disease show sustained remission after treatment with thionamides. This may possibly be secondary to a decrease in TSH-stimulating antibody levels by these drugs.

In the *titration regimen*, the initial doses of carbimazole (30–40 mg per day) or PTU (300–400 mg per day) are gradually reduced over 4–8 weeks (depending on thyroid function tests) to a maintenance dose of 5–15 mg per day of carbimazole or 50–150 mg per day of PTU. A higher initial dose of carbimazole (60 mg per day) or PTU (200 mg three times a day) is occasionally required in severely thyrotoxic patients.

The antithyroid drug dose is titrated down at monthly follow-up visits, using the free T_4/T_3 levels as a guide. It takes longer (up to several months) for suppressed TSH levels to increase. Treatment is continued for 12–18 months with regular monitoring of thyroid function tests.

In the *block and replacement* regimen, carbimazole 40 mg per day or PTU 400 mg per day is started, and T_4 (usually 100 μg) is added when free T_4 is in the normal range (usually after about 4 weeks). This regimen is given for 18 months and requires fewer follow-up visits. The block and replacement regimen is contraindicated in pregnancy because levothyroxine crosses the placenta less well than antithyroid drugs, resulting in fetal hypothyroidism and goitre.

A rare but significant complication of antithyroid drugs is *agranulocytosis*, which usually occurs within the first 3 months of treatment in 0.1–0.5% of patients. Patients must be given written instructions to stop their antithyroid drug and tell their doctor immediately if they develop fever, a sore throat, mouth ulcers or any signs of infection. Patients should have their full blood count checked. Mild neutropenia $(1–1.5 \times 10^9/L)$ is common in patients on antithyroid drugs. However, in patients with a neutrophil count of less than $1 \times 10^9/L$, antithyroid drugs should be discontinued. Such patients need radio-iodine or urgent surgery. In the short term, beta-blockers may be used to control the symptoms.

The cut-off for intervention is controversial. Patients with a neutrophil count of less than $0.5 \times 10^9/L$ and a sore throat may require admission and treatment with granulocyte colony-stimulating factor and antibiotics.

Rashes and pruritus are common side-effects of antithyroid drugs and may be treated with antihistamines without stopping treatment. Occasionally, one antithyroid drug may need to be substituted with another. Other side-effects include macular rash (1–5%), nausea, vomiting, abnormal taste/smell, arthralgia, pruritus, lymphadenopathy and deranged liver function tests (cholestatic or hepatitis). PTU may rarely be associated with antineutrophil cytoplasmic antibody positive vasculitis.

Follow-up

In both the regimens described above, drugs are discontinued after 18 months of treatment, and thyroid function tests are checked at intervals (e.g. 6-weekly for 6 months, 6-monthly for 2 years and then annually) or sooner if the patient develops symptoms suggestive of relapse. Around 70% of relapses occur in the first year; relapse is more likely in patients with a large goitre and high free T_3 levels at the time of diagnosis. Those who relapse (50% of females, 95% of males) need further definitive treatment in the form of radio-iodine or surgery (thyroidectomy). Those who cannot have definitive treatment require lifelong antithyroid drug treatment. Autoimmune hypothyroidism may occur in 15% of patients with Graves' disease.

Radio-iodine

Radio-iodine (^{131}I) is given orally as a capsule or solution. It is concentrated in the thyroid, and its beta-emissions result in cell damage and death over a period of 6–18 weeks. Antithyroid drugs should be discontinued (about 3 days) before radio-iodine to allow uptake of the isotope by the thyroid gland.

Some centres use a fixed dose (370 or 555 MBq) to ablate the thyroid gland in Graves' disease; others vary the dose (200–600 MBq) according to the size of the thyroid gland and the 24-hour radio-iodine uptake result. Higher doses of radio-iodine (e.g. 600–800 MBq) are used to treat toxic adenoma or toxic multinodular goitre. In patients with renal failure, doses of radio-iodine must be significantly reduced.

Most endocrinologists prefer to delay radio-iodine treatment in patients with moderate-to-severe ophthalmopathy until their eye disease has been stable for at least 1 year. Radio-iodine is occasionally given with prednisolone cover (25–30 mg per day withdrawn over 6–12 weeks).

Complications and advice for patients
Radio-iodine destroys fetal thyroid and is contraindicated in pregnancy and breast-feeding. Pregnancy is safe 4 months after radio-iodine. Patients must avoid close contact with small children for several weeks depending on the radio-iodine dose. Therefore radio-iodine may not be an option for those patients who cannot comply with the restrictions.

Most studies suggest that radio-iodine is associated with the appearance or exacerbation of Graves' ophthalmopathy. Radio-iodine therapy is followed by a transient increase in serum TSH receptor antibodies, which might be important in initiating or exacerbating ophthalmopathy.

Radio-iodine may occasionally cause transient thyroiditis and sialoadenitis. Radio-iodine therapy for hyperthyroidism does not increase the overall risk of malignancy.

Follow-up
Antithyroid drugs may need to be started shortly after radio-iodine treatment in those who develop a transient thyroiditis. A total of 10% of patients develop permanent hypothyroidism during the first year and 2–3% annually thereafter. Therefore patients should be followed up with repeat thyroid function tests regularly in the first year and then annually. It is common practice to wait 4–6 months before repeating radio-iodine treatment in patients with persistent thyrotoxicosis because remission commonly occurs during this period.

Surgery

Surgery is an unpopular therapy for Graves' hyperthyroidism, and the extent of surgery for Graves' hyperthyroidism is controversial. More aggressive surgery (thyroid remnants <4 g) is associated with a higher rate of hypothyroidism. Less aggressive surgery is associated with a higher rate of recurrent overt/subclinical hyperthyroidism. Surgery is more popular for patients with toxic multinodular goitre and toxic adenomas (see above).

Recurrence rates are about 2–4% in the best centres. The prevalence of hypothyroidism may be up to 80% several years after surgery. Other surgical complications (<1%) include hypoparathyroidism, recurrent laryngeal nerve damage and laryngeal oedema (due to bleeding into the neck).

Preparation of thyrotoxic patients for thyroidectomy
Preparation includes administration of a beta-blocker, antithyroid drugs and an excess of iodide/iodine, for example potassium iodide 60 mg three times a day or Lugol's iodine 0.3 mL three times a day. Iodide excess is given for 10 days before surgery to inhibit thyroid hormone synthesis (the Wolff–Chaikoff effect) and probably reduce perioperative blood loss. If the window at 10 days is missed, recurrent thyrotoxicosis occurs (the Jod–Basedow effect). PTU should be administered an hour before any iodide to prevent organification of the administered iodine.

Surgery is chosen over radio-iodine in:
- patients with large goitres causing upper airway obstruction or dysphagia
- patients who cannot take antithyroid drugs (e.g. due to allergy/agranulocytosis) and are either pregnant or have moderate/severe Graves' ophthalmopathy (which may be exacerbated by radio-iodine).

Graves' ophthalmopathy

Urgent ophthalmology review is needed in cases of visual impairment or corneal damage.

Patients should be reviewed by surgeons specialized in orbital, oculoplastic and strabismus surgery depending on their presentation. Patients must be advised to stop smoking. The treatment of Graves' ophthalmopathy depends on the severity of symptoms:
- for mild symptoms:
  — artificial tears during the day and ointments at night
  — eye shades
  — elevation of the head of the bed
  — advice to avoid sleeping on the face
- for congestive ophthalmopathy with visual impairment:
  — i.v. methylprednisolone (1 g daily for 3 days) or high-dose prednisolone
  — decompression surgery
  — radiotherapy.

Orbital radiotherapy is contraindicated in patients with diabetic retinopathy. Surgical correction may also be performed for cases of diplopia or cosmetic disability. Hypothyroidism (e.g. after radioactive iodine, overtreatment with drugs) is a risk factor for developing or worsening eye disease and must be promptly corrected.

Pretibial myxoedema

Pruritus or discomfort may be treated with topical steroid ointment such as fluocinolone covered by an occlusive dressing. Systemic corticosteroid therapy may occasionally be given for resistant cases.

Special circumstances

Thyroid storm (thyrotoxic crisis)

General supportive treatments include:
- close monitoring in the high-dependency or intensive therapy unit
- i.v. fluids, paracetamol and cooling. Avoid aspirin (as it displaces T_4 from thyroid-binding globulin)
- antiarrhythmics; when anticoagulation is given for atrial fibrillation, remember that thyrotoxic patients are very sensitive to warfarin
- treating the precipitating cause, for example antibiotics for infection
- chlorpromazine (50–100 mg intramuscularly) is useful for the treatment of agitation and hyperpyrexia
- monitoring glucose (as liver glycogen stores are depleted during thyroid storm).

Specific treatments include:
- *PTU:* a 600 mg loading dose, and then 200 mg 4-hourly orally or via a nasogastric tube
- *propranolol:* 60–80 mg 4-hourly orally. Caution should be taken with complicating cardiac failure
- *hydrocortisone:* 100 mg i.v. four times a day (it inhibits the peripheral conversion of T_4 to T_3)
- *potassium iodide:* 60 mg four times a day via a nasogastric tube (it blocks thyroid hormone release). It must be commenced 6 hours after starting PTU. Alternatively, Lugol's iodine 1 mL four times daily may be given and should be started at least 1 hour after the first dose of PTU. Potassium iodide can be given for a maximum of 14 days followed by definitive treatment.

Thyrotoxicosis and atrial fibrillation

Left atrial enlargement (a risk factor for thrombus formation) is seen in about 90% of hyperthyroid patients with atrial fibrillation; therefore these patients should usually be anticoagulated. Around 60% of hyperthyroid patients with atrial fibrillation cardiovert back to sinus rhythm when the hyperthyroidism is treated.

Subclinical hyperthyroidism

In exogenous subclinical hyperthyroidism, the levothyroxine dose should be reduced to maintain a normal serum TSH (except in those with previous thyroid cancer in whom suppressed TSH is required). There is no consensus about the management of endogenous subclinical hyperthyroidism. The following recommendations are consistent with those of a clinical consensus group from the Endocrine Society, American Thyroid

Association and American Association of Clinical Endocrinologists:

- In elderly patients and postmenopausal women not on hormone replacement who have a high risk of complications of hyperthyroidism (i.e. osteoporosis or atrial fibrillation):
  - If **TSH** <0.1, treat for hyperthyroidism, for example with radio-iodine
  - If **TSH** 0.1–0.3, consider treatment if the thyroid radioisotope scan shows an area of high uptake or if bone density is low.
- In younger patients with a lower risk of complications of hyperthyroidism:
  - If **TSH** <0.1, consider treatment if the thyroid radioisotope scan shows an area of high uptake or if the bone density is low
  - If **TSH** 0.1–0.3, follow-up every 6 months.

Subacute and postpartum thyroiditis

Mild thyroiditis is treated with non-steroidal anti-inflammatory drugs. Moderate or severe thyroiditis may require steroids (prednisolone 40 mg per day for 1 week followed by gradual withdrawal over 4–6 weeks). The symptoms of patients with postpartum thyroiditis may be controlled with propranolol. Patients should be followed up as there is a risk of developing hypothyroidism.

Amiodarone-induced thyrotoxicosis

The decision to continue or stop amiodarone should be made by a cardiologist. Type 1 thyrotoxicosis usually responds to antithyroid drugs, and type 2 thyrotoxicosis responds to prednisolone (40 mg once daily continued for about 8 weeks before tapering). If the type of the hyperthyroidism is uncertain, prednisone (40 mg per day) and carbimazole (40 mg per day) are given initially. A rapid response suggests type 2 thyrotoxicosis, and carbimazole can then be tapered. A poor initial response suggests type 1 disease, and steroids can be tapered.

Thyroid hormone resistance

An important differential diagnosis of secondary hyperthyroidism is thyroid hormone resistance. Patients with this condition have a similar thyroid function profile to those with TSH-secreting pituitary tumours (TSHomas), i.e. high free T_4/T_3 levels and an inappropriately normal or elevated serum TSH.

Thyroid hormone resistance is characterized by reduced responsiveness of the tissues to thyroid hormone. It results from mutations in the gene for the beta form of the thyroid hormone receptor in 90% of patients. The mutations may be inherited (mostly as autosomal dominant) or occur de novo. Thyroid hormone resistance has been detected in 1 in 50 000 live births, and affects males and females equally.

The severity of thyroid hormone resistance may vary in different tissues (pituitary and peripheral tissues) in the same patient and among different patients having the same mutation. Most patients

Table 3.1 Features that help differentiate thyroid hormone resistance from thyroid-stimulating hormone (TSH) secreting adenomas

TSH-secreting adenomas	Thyroid hormone resistance
Often clinically thyrotoxic	Usually euthyroid (except those with selective pituitary resistance who are thyrotoxic)
High serum SHBG (85%)	Normal serum SHBG
High serum alpha subunit of TSH	Normal serum alpha subunit of TSH
TSH levels do not increase in response to TRH	TSH levels increase in response to TRH
TSH levels less likely to fall in response to T_3	TSH levels more likely (90%) to fall in response to T_3
Pituitary tumour may be seen on magnetic resonance imaging (but remember that a pituitary incidentaloma may be detected in up to 10% of normal subjects)	Identification of known mutations in the thyroid hormone receptor beta gene confirms the diagnosis

SHBG, sex hormone-binding globulin; TRH, thyrotrophin-releasing hormone.

have few or no symptoms and signs of thyroid dysfunction. However, patients may have some of the following features:

- goitre (65–95%)
- tachycardia (16–80%), probably due to unopposed activation of the alpha form of the thyroid hormone receptor
- attention deficit hyperactivity disorder, emotional disturbances, learning disability
- growth retardation, delayed bone maturation
- recurrent ear and throat infections, sensorineural hearing loss.

Table 3.1 summarizes the features that help differentiate thyroid hormone resistance from TSHomas.

In most patients with resistance to thyroid hormone, treatment is not required as the increase in thyroid hormone secretion compensates for the partial tissue resistance. However, levothyroxine replacement is required in those with prior destructive antithyroid therapy (i.e. radio-iodine or surgery). Thyrotoxic patients with selective pituitary resistance to thyroid hormone may be treated with beta-blockers and triiodothyroacetic acid (TRIAC).

Key points:

- 'Thyrotoxicosis' refers to an excess of circulating free T_4 and/or free T_3. Thyrotoxicosis may be due to either increased thyroid hormone synthesis (hyperthyroidism) or increased thyroid hormone release from an inflamed thyroid gland (thyroiditis).
- Primary hyperthyroidism is characterized by a raised free T_4 and/or T_3 and low TSH.
- Secondary hyperthyroidism is characterized by raised T_4 and T_3 due to increased TSH secretion from a pituitary tumour.
- Graves' disease accounts for 70–80% of all cases of hyperthyroidism. Toxic multinodular goitre is the most common cause of hyperthyroidism in the elderly.
- Thyrotoxic patients may present with heat intolerance, anxiety, irritability, weakness, palpitations (atrial fibrillation or sinus tachycardia), exertional breathlessness, increased appetite, weight loss, oligomenorrhoea and osteoporosis.
- Clinical signs specific to Graves' disease include ophthalmopathy, pretibial myxoedema and thyroid acropachy.
- Treatment options for hyperthyroidism include antithyroid drugs, radio-iodine and surgery (thyroidectomy).
- A rare but significant complication of antithyroid drugs is agranulocytosis.

Chapter 4

Goitre, thyroid nodules and cancer

Goitre and thyroid nodules

A *goitre* is an enlarged thyroid gland and may be diffuse or nodular (consisting of a solitary or multiple nodules). Box 4.1 summarizes the differential diagnosis of goitre.

Box 4.1 Differential diagnosis of goitre

Thyrotoxic patients
Graves' disease
Multinodular goitre
Solitary adenoma
Thyroiditis (subacute or painless)

Hypothyroid patients
Hashimoto's thyroiditis

Euthyroid patients
Simple goitre (non-toxic)
Malignancy: thyroid carcinoma, lymphoma
Riedel's thyroiditis

Epidemiology

The prevalence of goitres and thyroid nodules was reported as 15% by the Whickham survey in North East England. Goitres are clinically visible in 7% of

Lecture Notes: Endocrinology and Diabetes. By A. Sam and K. Meeran. Published 2009 by Blackwell Publishing. ISBN 978-1-4051-5345-4.

the population (Fig. 4.1) and are palpable (and not visible) in 8%. They are four times more common in females. Prevalence increases with age, iodine deficiency and previous exposure to ionizing radiation. The Himalayas and the Andes are the most important goitrous areas in the world today. Iodine deficiency is also seen in central areas of Asia, Africa and Europe.

Fewer than 5% of thyroid nodules are cancerous. Thyroid nodules are more likely to be cancerous in males. However, as thyroid nodules are more common in females, they are more frequently affected by thyroid cancer than males. The challenge for the endocrinologists is to identify those few patients who have cancerous thyroid nodules.

Clinical presentations

A mass in the neck noticed by the physician, the patient or relatives may be the only presenting complaint.

Features in the history and examination that raise the suspicion of malignancy include:
- age <20 or >60 years
- recent rapid enlargement of a thyroid nodule
- local compressive symptoms: dysphagia, dyspnoea, hoarseness, stridor
- family history of thyroid cancer or multiple endocrine neoplasia (MEN)
- history of exposure to radiation
- lymphadenopathy.

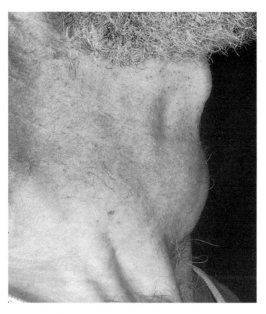

Figure 4.1 Goitre.

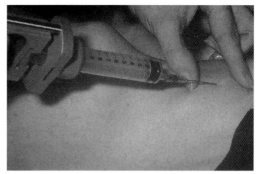

Figure 4.2 Fine needle aspiration of a thyroid nodule.

In addition, a history of Hashimoto's thyroiditis raises incidence of lymphoma. Papillary thyroid carcinoma may be associated with some rare inherited syndromes such as familial adenomatous polyposis, Gardner's syndrome (autosomal dominant disease characterized by gastrointestinal polyps, multiple osteomas, skin and soft tissue tumours) and Cowden's disease (an autosomal dominant condition characterized by multiple hamartomas and an increased risk of early-onset breast and thyroid cancer).

Thyroid examination should include the following steps:

• *Inspection*: ask the patient to swallow (the goitre moves upward).

• *Palpation*: examine the goitre with the patient swallowing—the goitre moves upward. This may be lost in anaplastic carcinoma and Riedel's thyroiditis (a rare chronic inflammatory disease of the thyroid gland characterized by a dense fibrosis replacing normal thyroid parenchyma, which results in a 'woody' goitre). Determine the size, whether the goitre is nodular or diffusely enlarged, soft or hard, or tender (e.g. in subacute thyroiditis or bleeding into a cyst) and the presence of lymph nodes.

• *Percussion* of the upper mediastinum (dull in retrosternal goitre).

• *Auscultation*: for a bruit (in hyperthyroidism) and inspiratory stridor (in cases of tracheal compression).

• *Determination of thyroid status* (look for features of hypothyroidism or thyrotoxicosis).

Investigations

Laboratory findings

Thyroid function tests

Thyroid function tests (thyroid-stimulating hormone [TSH] and free thyroxine [T_4]) should be requested to exclude thyrotoxicosis and hypothyroidism. Serum thyroglobulin levels are increased in both benign and malignant nodules, and can only be used in the follow-up of patients with treated differentiated (papillary and follicular) cancers. Calcitonin should be measured when medullary cell carcinoma is suspected (usually after fine needle aspiration cytology results).

Patients with suspected tracheal obstruction should have respiratory flow–volume loop studies.

Fine needle aspiration and cytology

All patients should have fine needle aspiration of the thyroid nodule for cytological examination (Fig. 4.2).

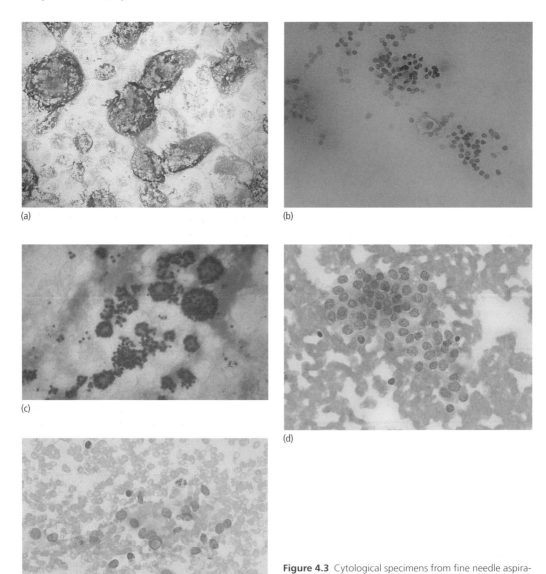

Figure 4.3 Cytological specimens from fine needle aspiration of thyroid nodules. (a) Non-diagnostic: thick blood with no thyroid cells (Thy1). (b) Non-neoplastic (Thy2), (c) Follicular neoplasm: may be an adenoma or carcinoma (Thy3). (d) Suspicious of malignancy (Thy4). (e) Diagnostic of malignancy (Thy5).

The cytologist's report may be one of the following (Fig. 4.3):

- Non-diagnostic
- Non-neoplastic (abundant colloid, features compatible with multinodular goitre or thyroiditis)
- Follicular lesions: adenoma or carcinoma
- Suspicious of malignancy
- Diagnostic for malignancy.

Ultrasound-guided fine needle aspiration should be performed where there is high suspicion of malignancy (history of radiation, MEN type 2 (see

Chapter 32), suspicious ultrasound features, presence of cervical lymph nodes).

Imaging

There are no ultrasonographic findings that are specific for thyroid carcinoma. However, features that raise suspicion of malignancy include hypoechogenicity, irregular border, microcalcifications and increased colour Doppler flow.

A radioisotope uptake scan should be performed in all patients with suppressed TSH. ^{99}Technetium pertechnetate is more commonly used than ^{123}iodine as it is cheaper and more readily available. Some endocrinologists also perform a thyroid uptake scan in cases of indeterminate fine needle aspiration cytology (10% of cases).

Malignant nodules are more likely to be cold (i.e. not to take up radioisotope). However, most (80%) cold nodules are benign (e.g. colloid nodules, haemorrhage, cysts or inflammatory lesions such as Hashimoto's thyroiditis) (Fig. 4.4). Hot nodules are associated with a low incidence of thyroid cancer. However, the presence of hot nodules does not exclude malignancy.

Clinical suspicion of a retrosternal goitre causing tracheal compression may be confirmed by computed tomography (CT) or magnetic resonance imaging (MRI) of the neck and thoracic inlet (Fig. 4.5).

Treatment

Toxic multinodular goitre/solitary nodule

For a detailed discussion of the treatment of toxic multinodular goitre and solitary nodules, see Chapter 3.

Non-toxic goitre/thyroid nodules

Following fine needle aspiration of thyroid nodules and cytological examination, all patients should be discussed at a specialist thyroid multidisciplinary meeting.
• Patients with non-diagnostic cytology need repeat ultrasound-guided fine needle aspiration immediately.
• Patients with suspicious or malignant cytology should be offered surgery.
• Patients with benign cytology should be followed up clinically with palpation (and with ultrasound if a nodule is not easily palpable). Some guidelines recommend repeat fine needle aspiration after 6 months to reduce false-negative rates.

Surgery may also be offered in the presence of symptoms caused by local compression or significant cosmetic disfigurement.

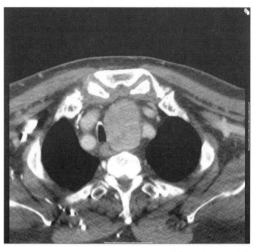

Figure 4.5 Computed tomography scan showing an enlarged left thyroid lobe extending into the mediastinum and indenting the trachea at the level of origin of the large vessels of the aortic arch.

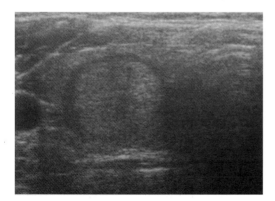

Figure 4.4 Neck ultrasound scan showing a benign thyroid nodule.

Box 4.2 Classification of thyroid carcinoma

Papillary (70–80%)
Follicular (15%)
Anaplastic (5%)
Medullary (5–10%)
Lymphoma (5–10%)

Thyroid cancer

Epidemiology

Thyroid cancer (Box 4.2) is the most common endocrine malignancy. It comprises less than 1% of all cancers and fewer than 0.5% of cancer deaths. The incidence of thyroid cancer has increased since 1980, partly due to an increase in the sensitivity of diagnostic methods.

Aetiology

Environmental factors

Exposure to ionizing radiation, particularly at a young age, increases the risk of thyroid nodules (both benign and malignant). The incidence of follicular carcinomas may have been reduced by iodine supplementation.

Genetic factors

Papillary thyroid carcinomas are associated with rearrangements of two genes—*RET* and *NTRK1*—and the formation of chimeric genes. The new 5′ end of the chimeric gene results in expression of the active tyrosine kinases in thyroid epithelial cells. This presumably activates growth pathways, causing papillary carcinomas in some patients. Mutations in *BRAF* (encoding a serine/threonine kinase) have also been implicated in the pathogenesis of papillary thyroid carcinoma. Activating point mutations of the *RAS* gene are found in follicular adenomas and carcinomas. *PPARG–PAX8* rearrangements are only found in follicular carcinomas. Inactivating point mutations of the *p53*

gene are found in poorly differentiated and anaplastic thyroid carcinomas.

Papillary thyroid cancer

Papillary thyroid cancer is the most common thyroid cancer (70–85%). It is more common in young women (30–50 years). Papillary thyroid carcinoma is often multifocal. In some patients, this may represent intraglandular metastases from the primary tumour. About 15–20% show local extrathyroidal invasion. Papillary carcinomas metastasize via the lymphatics to the regional lymph nodes (clinically evident in about one third of patients at presentation) and distantly, for example to the lungs and bones (2–10% at diagnosis).

Papillary carcinomas are typically unencapsulated. They are characterized by papillae consisting of one or two layers of tumour cells surrounding a fibrovascular core. The cells and nuclei are large, and their cytoplasm has a 'ground glass' appearance. Nucleoli are prominent, and the nuclei have clefts, grooves and 'holes' due to intranuclear cytoplasmic inclusions ('Orphan Annie eyes'). About 50% of papillary carcinomas contain calcified psammoma bodies, the scarred remnants of tumour papillae that presumably infarcted.

There are several variant forms of papillary carcinoma including follicular, columnar cell, tall cell and diffuse sclerosing variant.

Follicular carcinoma

This type of epithelium-derived thyroid carcinoma shows follicular differentiation and capsular or vascular invasion. The peak incidence of follicular carcinomas is between ages 40 and 60 years. Fine needle aspiration specimens may show microfollicles with varying nuclear atypia and little colloid. However, it is difficult to differentiate between benign follicular adenomas and malignant follicular carcinomas on cytology. The distinction between follicular adenoma and carcinoma can only be made through histological identification of capsule and/or vascular invasion (Fig. 4.6), and therefore surgery is recommended. Follicular carcinomas may be minimally or widely invasive.

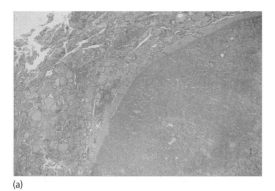

(a)

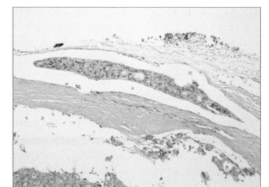

(b)

Figure 4.6 (a) Follicular adenoma. (b) Follicular carcinoma: a capsular blood vessel with tumour in the lumen is indicative of vascular invasion.

Spread is more likely to be haematogenous (to lung and bones) than to regional lymph nodes.

Hurthle cell carcinoma is a variant of follicular thyroid carcinoma and is characterized by the presence of oncocytic cells, which have an abundant oxyphillic cytoplasm (due to the accumulation of altered mitochondria) and round oval nuclei with prominent nucleoli.

Medullary cell carcinoma

See Chapter 32.

Anaplastic carcinoma

Anaplastic thyroid carcinoma occurs more frequently in older patients (60–80 years of age).

Patients usually present with a rapidly enlarging neck mass. The spread is haematogenous, and distant metastases are found in 15–50% of patients at initial disease presentation.

Thyroid lymphoma

Thyroid lymphoma may be part of a systemic disease or may primarily involve the thyroid gland. The risk of thyroid lymphoma is increased in patients with autoimmune thyroiditis.

Treatment

Papillary and follicular carcinoma

Treatment includes initial *thyroidectomy*, postoperative *TSH suppression* with thyroxine and, in high-risk patients, postoperative *radio-iodine ablation*.

Surgery
Surgery is the primary treatment and should be performed by an experienced thyroid surgeon to minimize the risk of hypoparathyroidism and recurrent laryngeal nerve injury. Total thyroidectomy is appropriate when the primary tumor is 1.0 cm or more, or if there is extra-thyroidal extension or metastasis. This aggressive initial surgical approach is associated with lower rates of local and regional recurrence and overall mortality.

Lobectomy plus isthmusectomy may be appropriate for tumours of less than 1.0 cm confined to one lobe of the gland. Lymph node status should be assessed by neck ultrasound scans, and regional neck dissection is carried out in cases of central or lateral nodal involvement.

TSH suppression
After initial surgery, all patients should receive thyroxine to prevent hypothyroidism and to minimize potential TSH stimulation of tumour growth. The dose of levothyroxine should be adjusted by 25 μg every 6 weeks until the serum TSH is below 0.1 mU/L. Most patients require 175–200 μg daily. A lower level of TSH suppression may be appropriate in those with heart disease or low bone mineral density.

Radio-iodine

Thyroid follicular cells can take up radio-iodine (^{131}I), which causes cell death by the emission of beta rays. Postoperatively (at about 4–6 weeks), radio-iodine ablation is given to high-risk patients (those aged ≥45 years, tumours >3–4 cm, aggressive histological variants, extra-thyroidal disease with direct invasion or metastases). The need for radio-iodine ablation in low-risk patients is controversial.

Radio-iodine ablation destroys residual normal thyroid as well as microscopic malignant tissue and improves the specificity of subsequent radio-iodine scans and serum thyroglobulin for detecting recurrent or metastatic cancer. Follow-up scanning with ^{123}I and further radio-iodine treatment with ^{131}I in cases of positive uptake is done 6–12 months after initial radio-iodine and is repeated until the patient has a negative scan.

Prior to the diagnostic or therapeutic use of radio-iodine, thyroid hormone replacement should be withdrawn to allow an increase in serum TSH, which stimulates thyroid tissue to take up radio-iodine. Thyroxine is stopped 6 weeks prior to radio-iodine scan/ablation and is replaced with the shorter-acting triiodothyronine (T_3; 20 µg two or three times daily, or lower doses in elderly patients). T_3 has a shorter half-life and can be stopped 10 days before radio-iodine scanning or treatment. This minimizes the duration and symptoms of hypothyroidism. Patients are also advised to avoid foods with a high iodine content for at least 2 weeks before radio-iodine scanning.

Patients who do not tolerate hypothyroidism (e.g. those with congestive cardiac failure or sleep apnoea) may be given recombinant TSH prior to radio-iodine scanning. This obviates the need for thyroid hormone withdrawal.

Complications of radio-iodine include radiation thyroiditis, painless neck oedema, sialoadenitis, tumour haemorrhage or oedema, and nausea. An increased risk of secondary malignancies has been reported.

The radio-iodine doses given in thyroid cancer are much higher than those given in hyperthyroidism, and patients may be isolated after treatment. However, some studies suggest that instructions to the patient to sleep alone, drink fluids liberally and avoid prolonged close personal contact with family members for 2 days after the treatment may be sufficient.

Anaplastic thyroid carcinoma

The treatment of anaplastic thyroid carcinoma includes total thyroidectomy with lymph node clearance, chemotherapy (e.g. doxorubicin and cisplatin) and external beam irradiation.

Thyroid lymphoma

Disease limited to the thyroid is treated with radiotherapy.

Prognosis of thyroid cancer

Poor prognostic factors in differentiated thyroid carcinomas include age (≥45 years), male gender, family history, tumour size, local extension, lymph node and distant metastases, and aggressive histological variants.
- *Papillary cancer* has a 10-year mortality of 5% and a 10-year recurrence rate of 10%.
- *Follicular carcinomas* have a 10-year mortality of 15%. An aggressive variant of follicular carcinoma (Hurthle cell carcinoma), which fails to concentrate radio-iodine, has a 10-year mortality of 25%.
- *Anaplastic carcinoma* has a mean survival of 6 months.

Follow-up and monitoring

Most recurrences of differentiated thyroid carcinoma happen within the first 5 years after initial treatment. However, recurrences may occur many years later (particularly in papillary carcinoma). All patients should have periodic physical examinations and serum thyroglobulin (and thyroglobulin antibody) measurements.

Serum thyroglobulin

If initial surgery and thyroid remnant ablation are successful, the serum thyroglobulin concentration should be very low (<2 ng/mL). Serum thyroglobulin levels are elevated in 95% of patients with tumour recurrences. The laboratory should always test for anti-thyroglobulin antibodies. Anti-thyroglobulin antibodies interfere with the assay for thyroglobulin, so serum thyroglobulin cannot be used to monitor patients with these antibodies. These patients may need more frequent imaging studies during early follow-up.

Further imaging

If there is evidence of recurrence from clinical examination or tests, further imaging using radio-iodine uptake scanning, ultrasonography, CT or MRI, skeletal X-rays or skeletal radionuclide imaging may be indicated to identify sites of disease. In patients with evidence of distant metastases, fluorodeoxyglucose positron emission tomography (PET) scanning may provide useful prognostic information.

Key points:

- Goitre (enlargement of the thyroid gland) affects up to 15% of the population.
- Patients with goitre may be euthyroid, hypothyroid or thyrotoxic.
- Features that raise suspicion of malignancy in a thyroid nodule include rapid enlargement, symptoms of local compression, a family history of thyroid cancer, radiation exposure and lymphadenopathy.
- Thyroid carcinoma is classified into papillary, follicular, anaplastic, medullary and lymphoma.
- The treatment of differentiated thyroid carcinoma includes surgery, TSH suppression with thyroxine and radio-iodine ablation (in high-risk patients).

Chapter 5

Adrenal anatomy and physiology

The adrenal glands are small Y-shaped glands located extraperitoneally at the upper poles of the kidneys (Fig. 5.1). The arterial blood supply arises from the renal arteries, aorta and inferior phrenic artery. Venous drainage is via the central vein into the inferior vena cava on the right, and into the left renal vein on the left.

The adrenal glands consist of an outer *cortex* (90%) surrounding an inner *medulla* (10%). The adrenal cortex is derived from mesodermal tissue, whereas the adrenal medulla is derived from neuroectodermal tissue (embryonic neural crest). The cortex has three layers or 'zones' (Fig. 5.2):

- The *zona glomerulosa* secretes mineralocorticoids (aldosterone: 100–150 μg per day).
- The *zona fasciculata* secretes glucocorticoids (cortisol: 10–20 mg per day).
- The *zona reticularis* secretes androgens (mainly dehydroepiandrosterone: DHEA).

The adrenal medulla is composed of *chromaffin cells*, which produce catecholamines (adrenaline, noradrenaline, dopamine) from the amino acid tyrosine. Chromaffin cells are so named because they can be visualized by staining with chromium salts. Catecholamine secretion is stimulated by preganglionic sympathetic nerves.

Lecture Notes: Endocrinology and Diabetes. By A. Sam and K. Meeran. Published 2009 by Blackwell Publishing. ISBN 978-1-4051-5345-4.

The pathways of steroid hormone biosynthesis in the adrenal glands are shown in Fig. 5.3.

Aldosterone

Aldosterone secretion is stimulated by the *renin–angiotensin system* and elevated serum potassium. Renin is synthesized and stored in the juxtaglomerular apparatus in the kidney. Renin cleaves angiotensinogen (synthesized in the liver) to angiotensin I (a decapeptide); this is then converted to angiotensin II by angiotensin-converting enzyme on the luminal surface of capillaries in the lungs. Angiotensin II stimulates aldosterone secretion, resulting in sodium retention and potassium loss in the kidney. Renin release is stimulated by reduced renal perfusion pressure and blood flow, reduced sodium concentration in the renal tubules (sensed by macula densa cells) and increased renal sympathetic activity.

Effects

Aldosterone is a lipid-soluble hormone that crosses plasma membranes and binds to intracellular receptors. The hormone–receptor complex increases the expression of certain genes and upregulates the synthesis of sodium channels and sodium/potassium (Na/K) ATPase in the distal renal tubular cells. Aldosterone increases sodium

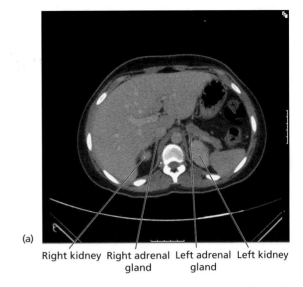

(a)

Right kidney Right adrenal Left adrenal Left kidney
                  gland   gland

Inferior
vena cava

Aorta

Right adrenal
gland

Left adrenal
gland

Right kidney

Left kidney

Right crus
of diaphragm

Left crus
of diaphragm

(b)

Figure 5.1 (a) Typical appearance of the adrenal glands on an abdominal computed tomography scan. (b) Diagram illustrating the cross-sectional anatomy of the adrenal glands.

and water reabsorption and potassium secretion in the kidney. It also stimulates hydrogen ion secretion into the tubular lumen by cells in the collecting ducts.

Cortisol

Cortisol release is stimulated by *adrenocorticotrophic hormone* (ACTH) released from the anterior pituitary (Fig. 5.4). ACTH secretion is stimulated by hypothalamic *corticotrophin-releasing hormone* (CRH). Cortisol in turn inhibits ACTH and CRH production (negative feedback).

Activation of the ACTH receptor on the plasma membrane of cells in the zona fasciculata results in the activation of adenylate cyclase and hence increased cyclic AMP levels. This leads to the stimulation of steroidogenic acute regulatory protein (StAR), which mediates the transport of cholesterol through the cytosol to the inner mitochondrial membrane, where it is converted to pregnenolone. This is the rate-limiting step in cortisol synthesis

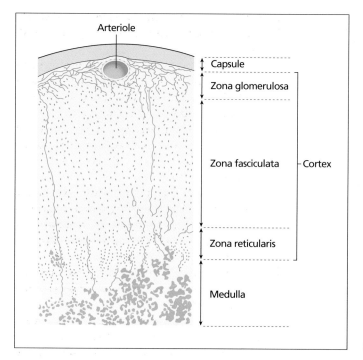

Figure 5.2 Adrenal histology.

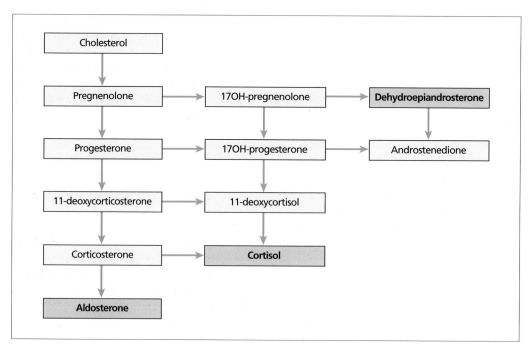

Figure 5.3 Biosynthesis of adrenal steroid hormones.

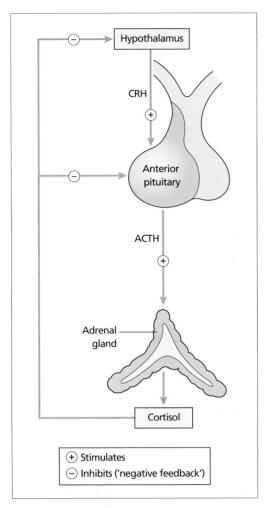

Figure 5.4 Hypothalamic–pituitary–adrenal axis.

sequences and regulate the expression of certain genes. Cortisol increases hepatic *gluconeogenesis* by:

● enhancing the expression of enzymes involved in gluconeogenesis such as glucose-6-phosphatase and phosphoenolpyruvate carboxykinase (the rate-limiting enzyme in gluconeogenesis)

● increasing the availability of substrates, for example glucogenic amino acids and glycerol, by stimulating proteolysis (in skeletal muscle) and lipolysis respectively.

Cortisol also has an important role in the maintenance of hepatic glycogen stores by activating the enzyme glycogen synthase and inactivating the glycogen-mobilizing enzyme glycogen phosphorylase.

Glucocorticoids inhibit glucose uptake and utilization by the peripheral tissues (adipocytes and skeletal muscle).

In humans with chronic cortisol excess, a redistribution of body fat occurs with relative sparing of the extremities and marked fat deposition in the dorsocervical and supraclavicular regions, trunk, anterior mediastinum and mesenteries. Cortisol also increases appetite.

Cortisol has inhibitory effects on T cell- and B cell-mediated immune responses as well as suppressive effects on monocytes and neutrophils. Cortisol also promotes the transcription of genes coding for *anti-inflammatory* products, and inhibits both the synthesis and the secretion of inflammatory cytokines.

(Fig. 5.3). Activation of adenylate cyclase also results in upregulated gene expression of other enzymes involved in steroid synthesis.

Cortisol secretion normally reflects that of ACTH, and is therefore also pulsatile with a circadian rhythm.

Effects

Cortisol is a lipid-soluble hormone that crosses plasma membranes and binds to intracellular receptors, which in turn bind to specific DNA

Adrenal androgens

Adrenal androgens are produced in the zona reticularis. Their synthesis is under the control of ACTH.

DHEA is converted to DHEA-sulphate (DHEA-S) in the adrenals and liver, both of which contain a sulphotransferase. In the adrenal glands and peripheral tissues, small amounts of DHEA and DHEA-S are converted to more active androgens such as androstenedione, testosterone and 5-dihydrotestosterone, and oestrogens such as oestradiol and oestrone.

These hormones exert their androgenic and oestrogenic effects via androgen and oestrogen receptors respectively. Androgen (and oestrogen) receptors are nuclear receptors that bind to specific DNA sequences and regulate the expression of certain genes.

In women, the adrenal production of DHEA and DHEA-S contributes substantially to overall androgen levels. In men, the adrenal contribution is very small compared with that of the testes.

Key points:

- The adrenal glands are located at the upper poles of the kidneys.
- The adrenal glands consist of an outer cortex (90%) surrounding an inner medulla (10%).
- The adrenal cortex has three 'zones': the zona glomerulosa secretes aldosterone; the zona fasciculata secretes cortisol; and the zona reticularis secretes adrenal androgens.
- The adrenal medulla produces catecholamines: adrenaline (80%) and noradrenaline (20%).
- Aldosterone secretion is stimulated by the renin–angiotensin system and elevated serum potassium.
- Cortisol release is stimulated by ACTH from the anterior pituitary.
- Cortisol, aldosterone and adrenal androgens are lipid-soluble hormones. They cross the plasma membrane and bind to intracellular nuclear receptors that bind in turn to specific DNA sequences and regulate the expression of certain genes.

Chapter 6

Adrenal insufficiency

Adrenal insufficiency refers to a reduced production of the hormones secreted by the adrenal cortex. Adrenal insufficiency may be 'primary' due to a disease affecting the adrenal cortex (*Addison's disease*), or 'secondary' due either to pituitary/hypothalamic disease or long-term steroid use and suppression of the hypothalamic–pituitary–adrenal (HPA) axis.

Epidemiology

The prevalence of Addison's disease is about 120 per million. Isolated autoimmune adrenal insufficiency occurs predominately in males during the first two decades of life, equally in males and females in the third decade, and predominately in females thereafter (80%). The reason for these sex differences is unknown. In contrast, 70% of patients with autoimmune adrenal insufficiency as part of one of the autoimmune polyglandular syndromes are female.

Aetiology

The most common cause of primary adrenal insufficiency is *autoimmune* adrenalitis (up to 80% of cases). In these patients, there is evidence of both humoral and cell-mediated immune mechanisms directed at the adrenal cortex. Up to 75% of patients with autoimmune primary adrenal insufficiency have antibodies against steroidogenic enzymes (most often 21-hydroxylase) and all three zones of the adrenal cortex. The first evidence of autoimmune adrenal insufficiency is an increase in plasma renin activity, suggesting that the zona glomerulosa failure and reduction in aldosterone occur first. Zona fasciculata dysfunction becomes evident several months to years later.

About 50% of patients with autoimmune adrenal insufficiency have one or more other autoimmune endocrine disorders. On the other hand, patients with the more common autoimmune endocrine disorders, such as type 1 diabetes mellitus or Graves' disease, rarely develop adrenal insufficiency.

Autoimmune adrenal insufficiency may rarely be part of autoimmune polyglandular syndromes (APS):

- *APS type 1* is an autosomal recessive disorder caused by mutations in the *AIRE* gene, which encodes a nuclear transcription factor. APS type 1 is characterized by chronic mucocutaneous candidiasis and hypoparathyroidism (appearing by the early 20s) followed by Addison's disease (in 60%).
- *APS type 2* or Schmidt's syndrome may be inherited in an autosomal recessive, dominant or polygenic manner and is characterized by Addison's disease (100%), autoimmune thyroid disease and diabetes mellitus.

Lecture Notes: Endocrinology and Diabetes. By A. Sam and K. Meeran. Published 2009 by Blackwell Publishing. ISBN 978-1-4051-5345-4.

Box 6.1 Causes of primary adrenal insufficiency

Autoimmune

Infection
Tuberculosis, fungal (histoplasmosis, cryptococcosis), cytomegalovirus (in AIDS)

Infiltration
Metastases (lung, breast, kidney), lymphoma, amyloidosis, haemochromatosis

Infarction
Due to thrombosis caused by thrombophilia (e.g. antiphospholipid syndrome)

Haemorrhage
Waterhouse–Friderichsen syndrome due to meningococcal septicaemia, anticoagulants

Adrenoleukodystrophy

Adrenal dysgenesis
Congenital adrenal hypoplasia (due to mutations of the *NR0B1* gene on the X chromosome, encoding a nuclear receptor protein called DAX1), mutations in SF1 gene

Iatrogenic
Adrenal suppressors (ketoconazole, etomidate), bilateral adrenalectomy

Primary hypogonadism occurs in both types of APS, and ovarian failure is more frequent than testicular failure.

Tuberculosis is the second most common cause of 'Addison's disease'. Rarer causes of adrenal insufficiency are listed in Box 6.1.

The adrenal glands are a relatively common site of metastases. However, adrenal insufficiency with metastases is much less common.

Adrenoleukodystrophy is a rare X-linked disorder, caused by mutations in the *ABCD1* gene that result in the prevention of normal transport of very long chain fatty acids into peroxisomes (for beta-oxidation) and their accumulation in the central nervous system and adrenal cortex. Patients may present in childhood with increasing cognitive and behavioural abnormalities, blindness and the development of quadriparesis.

Adrenoleukodystrophy consists of a spectrum of phenotypes that includes adrenomyeloneuropathy. Adrenomyeloneuropathy typically presents in adult males between 20 and 40 years of age with adrenal insufficiency, spastic paraparesis, abnormal sphincter control or cerebellar signs.

For causes of secondary adrenal insufficiency see Chapter 12.

Chronic glucocorticoid use and HPA axis suppression

The following groups of patients are likely to have adrenal insufficiency secondary to HPA axis suppression by long-term glucocorticoid use:
- those who have received a glucocorticoid dose equivalent to or more than 20 mg of prednisolone per day for more than 3 weeks
- those who have received an evening or bedtime dose of prednisone for more than a few weeks
- those who have a Cushingoid appearance.

Clinical presentations of primary adrenal insufficiency

The insidious onset and non-specific symptoms usually result in a delay in diagnosis. Adrenal insufficiency may therefore be undetected until an acute illness or other stress precipitates an adrenal crisis.

Patients may have symptoms and signs of glucocorticoid, mineralocorticoid and, in women, androgen deficiency. Patients with secondary adrenal insufficiency usually have normal mineralocorticoid function as mineralocorticoids are regulated by the renin–angiotensin system rather than adrenocorticotrophic hormone (ACTH).

Clinical presentations of primary adrenal insufficiency are summarized in Box 6.2.

Adrenal crisis

Adrenal crisis most commonly presents as *shock*. Acute adrenal crisis may be seen in patients with:
- previously undiagnosed adrenal insufficiency who have been subject to acute stress or illness, for example infection
- known adrenal insufficiency who have not increased their steroid dose during an infection or other illness, or have been vomiting

---

> **Box 6.2 Clinical presentations of primary adrenal insufficiency**
>
> **Acute adrenal crisis**
>
> **General**
> Malaise, fatigue, weakness, anorexia, weight loss
>
> **Gastrointestinal**
> Nausea, vomiting, abdominal pain, diarrhoea
>
> **Hypotension**
> Postural hypotension, improved blood pressure in hypertensive patients
>
> **Metabolic**
> Hyponatraemia, hyperkalaemia, hypoglycaemia, hypercalcaemia
>
> **Skin**
> Hyperpigmentation (generalized, palmar creases, nails, buccal, scars, nails), associated vitiligo
>
> **Musculoskeletal**
> Myalgia, arthralgia, flexion contractures of legs (rare), calcification of the auricular cartilages in men
>
> **Psychiatric**
> Impairment of memory, confusion, depression, psychosis

- those with HPA suppression caused by the long-term use of glucocorticoids (oral and occasionally inhaled) who suddenly stop their treatment
- bilateral adrenal infarction or haemorrhage
- pituitary apoplexy (infarction) resulting in acute cortisol deficiency.

General

Patients with adrenal insufficiency often have non-specific symptoms such as malaise, fatigue, lethargy, weakness, anorexia and weight loss.

Gastrointestinal

Patients may complain of nausea, occasionally vomiting, abdominal pain and diarrhoea that may alternate with constipation. The cause of gastrointestinal symptoms in adrenal insufficiency is not fully understood but may be related to electrolyte abnormalities.

Hypotension

Adrenal insufficiency can present with *postural hypotension* (causing postural dizziness), low blood pressure or improved blood pressure in patients with pre-existing hypertension. This is mainly due to volume depletion resulting from aldosterone deficiency. Glucocorticoid deficiency can contribute to hypotension by causing decreased vascular responsiveness to the vasoconstrictor effect of noradrenaline and angiotensin II.

Skin

In primary adrenal insufficiency, lack of cortisol negative feedback causes an increase in the hypothalamic precursor protein proopiomelanocortin (POMC) and its cleavage products, including ACTH and alpha-melanocyte-stimulating hormone. The latter increases the melanin content of the skin, resulting in *hyperpigmentation*.

Hyperpigmentation may be generalized, particularly in areas exposed to light or pressure (e.g. elbows, knees, spine, knuckles, brassiere straps). It may also be seen in the palmar creases, nails (longitudinal bands of darkening), buccal mucosa (Fig. 6.1) and scars acquired when primary adrenal insufficiency is present and untreated. The hyperpigmentation usually disappears after a few months of treatment with glucocorticoids. However, scars never fade because the melanin is trapped in fibrous connective tissue.

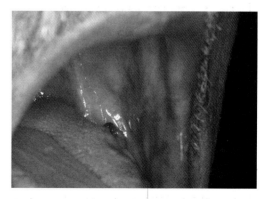

Figure 6.1 Buccal pigmentation in a patient with Addison's disease.

Associated vitiligo (areas of depigmented skin) is seen in 10–20% of patients with Addison's disease. Vitiligo results from autoimmune destruction of dermal melanocytes.

Electrolyte abnormalities

Hyponatraemia is seen in 90% of patients and is due to sodium loss caused by mineralocorticoid deficiency, and increased antidiuretic hormone secretion caused by cortisol deficiency (resulting in reduced renal water clearance). Patients may present with salt craving.

Hyperkalaemia occurs in 60% of patients. It is associated with mild hyperchloraemic acidosis and is due to mineralocorticoid deficiency.

Patients may have an elevated urea (and possibly creatinine) due to dehydration. Hypercalcaemia may rarely occur in Addison's disease.

Hypoglycaemia

Hypoglycaemia is rare in adults in the absence of infection or alcohol ingestion. It may occur after prolonged fasting or, rarely, several hours after a high-carbohydrate meal. It is more common in patients with secondary adrenal insufficiency caused by isolated ACTH deficiency.

Addison's disease should be suspected in patients with type 1 diabetes mellitus in whom insulin requirements decrease.

Reduced adrenal androgens in women

In women, the adrenal cortex is the primary source of androgens in the form of dehydroepiandrosterone (DHEA) and DHEA sulphate. Women with adrenal insufficiency may have decreased pubic and axillary hair and loss of libido due to reduced adrenal androgens.

Clinical presentations of secondary adrenal insufficiency

Many of the symptoms such as weakness, fatigue, myalgia and arthralgia are the same as those for primary adrenal insufficiency. The major exceptions are that in secondary adrenal insufficiency:

- there is no hyperpigmentation (due to ACTH deficiency)
- there is no dehydration or hyperkalaemia (reflecting the presence of aldosterone)
- gastrointestinal symptoms are less common (suggesting that electrolyte disturbances may be involved in their aetiology)
- hypoglycaemia is more common (possibly because patients tolerate their illness longer due to an absence of dehydration and hypotension, and present with symptoms of chronic glucocorticoid deficiency rather than mineralocorticoid deficiency)
- there may be clinical manifestations of a pituitary or hypothalamic tumour, such as a headache, visual field defects or symptoms and signs of deficiency of other anterior pituitary hormones.

Investigations

Initial blood tests at presentation may show:
- hyponatraemia
- hyperkalaemia
- acidosis (normal anion gap)
- high urea
- mild hypercalcaemia
- eosinophilia
- hypoglycaemia (rare in adults).

Patients with Addison's disease may have low free thyroid hormone levels and elevated thyroid-stimulating hormone. This may either be a direct effect of glucocorticoid deficiency or due to associated primary autoimmune hypothyroidism. Thus thyroid function tests must be rechecked after adrenal insufficiency has been treated.

9 a.m. cortisol and short ACTH stimulation test

A 9 a.m. serum cortisol level of less than 100 nmol/L is diagnostic of adrenal insufficiency. Adrenal insufficiency is unlikely if the 9 a.m. cortisol is more than 550 nmol/L.

Patients with an 8–9 a.m. cortisol of between 100 and 550 nmol/L should have a *short ACTH stimulation test*. 250 µg of synthetic ACTH (amino acids 1–24) is given intramuscularly and serum cortisol is measured at time 0 (just before the injection) and 30 and 60 minutes after the synthetic ACTH has been given. A normal response to the short ACTH stimulation test is a peak cortisol of over 550 nmol/L. An abnormal response is consistent with primary or secondary adrenal failure and should be investigated further (see below).

If the patient is already on hydrocortisone, this should be stopped 20–24 hours before the short ACTH stimulation test. This is because the exogenous hydrocortisone may be measured as cortisol by the assay. In patients in whom discontinuing steroids is not thought to be safe, hydrocortisone (or prednisolone) should be substituted by an equivalent dose of dexamethasone, which does not interfere with the cortisol assay (0.75 mg of dexamethasone is given for every 5 mg of prednisolone or 20 mg of hydrocortisone).

Oestrogens should be discontinued for 6 weeks before the test. This is because the assay measures total cortisol level, and oestrogens increase cortisol-binding globulin (CBG) and result in higher total cortisol level measurements.

False-negative results may be seen in acutely unwell patients, in whom levels of CBG may be low. The assay for cortisol measures total cortisol levels (i.e. free cortisol plus cortisol bound to CBG). Thus total cortisol levels measured following the ACTH stimulation test may be misleadingly low (due to low CBG) even though free cortisol levels may be normal or even high.

A normal response does not exclude the diagnosis of secondary adrenal insufficiency, particularly if the secondary adrenal insufficiency is recent (e.g. within 2 weeks after pituitary surgery). This is because, in these patients, the adrenals have not yet become completely atrophic, and are still capable of responding to ACTH stimulation. In these patients, an insulin tolerance test (i.e. stimulation of ACTH and subsequently cortisol release by insulin-induced hypoglycaemia) is the preferred test.

Chronic glucocorticoid use and HPA axis suppression

In patients who have been on long-term glucocorticoids, a short ACTH stimulation test should be performed if:

- abrupt discontinuation is required
- the patient is facing an acute stress, for example surgery
- there is difficulty in reducing the dose below 5 mg per day because of non-disease-related symptoms.

Determining the level of defect

Once adrenal insufficiency has been diagnosed, it should be determined whether it is primary or secondary.

Basal plasma ACTH

Basal plasma ACTH levels should be measured at the beginning of the short ACTH stimulation test (i.e. before synthetic ACTH is given). ACTH is unstable in blood at room temperature. Thus the specimen for plasma ACTH is collected in an EDTA tube and is sent to the laboratory on ice immediately. Raised ACTH (>200 ng/L) in the presence of an impaired cortisol response is consistent with primary adrenal insufficiency. ACTH levels less than 10 ng/L are consistent with a diagnosis of secondary adrenal insufficiency.

ACTH secretion is suppressed by glucocorticoid therapy. Thus blood samples for ACTH must be drawn before starting glucocorticoids. In patients who are already on hydrocortisone, the test should be done at least 24 hours after the last dose of hydrocortisone, and longer after long-acting glucocorticoids such as dexamethasone if this is thought to be safe clinically.

Prolonged ACTH stimulation test

A prolonged ACTH stimulation test may be used to distinguish primary from secondary adrenal insufficiency. In primary adrenal insufficiency, the adrenal glands are partially or completely destroyed. They are already exposed to maximal levels of endogenous ACTH, and cannot respond to additional ACTH. However, in secondary adrenal insufficiency, the atrophic adrenal glands recover cortisol secretory capacity when chronically exposed to ACTH.

A dose of 1 mg of depot synthetic ACTH is given intramuscularly, and serum cortisol is measured at time 0 (before synthetic ACTH injection) and at 30 minutes, 1, 2, 4, 6, 8 and 24 hours. A normal response is an elevation in serum cortisol to over 900 nmol/L. Patients with primary adrenal insufficiency show no increase after 6 hours, whereas in secondary adrenal insufficiency a continuous increase is seen. Patients who are already on glucocorticoids should have their last dose 24 hours before the start of the test.

Metyrapone test

The metyrapone test may occasionally be used if partial ACTH deficiency is suspected. Metyrapone blocks the final step in cortisol biosynthesis, resulting in reductions in cortisol concentration and stimulation of ACTH secretion due to reduced negative feedback. Hypocortisolaemia is a weaker stimulus to ACTH secretion than hypoglycaemia, and thus the metyrapone test will detect partial ACTH deficiency that may be missed by the insulin tolerance test.

Determining the aetiology

The investigations for determining the aetiology of primary adrenal insufficiency are discussed below. Patients with secondary adrenal insufficiency should have a pituitary magnetic resonance imaging scan to exclude a tumour or other mass lesion, and further pituitary function tests (see Chapter 12).

Adrenal antibodies

Antibodies to enzymes of the adrenal cortex are found in more than 90% of the patients with recent-onset adrenal autoimmunity. 21-Hydroxylase antibodies are the major component of adrenal cortex antibodies.

Imaging

If there is clinical suspicion of tuberculosis, chest and abdominal radiographs should be performed to look for apical shadowing and adrenal calcification respectively. Abdominal computed tomography (CT) may show adrenal enlargement with or without calcification in patients with tuberculosis, infiltration or metastatic disease. In autoimmune adrenalitis, the adrenal glands are often small and atrophic.

Other tests

Other tests may be done depending on the suspected causes of adrenal insufficiency. These may include, for example, serological or microbiological investigations for infections (e.g. urine culture for *Mycobacterium tuberculosis*, tuberculin skin testing, complement fixation titres for *Histoplasma capsulatum*), thrombophilia screen (including antiphospholipid antibodies), plasma concentration of very long chain fatty acids (elevated in adrenoleukodystrophy) and percutaneous CT-guided biopsy.

Detecting other autoimmune diseases

Patients with autoimmune adrenal failure should be investigated for:
- diabetes mellitus: fasting glucose
- thyroid disease: free thyroxine/triiodothyronine and thyroid-stimulating hormone
- parathyroid dysfunction: calcium and phosphate (and parathyroid hormone if hypocalcaemic)
- pernicious anaemia: parietal cell antibodies
- primary gonadal failure: luteinizing hormone, follicle-stimulating hormone, testosterone (in men), oestradiol (in women).

Treatment

Addisonian crisis

Adrenal crisis is a life-threatening emergency and requires immediate treatment.

Blood for serum cortisol, ACTH, renin and serum urea and electrolytes should be drawn and therapy should be started immediately:
- *Fluids*: 1–3 L of 0.9% saline should be infused intravenously within the first 12–24 hours based on an assessment of volume status and urine

output. Hypoglycaemia (if present) must be corrected with intravenous (i.v.) dextrose.

- *Glucocorticoids*: In a patient without a previous diagnosis of adrenal insufficiency, dexamethasone (4 mg i.v.) is preferred as, unlike hydrocortisone, it is not measured by serum cortisol assays. Patients with known adrenal insufficiency should be treated with hydrocortisone 100 mg intramuscularly or i.v. 6-hourly. Mineralocorticoid replacement is not useful acutely because it takes several days for its sodium-retaining effects to appear, and adequate sodium replacement can be achieved by intravenous saline alone. Unless there is a major complicating illness, parenteral glucocorticoid therapy can be tapered over 1–3 days and changed to an oral maintenance dose.

- The *precipitating cause* of the adrenal crisis (e.g. bacterial infection or viral gastroenteritis) should be treated appropriately.

Once the patient's condition is stable, the diagnosis can be confirmed in patients not known to have adrenal insufficiency with a short ACTH stimulation test.

Long-term treatment

Glucocorticoid replacement

Hydrocortisone is the logical option for glucocorticoid replacement because it is the glucocorticoid the adrenals make. A daily regimen of 10 mg in the morning, 5 mg at noon and 5 mg in the evening is probably the 'best-guess' starting dose.

Cortisol has a plasma half-life of less than 2 hours. The traditional hydrocortisone regimen of 20 mg in the morning and 10 mg in the evening is suboptimal. This is because it may result in low cortisol levels and low quality of life scores in the late afternoon. In addition, hydrocortisone production rates in normal individuals are lower than previously believed. Over-replacement may result in Cushing's syndrome. Thus the total daily dose should not exceed 20 mg (except at times of intercurrent illness).

It is essential that patients are provided with:
- information regarding the doubling of hydrocortisone dose at times of intercurrent illness

- an emergency intramuscular hydrocortisone supply (to be given at times of vomiting on their way to hospital)
- a steroid card and MedicAlert bracelet.

It must be remembered that glucocorticoid replacement may unmask underlying central diabetes insipidus, leading to marked polyuria.

Mineralocorticoid replacement

Fludrocortisone is given orally in a usual dose of 100 µg per day. Patients receiving hydrocortisone (which has some mineralocorticoid activity) may require a lower dose of fludrocortisone (e.g. 50 µg per day). However, patients receiving prednisolone or dexamethasone (which have no mineralocorticoid activity) may require up to 200 µg per day of fludrocortisone. The mineralocorticoid dose may have to be increased in the summer, when salt loss in perspiration increases.

Patients with essential hypertension and primary adrenal insufficiency should be treated by dietary sodium restriction and a lower dose of fludrocortisone. Fludrocortisone cannot usually be discontinued without risking sodium depletion. If an antihypertensive drug is needed, diuretic drugs and spironolactone should not be used, as they simply counteract the action of fludrocortisone.

Mineralocorticoid replacement is not required in patients with secondary adrenal insufficiency as ACTH is not an important regulator of aldosterone release.

Androgen replacement

Clinical trial data suggest that DHEA replacement in women may be beneficial for mood and psychological well-being. However, there is insufficient evidence to recommend therapy in all patients with adrenal insufficiency, particularly in men. In women with adrenal insufficiency (primary or secondary), DHEA therapy (25–50 mg daily) may be tried only for those who have a significantly impaired sense of well-being or mood despite optimal glucocorticoid and mineralocorticoid replacement. If no obvious benefit has been seen after 6 months, or if adverse effects such as acne occur, DHEA is discontinued.

Treatment of the underlying disorder

Patients with causes other than autoimmune adrenalitis (e.g. adrenal tuberculosis or adrenoleukodystrophy) should be referred to the appropriate specialists.

HPA axis suppression

Patients who are likely to have HPA axis suppression due to the chronic use of glucocorticoids (e.g. for inflammatory diseases), should wear a Medic-Alert bracelet and carry a 'steroid card' and arguably a hydrocortisone ampoule.

If withdrawal from glucocorticoids is indicated, the dose must be reduced *gradually*. The goal of tapering is to prevent both recurrent activity of the underlying disease and symptoms of cortisol deficiency:

- For prednisone doses of 20–60 mg per day: reduce by 5 mg per day every 1–2 weeks.
- For prednisone doses of 10–19 mg per day: reduce by 2.5 mg per day every 1–2 weeks.
- For prednisone doses of 5–9 mg per day: reduce by 1 mg per day every 1–2 weeks.
- For prednisone doses below 5 mg per day: reduce by 0.5 mg per day every 1–2 weeks.

Follow-up and monitoring

Glucocorticoid replacement

The adequacy of treatment is monitored by *clinical assessment* and laboratory tests. The glucocorticoid dose should be increased if symptoms of cortisol deficiency are present. However, if increasing the dose does not promptly ameliorate the symptoms, the patient has other causes and the lower steroid dosage should be resumed. The glucocorticoid dose may be high if the patient develops excessive weight gain, facial plethora, osteoporosis or other symptoms or signs of Cushing's syndrome.

Some endocrinologists use *hydrocortisone day curves* to adjust the dose and timing of hydrocortisone replacement therapy. Blood is taken in the morning and before and 1 hour after the lunchtime and evening doses. The aim is to achieve adequate cortisol levels throughout the day (peak <900 nmol/L and trough >50–100 nmol/L). Once adequate levels have been achieved, this rarely needs to be repeated. All oestrogens should be stopped 6 weeks prior to the test as they increase CBG levels and result in misleadingly high measured total cortisol levels.

Mineralocorticoid replacement

The adequacy of mineralocorticoid replacement should be monitored by asking about symptoms of postural hypotension and measuring *lying and standing blood pressure* and serum urea and electrolytes. Postural hypotension suggests underreplacement. Hypertension, oedema and hypokalaemia suggest over-replacement.

Annual measurement of *plasma renin activity* (PRA) is useful until the patient is on a stable dose of fludrocortisone. The fludrocortisone dose is adjusted to lower the PRA to the upper-normal range. However, in asymptomatic patients with normal serum electrolytes but a high PRA, the dose of fludrocortisone should not be raised to normalize PRA as patients may develop hypokalaemia and oedema.

Key points:

- The most common cause of primary adrenal insufficiency is autoimmune adrenalitis.
- The insidious onset and non-specific symptoms usually result in a delay in diagnosis.
- Physical signs of Addison's disease include postural hypotension and hyperpigmentation.
- Laboratory tests in Addison's disease may show hyponatraemia and hyperkalaemia.
- Patients with suspected Addison's disease should have a short ACTH stimulation test.
- Addisonian crisis is treated with i.v. fluids (0.9% saline) and intramuscular hydrocortisone.
- The long-term treatment of Addison's disease includes oral hydrocortisone and fludrocortisone replacement.
- Patients must be advised to carry a steroid card and a MedicAlert bracelet, and to double their hydrocortisone dose at times of intercurrent illness.
- If withdrawal from glucocorticoids is indicated in patients who are likely to have HPA axis suppression due to long-term glucocorticoid use, the dose must be reduced gradually.

Chapter 7

Primary hyperaldosteronism

Primary hyperaldosteronism is characterized by an excessive autonomous secretion of aldosterone resulting in a suppression of plasma renin activity. The two main causes of primary hyperaldosteronism are *unilateral adenoma* secreting excess aldosterone, and *bilateral hyperplasia* of the adrenal cortex.

Secondary hyperaldosteronism is due to increased plasma renin activity and may be seen in conditions associated with reduced renal perfusion such as renal artery stenosis, congestive cardiac failure and cirrhosis.

Epidemiology

The prevalence of primary hyperaldosteronism in hypertensive patients is 1–2%. Aldosterone-producing adenomas occur more commonly in women (2:1 ratio) and in younger patients (<50 years). Bilateral adrenal hyperplasia occurs more commonly in men and usually presents at an older age. Adrenal carcinomas are more common in females and are usually seen in 50–70-year olds.

Aetiology

Primary hyperaldosteronism may be due to a unilateral aldosterone-producing adenoma (70%) or

Lecture Notes: Endocrinology and Diabetes. By A. Sam and K. Meeran. Published 2009 by Blackwell Publishing. ISBN 978-1-4051-5345-4.

bilateral hyperplasia of the adrenal cortex (30%). Rarely, hyperaldosteronism may be secondary to glucocorticoid-suppressible hyperaldosteronism (1–3%) or an aldosterone-producing adrenal carcinoma.

Aldosterone stimulates sodium reabsorption and potassium and hydrogen loss by acting on the distal renal tubules. Therefore excessive aldosterone secretion results in sodium and water retention, hypertension, hypokalaemia and metabolic alkalosis.

Aldosterone-producing adenomas (Conn's syndrome) are usually 0.5–2 cm in size and have a yellow colour due to their high cholesterol content (Fig. 7.1). These adenomas express very high levels of aldosterone synthase and usually produce greater levels of aldosterone than bilateral adrenal hyperplasia. Although aldosterone production is autonomous, it is sensitive to adrenocorticotrophic hormone (ACTH) (rather than angiotensin II) in the majority of aldosterone-producing adenomas.

In *bilateral adrenal hyperplasia* (also known as idiopathic hyperaldosteronism), the adrenal zona glomerulosa (which produces aldosterone) is very sensitive to angiotensin II (and usually not ACTH). The hyperplasia may be macro- or micronodular.

Glucocorticoid-suppressible hyperaldosteronism is a rare autosomal dominant condition caused by a mutation that results in a chimeric gene containing the promoter region of the gene encoding 11β-hydroxylase (which catalyzes the conversion of 11-deoxycortisol to cortisol) and the coding

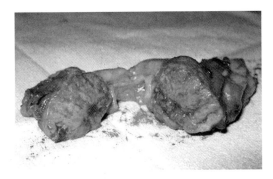

Figure 7.1 Bisected Conn's adenoma.

sequences of the gene for aldosterone synthase. This results in an ACTH-dependent activation of aldosterone synthase, which is expressed in the zona fasciculata as well as zona glomerulosa. Glucocorticoid-suppressible hyperaldosteronism is usually associated with bilateral adrenal hyperplasia.

Aldosterone-producing carcinomas are often over 4 cm in diameter at presentation. They are usually associated with the hypersecretion of cortisol, androgens and oestrogens, as well as high levels of aldosterone.

Clinical presentations

Patients usually present with *hypertension* and *hypokalaemia.*

Hypertension is often asymptomatic. Hypokalaemia may cause fatigue, muscle weakness, cramps, polydipsia and polyuria (due to hypokalaemia-induced nephrogenic diabetes insipidus). Serum potassium may be normal in 50% of patients. A low-sodium diet may mask hypokalaemia as reduced sodium delivery to the distal nephron diminishes aldosterone-induced potassium loss.

Early haemorrhagic strokes are characteristic in patients with glucocorticoid-suppressible hyperaldosteronism.

Investigations

Primary hyperaldosteronism should be excluded in hypertensive patients with:

- a young age of onset (<40 years)
- severe or resistant hypertension
- hypokalaemia: spontaneous or diuretic-induced hypokalaemia that does not respond to potassium replacement.

Screening tests

Nearly all patients have a serum potassium level below 4 mmol/L. A 24-hour urine collection (72 hours after stopping diuretics) may show inappropriate potassium wasting (>30 mmol/L in a patient with hypokalaemia). Serum sodium levels usually remain normal because of the parallel increase in the water content of the blood.

The initial screening test is measurement of *plasma aldosterone concentration* and *plasma renin activity.* A raised plasma aldosterone concentration to renin activity ratio suggests primary hyperaldosteronism. The cut-off for a 'high' ratio is dependent on the plasma renin activity assay and is therefore laboratory dependent.

Two things must be done before measuring the 'aldosterone-to-renin' ratio:

- Several antihypertensives should be stopped. Spironolactone, eplerenone, angiotensin-converting enzyme (ACE) inhibitors, angiotensin receptor blockers and diuretics increase plasma renin activity. Beta-blockers suppress renin release, and calcium channel blockers may reduce aldosterone levels. The duration of wash-out is 6 weeks for spironolactone and 2 weeks for most other antihypertensives. If antihypertensive therapy is required, an alpha-blocker (e.g. doxazosin) may be used.
- Hypokalaemia should be corrected (with oral potassium chloride supplementation) as it reduces aldosterone secretion.

A false-negative result may be seen in chronic renal failure.

Confirmatory tests

Salt loading

The response in normal people following a sodium load is aldosterone suppression. Failure of aldosterone suppression following a sodium load confirms primary hyperaldosteronism.

Oral sodium chloride (two 1g sodium chloride tablets taken three times a day with food) is given. On the third day, a 24-hour urine specimen is collected for measurement of aldosterone, sodium and creatinine. Urine aldosterone excretion of greater than 39 nmol per day is consistent with hyperaldosteronism. The 24-hour urine sodium excretion should exceed 200 mmol to document adequate sodium loading. Urine creatinine is measured to ensure adequate urine collection. Remember that sodium loading causes increased urinary potassium loss and hypokalaemia. Therefore serum potassium should be measured daily, and hypokalaemia must be corrected.

Alternatively, intravenous 0.9% sodium chloride (2 L over 4 hours) may be given. A plasma aldosterone level of over 277 pmol/L is consistent with primary hyperaldosteronism.

Captopril suppression test

This involves the oral administration of 25–50 mg of captopril (an ACE inhibitor), which suppresses aldosterone levels in normal people. An inability to reduce plasma aldosterone levels after administration of captopril suggests primary hyperaldosteronism.

Determining the cause

The cause must be determined because of significant treatment implications. Unilateral adenomas can be surgically cured, whereas bilateral adrenal hyperplasia requires lifelong pharmacotherapy with aldosterone antagonists. The specific pitfalls of different biochemical and radiological tests need to be considered.

Postural test

Plasma aldosterone concentration, renin activity and cortisol are measured in the morning (8 a.m., after overnight recumbency) in the supine position and after 4 hours of maintaining an upright posture (at noon).

In patients with *bilateral hyperplasia* (in which aldosterone release is renin mediated), aldosterone levels increase (>33%) at noon. This is because an upright posture leads to pooling of blood in the lower extremities and effective volume depletion, resulting in activation of the renin–angiotensin–aldosterone axis.

In patients with *adrenal adenomas* (in which aldosterone secretion is usually ACTH mediated), aldosterone levels are lower at noon. This is because the circadian secretion of pituitary ACTH release reaches a nadir during the day. Hence, a low midday aldosterone level, or failure to rise by more than 33% from baseline, is suggestive of an adenoma. However, this test is rarely used on its own to confirm the presence of an adenoma because up to 20% of these tumours are actually more responsive to angiotensin II than ACTH and will therefore give a false-negative result.

Imaging

Imaging should be done only after biochemical confirmation of primary hyperaldosteronism since non-functioning adrenal 'incidentalomas' are common. High-resolution computed tomography (CT) or magnetic resonance imaging may show a unilateral adenoma (and rarely carcinomas, which are usually >4 cm in size) with a normal contralateral adrenal gland. In bilateral hyperplasia, the adrenal glands may be enlarged or of normal size. Adrenal imaging identifies most adenomas of over 0.5 cm. It should be noted that patients with primary hyperaldosteronism and a normal CT scan or bilateral adrenal nodules on CT may be found to have a unilateral source of aldosterone following adrenal vein sampling. A unilateral adenoma seen on CT may be found to be a non-functioning adenoma in a patient with bilateral hyperplasia.

Adrenal vein sampling

In patients for whom surgery is practical and feasible, adrenal vein sampling should be performed to differentiate between a unilateral aldosterone-producing adenoma and bilateral hyperplasia.

Although modern-day radiological techniques offer excellent resolution, it is still possible for a small adenoma to be missed and, conversely, for a unilateral adrenal lesion seen on CT to be a non-functioning 'incidentaloma' in a patient with bilateral hyperplasia.

The 'gold standard' test to distinguish between an adenoma and hyperplasia is adrenal vein sampling by an experienced radiologist. A bolus of tetracosactrin (250 µg) may be given 20 minutes prior to sampling. Aldosterone and cortisol levels are measured from the right and left adrenal veins and inferior vena cava. During the procedure, cortisol is measured to ensure correct catheterization of the adrenal veins (an adrenal vein to inferior vena cava cortisol ratio of 3:1 ensures proper placement of the catheter into the adrenal vein). A unilateral aldosterone-producing adenoma produces a ratio of aldosterone to cortisol that is 4–5 times greater than that of the opposite side.

With successful adrenal vein catheterization, the procedure is 95% successful in correctly distinguishing between bilateral hyperplasia and an adenoma. However, even in the best hands, correct placement of the cannula is achieved in only 75% of patients. The right adrenal vein in particular can be difficult to cannulate as it is short and enters the inferior vena cava at an acute angle. Other complications (groin haematoma, adrenal haemorrhage, adrenal vein dissection) are rare.

Radio-labelled cholesterol scanning

A Conn's tumour will take up radio-labelled cholesterol with no uptake on the contralateral side. Bilateral uptake suggests bilateral adrenal hyperplasia. This test requires a suppression of cortisol production with dexamethasone to avoid confusing normal cortisol production with bilateral hyperplasia.

Other investigations

Genetic testing for glucocorticoid-suppressible hyperaldosteronism should be done in patients with an onset of primary hyperaldosteronism at age less than 20 years, a history of stroke at age below 40 years or a family history of primary hyperaldosteronism.

Treatment

Bilateral adrenal hyperplasia

In bilateral adrenal hyperplasia, *spironolactone* (200–400 mg per day) is used to treat hypertension and hypokalaemia. The side-effects of spironolactone include gynaecomastia, impotence, menstrual irregularities, muscle cramps and gastrointestinal upset. Spironolactone may be changed to eplerenone if it causes intolerable side-effects. Patients who do not tolerate eplerenone may be started on amiloride (a potassium-sparing diuretic). Serum potassium, creatinine and blood pressure should be monitored frequently during the first 4–6 weeks of treatment. The clinical course and circumstances dictate the frequency of monitoring thereafter.

Other antihypertensives (e.g. ACE inhibitors and calcium channel blockers) may need to be added. It can take 4–8 weeks for the hypertension to respond to the treatments.

Aldosterone-producing adenomas

Aldosterone-producing adenomas are treated with *adrenalectomy* by an experienced endocrine surgeon. Laparoscopic adrenalectomy is increasingly being used as it is associated with reductions in postoperative morbidity, hospital stay and expense compared with open laparotomy.

Surgery may either cure hypertension (in about 50%) or make it more amenable to antihypertensive therapy in those who are not cured (usually the elderly or those with longstanding hypertension). Spironolactone given before surgery helps in correcting hypokalaemia. However, it should be stopped 2 days before the surgery to prevent mineralocorticoid deficiency after adrenalectomy. Patients with bilateral adrenal hyperplasia should not undergo adrenalectomy as the risks associated with bilateral adrenalectomy (including the need for lifelong glucocorticoid and mineralocorticoid replacement) outweigh the potential benefits.

Blood pressure control is often inadequate with subtotal adrenalectomy.

Glucocorticoid-suppressible hyperaldosteronism is treated with dexamethasone (0.25 mg in the morning and 0.5 mg at night). However, spironolactone may be used if dexamethasone is not tolerated due to side-effects.

Adrenal carcinoma is treated with surgery and postoperative mitotane. The prognosis is usually poor.

Other causes of endocrine hypertension

The causes of endocrine hypertension are summarized in Box 7.1. Cushing's syndrome, phaeochromocytoma, acromegaly, primary hyperparathyroidism and congenital adrenal hyperplasia are discussed in separate chapters.

11β-Hydroxysteroid dehydrogenase type 2 hypofunction (due to autosomal recessive mutations) or inhibition (by liquorice or carbenoxolone) causes hypertension, hypokalaemia and metabolic alkalosis. 11β-Hydroxysteroid dehydrogenase type 2 converts cortisol to cortisone, which does not bind to the mineralocorticoid receptor. Mutations in the gene encoding this enzyme result in a failure of conversion of cortisol to cortisone. Cortisol can therefore activate the mineralocorticoid receptor causing an '*apparent mineralocorticoid excess*'. This condition may be treated with dexamethasone to suppress endogenous cortisol, or with high-dose spironolactone/amiloride.

Liddle's syndrome is a rare autosomal dominant condition caused by mutations in the beta or gamma subunits of the renal epithelial sodium channels, resulting in a constitutive activation of sodium reabsorption in the collecting tubules. Amiloride (or triamterene) is the treatment of choice.

Box 7.1 Causes of endocrine hypertension

Primary hyperaldosteronism
Cushing's syndrome
Phaeochromocytoma
Acromegaly
Primary hyperparathyroidism

Low plasma renin activity and low plasma aldosterone levels occur in:
- congenital adrenal hyperplasia (11β-hydroxylase and 17α-hydroxylase deficiency)
- 11β-hydroxysteroid dehydrogenase type 2 defect (due to autosomal recessive mutations) or inhibition by liquorice or carbenoxolone
- Liddle's syndrome

Key points:

- Primary hyperaldosteronism is characterized by an excessive autonomous secretion of aldosterone, resulting in a suppression of plasma renin activity.
- Primary hyperaldosteronism may be due to a unilateral aldosterone-producing adenoma (70%) or bilateral hyperplasia of the adrenal cortex (30%).
- Patients usually present with hypertension and hypokalaemia.
- The initial screening test is measurement of plasma aldosterone concentration and plasma renin activity (after stopping interfering medications). Failure of suppression of aldosterone following salt loading confirms the diagnosis.
- The cause must be determined because of significant treatment implications. Adrenal vein sampling by an experienced radiologist is the 'gold standard' test to distinguish between an adenoma and hyperplasia.
- Bilateral adrenal hyperplasia is treated with spironolactone. Aldosterone-producing adenomas are treated with adrenalectomy by an experienced endocrine surgeon.

Chapter 8

Phaeochromocytomas and paragangliomas

Phaeochromocytomas are catecholamine-producing tumours that usually arise from the chromaffin cells of the adrenal medulla but are extra-adrenal in about 10% of cases. Extra-adrenal phaeochromocytomas are referred to as *paragangliomas*. However, the term 'paraganglioma' is also used to describe non-catecholamine-secreting tumours that are derived from parasympathetic paraganglia (e.g. carotid body chemodectomas).

The pattern of catecholamine secretion from phaeochromocytomas differs from that of normal adrenal medulla: phaeochromocytomas mainly secrete noradrenaline, whereas the normal adrenal medulla predominantly secretes adrenaline. Familial phaeochromocytomas are an exception and secrete large amounts of adrenaline.

Catecholamine-secreting tumours are rare and occur in fewer than 0.2 % of hypertensive patients. Around 10% of phaeochromocytomas are malignant, and 10% are bilateral.

Phaeochromocytomas may be familial in up to 30% of patients. Familial cases may be seen in patients with:
- multiple endocrine neoplasia (MEN) type 2a (associated with medullary thyroid carcinoma and hyperparathyroidism) and MEN type 2b (associated with medullary thyroid carcinoma and mucosal neuromas)

- von Hippel–Lindau (VHL) syndrome (associated with cerebellar or retinal haemangioblastomas, renal cell carcinoma and pancreatic tumours)
- mutations in the genes encoding subunits of the mitochondrial enzyme succinate dehydrogenase: *SDHB, SDHD, SDHC*
- neurofibromatosis type 1.

The approximate frequency of phaeochromocytoma in these disorders is 50% in MEN type 2, 10–20% in VHL syndrome and 2% in neurofibromatosis type 1.

Mutations in *VHL*, *SDHB* and *SDHD* may contribute to the pathogenesis of tumours via dysregulation of the hypoxia-inducible factor-1 (HIF-1) and HIF-2 transcription factors.

Clinical presentations

Patients with phaeochromocytomas usually have *paroxysmal* symptoms. The most common symptoms in patients with phaeochromocytomas are:
- headache (80%)
- sweating (70%)
- palpitations (70%).

Other presenting symptoms include:
- cardiorespiratory: chest pain and dyspnoea (20%), which may be due to myocardial ischaemia or heart failure
- gastrointestinal: nausea (40%), epigastric pain (20%), constipation (10%)

Lecture Notes: Endocrinology and Diabetes. By A. Sam and K. Meeran. Published 2009 by Blackwell Publishing. ISBN 978-1-4051-5345-4.

- neuropsychiatric: tremor (30%), weakness (30%), anxiety (20%)
- metabolic: hypercalcaemia, hypokalaemia.

Clinical signs in patients with phaeochromocytomas include:
- pallor (40%)
- tachycardia
- hypertension (paroxysmal or sustained)
- postural hypotension (due to reduced plasma volume).

Investigations

24-Hour urinary catecholamines and metanephrines

Patients with suspected phaeochromocytoma should be investigated with two or three measurements of 24-hour *urinary catecholamines*, i.e. adrenaline, noradrenaline and dopamine (sensitivity and specificity of 85%) and, if available, 24-hour urinary fractionated *metanephrines* (sensitivity 97%, specificity 64%).

The term 'metanephrines' describes two catecholamine metabolites produced by catechol-O-methyltransferase: normetanephrine and metanephrine. 'Fractionated metanephrines' refers to the measurement of normetanephrine and metanephrine separately.

Some phaeochromocytomas produce modest amounts of catecholamines and may not produce positive urine catecholamine test results. Also, many phaeochromocytomas secrete catecholamines episodically; therefore the urinary excretion of catecholamines may be normal between episodes. However, normetanephrine and metanephrine are produced continuously and independently of catecholamine release. Therefore their measurement may be a more sensitive test to diagnose phaeochromocytomas.

Urinary creatinine should be measured in the 24-hour collection to verify an adequate collection. Because catecholamines are more stable at low pH, urine should be collected in acid-containing bottles.

Urinary vanillylmandelic acid (a catecholamine metabolite) is now rarely measured as it has a low sensitivity (around 62%).

Plasma free metanephrines

In patients who are at high risk of phaeochromocytoma (i.e. familial syndromes or a previously surgically cured phaeochromocytoma or paraganglioma), plasma free metanephrine and normetanephrine should be measured if available. This test has a sensitivity of 99%, and a normal value excludes a symptomatic catecholamine-secreting neoplasm.

Free metanephrines are produced in the phaeochromocytoma tumour cells. Sulphate-conjugated metanephrines are formed predominantly in the gastrointestinal tissues.

Urinary free metanephrines are measured following a sulphate deconjugation step. Therefore the free metanephrines measured in urine are in fact the sum of free metanephrines and (previously) conjugated metanephrines. This may explain the higher sensitivity of plasma free metanephrine compared with urinary metanephrines.

False-positive results

Certain drugs should be tapered and discontinued at least 2 weeks before any biochemical tests (Box 8.1). If it is contraindicated to discontinue certain

---

Box 8.1 Medications that may increase measured catecholamines and metanephrines

Tricyclic antidepressants
Levodopa
Adrenergic receptor agonists (e.g. decongestants)
Amphetamines
Buspirone and most psychoactive agents (not selective serotonin reuptake inhibitors)
Phenoxybenzamine
Prochlorperazine
Ethanol
Caffeine, nicotine
Calcium channel blockers (may increase urinary catecholamines)
Paracetamol (may increase measured levels of fractionated plasma metanephrines in some assays)
Labetalol and methyldopa (may cause analytical interferences with high-performance liquid chromatography assays)

---

medications (e.g. antipsychotics) and the biochemical tests are abnormal, imaging is needed to exclude a catecholamine-secreting tumour.

The clinical circumstances in which catecholamines and metanephrines are measured must be assessed in each case. Catecholamine secretion may be appropriately increased in stress or illness (e.g. stroke, myocardial infarction, congestive cardiac failure, obstructive sleep apnoea, head injury).

Imaging

If the biochemical results are abnormal, imaging with computed tomography (CT) or magnetic res-

onance imaging (MRI) of the abdomen and pelvis is required to locate the tumour. Either test detects almost all sporadic tumours as most are 3 cm or larger. Around 90% of tumours will be visualized in the abdomen. If the tumour is not localized in the adrenals, whole-body imaging should be performed.

Both CT and MRI are sensitive (98–100%) but are only about 70% specific.

Computed tomography

Radiological features of the phaeochromocytomas on CT (Fig. 8.1a) include:

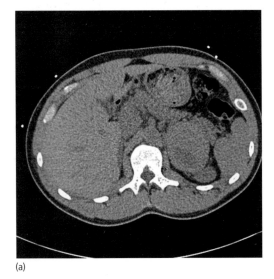

(a)

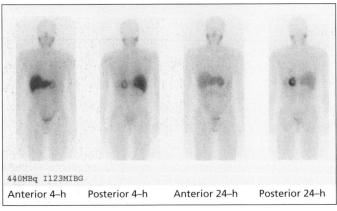

440MBq I123MIBG

Anterior 4–h   Posterior 4–h   Anterior 24–h   Posterior 24–h

(b)

Figure 8.1 (a) Computed tomography scan showing a left-sided phaeochromocytoma. (b) Radio-iodine-labelled MIBG scans in the same patient: anterior and posterior views 4 hours and 24 hours after injection. There is reduced uptake in the middle of the tumour due to necrosis.

- size >3 cm
- irregular/heterogeneous
- high (>20) Hounsfield unit (unit of X-ray attenuation) reading as they contain less fat.

There is a risk of exacerbation of hypertension if an intravenous contrast agent is given (which can be prevented by pre-treatment with alpha-adrenergic blockade).

Magnetic resonance imaging

Phaeochromocytomas appear hyperintense (compared with the liver) on *T2-weighted imaging*. With MRI, there is neither radiation nor dye. However, it is more expensive than CT.

MIBG scintigraphy

^{123}Iodine-metaiodobenzylguanidine (MIBG) is a compound resembling noradrenaline that is taken up by adrenergic tissue (Fig. 8.1b). An MIBG scan can detect tumours not detected by CT or MRI, or multiple tumours when CT or MRI is positive. MIBG scintigraphy is indicated in patients with large (>10 cm) adrenal phaeochromocytomas (increased risk of malignancy) or paragangliomas (increased risk of multiple tumours and malignancy).

MIBG scintigraphy may also be done if CT or MRI is negative and the diagnosis is still considered likely owing to clinical and biochemical evidence of phaeochromocytoma.

Screening for associated conditions

All patients with confirmed phaeochromocytomas should have screening tests/examinations for:
- MEN type 2: measure serum calcium and calcitonin
- VHL disease: ophthalmoscopy, MRI of the posterior fossa and renal ultrasound
- Neurofibromatosis type 1: a thorough clinical examination for neurofibromas, café-au-lait spots and axillary freckling.

Genetic testing

Genetic testing and counselling for mutations in *VHL, SDHB, SDHD* and *RET* genes should be considered (in a stepwise manner) in patients with:
- onset at a young age (<20 years)
- a family history of phaeochromocytoma or paraganglioma
- clinical findings suggestive of one of the familial disorders mentioned above
- bilateral adrenal phaeochromocytoma
- paraganglioma.

Treatment

Surgery

Surgical resection of the phaeochromocytoma (Fig. 8.2) may result in a resolution of hypertension in 75% of patients. Elective surgery has a mortality of less than 2%.

Phaeochromocytomas may be resected via an open adrenalectomy or a laparoscopic approach for patients with solitary intra-adrenal tumours less than 8 cm in diameter. For adrenal phaeochromocytomas, laparoscopic adrenalectomy by an experienced endocrine surgeon may be preferred because of the reduction in postoperative morbidity, hospital stay and expense compared with open laparotomy.

An anterior midline abdominal surgical approach is indicated for abdominal paragangliomas. Paragangliomas of the neck, chest (Fig. 8.3) and urinary bladder require specialized approaches.

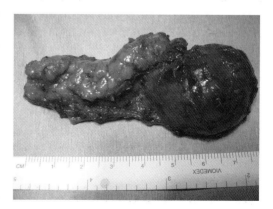

Figure 8.2 Resected phaeochromocytoma.

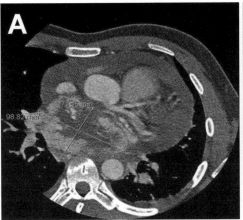
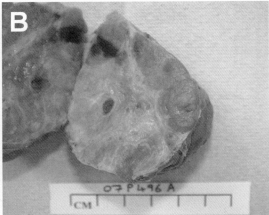

Figure 8.3 (a) Computed tomography scan showing a mediastinal paraganglioma. (b) Resected mediastinal paraganglioma.

Preoperative preparation

Inadequate preparation before surgery can cause hypertension during the surgery and hypotension postoperatively. All patients should receive an *alpha-blocker* (phenoxybenzamine) followed by a *beta-blocker* (propranolol) for at least 2–3 weeks before surgery. Patients should be warned of the side-effects of alpha-blockers, including postural hypotension and nasal stuffiness. The beta-blocker should always be started 2–3 days *after* the alpha-blocker in order to prevent unopposed alpha-stimulation causing a hypertensive crisis. Patients should be rehydrated (1 L of 0.9% saline) before alpha-blockade to prevent sudden hypotension on receiving the first dose of the alpha-blocker.

Treatment should be commenced in hospital, and pulse, blood pressure and haematocrit should be monitored closely as haemodilution may be caused by reversal of alpha-mediated vasoconstriction. Patients should also be adequately alpha- and beta-blocked prior to receiving any intravenous contrast.

Phenoxybenzamine

Phenoxybenzamine is started at 10 mg twice a day orally. The dose is increased by 10 mg daily. The usual dose is 1–2 mg/kg daily in two divided doses.

Intravenous phenoxybenzamine (0.5 mg/kg in 250 mL 5% dextrose over 2 hours) may be given for the 3 days prior to surgery to ensure complete preoperative alpha-blockade.

Propranolol

Propranolol is started at 40 mg three times a day 2–3 days after starting phenoxybenzamine. The dose may be increased to 80 mg three times a day as necessary to control the tachycardia (the goal being a heart rate of 60–80 beats per minute).

A calcium channel blocker (nicardipine) may be used to supplement the combined alpha- and beta-adrenergic blockade protocol when blood pressure control is inadequate, or to replace the adrenergic blockade protocol in patients with intolerable side-effects.

Perioperative hypertension and arrhythmias

Acute hypertensive crises may occur during an operation due to tumour handling. They should be treated with intravenous sodium nitroprusside started at a rate of 0.5 µg/kg per minute and adjusted every few minutes according to the blood pressure. Intravenous phentolamine and nicardipine are alternatives.

Perioperative cardiac arrhythmias are treated with lidocaine (50–100 mg intravenously) or esmolol.

Tumour devascularization may result in hypotension. This often responds to intravenous fluids but may require inotropes. Hypoglycaemia can occur in 10–15% of patients due to the removal of catecholamine suppression of insulin secretion, and is treated by intravenous dextrose.

Malignant phaeochromocytomas

A total of 10% of phaeochromocytomas are malignant. *SDHB* mutation carriers are more likely to develop malignant paragangliomas.

Surgical removal of the tumour to improve symptoms and survival is the primary treatment. Metastatic lesions should be resected if possible. Patients with malignant phaeochromocytomas need long term alpha- and beta-blockade.

Chemotherapy (with dacarbazine, cyclophosphamide and vincristine) may control the symptoms. Radiotherapy may be helpful in those with bony metastases. In initial studies, local tumour irradiation with ^{131}I-MIBG has been found to be of limited therapeutic value.

Malignant phaeochromocytomas are histologically and biochemically similar to benign ones. However, they are associated with local invasion or distant metastases, which may occur as long as 20 years after resection. Therefore patients should be followed up life-long to detect recurrence or metastases. Five-year survival for malignant phaeochromocytomas is about 44%.

Follow-up and monitoring

Twenty-four-hour urinary catecholamines should be measured about 2 weeks after surgery to assess cure (catecholamines may be elevated in the first 7–10 days postoperatively). Patients should be followed up life-long to detect recurrence. The recurrence rate of phaeochromocytomas is less than 10%. Five-year survival for benign tumours is about 96%.

Key points:

- Phaeochromocytomas are catecholamine-secreting tumours of the adrenal medulla.
- Patients may present with the triad of headache, sweating and palpitations.
- Patients with suspected phaeochromocytoma should have 24-hour urinary catecholamines and, if available, fractionated metanephrines measured.
- Those with abnormal biochemical tests should be further investigated with imaging (CT, MRI) to locate the tumour.
- All patients should receive an alpha-blocker (e.g. phenoxybenzamine) followed by a beta-blocker (propranolol) for at least 2–3 weeks before surgery. Preparation is critical and must include rehydration.
- Phaeochromocytomas are familial in up to 30% of patients.

Chapter 9

Congenital adrenal hyperplasia

Congenital adrenal hyperplasia (CAH) encompasses a group of autosomal recessive disorders caused by a deficiency of enzymes involved in the synthesis of adrenal steroids (Fig. 9.1).

The most common form of CAH is due to *21-hydroxylase deficiency* ('classic CAH').

Epidemiology

The incidence of classic CAH in the general population is 1 in 10000–15000. The incidence of the milder 'non-classic' (late-onset) form may be as high as 1 in 1000. The prevalence of the disorder is higher in Hispanic, Yugoslav and Eastern European Jewish women than in other ethnic groups. The other forms of CAH are very rare.

Aetiology

Classic CAH is caused by 21-hydroxylase (CYP21A2) enzyme deficiency and is an autosomal recessive condition. It is the most common form of CAH and accounts for 95% of cases of CAH. 21-hydroxylase deficiency causes:
- reduced aldosterone production
- reduced cortisol production resulting in increased adrenocorticotrophic hormone (ACTH)

Lecture Notes: Endocrinology and Diabetes. By A. Sam and K. Meeran. Published 2009 by Blackwell Publishing. ISBN 978-1-4051-5345-4.

secretion (due to reduced negative feedback), which stimulates the steroid synthesis pathway toward an increased production of adrenal androgens (dehydroepiandrosterone and androstenedione) and the substrate for the defective enzyme, i.e. 17-hydroxyprogesterone. Androstenedione is converted to testosterone in the peripheral tissues (e.g. liver). There is minimal synthesis of testosterone in the adrenal gland.

The non-classic form of CAH is due to reduced 21-hydroxylase activity caused by a classic mutation and a variant allele, or by two variant alleles.

Clinical presentations

In patients with 21-hydroxylase deficiency, three main clinical phenotypes have been described:
- Classic salt-losing
- Classic simple-virilizing
- Non-classic (late onset).

Presentation in infancy/childhood

Classic salt-losing (75%)

Male and female infants present with failure to thrive, dehydration, hyponatraemia and hyperkalaemia due to aldosterone deficiency.

Girls present with ambiguous genitalia (enlargement of the clitoris and labial fusion) caused

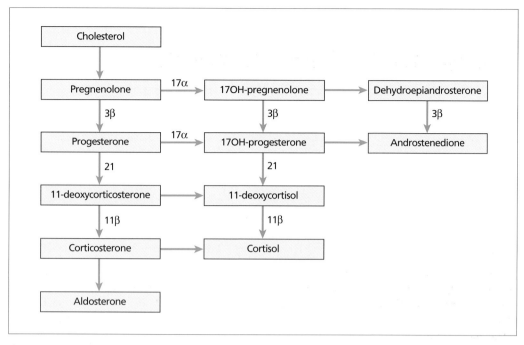

Figure 9.1 The adrenal steroid synthesis pathway and some of the enzymes involved: 3β, 3β-hydroxysteroid dehydroge-nase, 17α, 17α-hydroxylase, 21, 21-hydroxylase (CYP21A2), 11β, 11-hydroxylase.

by the effects of androgen excess on the development of the external genitalia in utero (female pseudohermaphrodism).

Boys may develop testicular masses ('adrenal rests') due to ectopic adrenal cells stimulated by ACTH hypersecretion. They are typically bilateral and may be diagnosed as early as 5 years, but usually present between the ages of 10 and 20 years (see 'Presentations in adolescents and adults' below).

Classic simple virilizing

In this form of CAH, aldosterone secretion is adequate, but cortisol is not synthesized efficiently.

Girls present with ambiguous genitalia (see above).

Boys present at 2–4 years of age with early virilization and signs of puberty (pubic hair, growth spurt, adult body odour). Boys may also develop testicular adrenal rests (see below).

Presentations in adolescents and adulthood

Reproduction

In *females*, fertility rates may be reduced by hyperandrogenaemia due to inadequate glucocorticoid therapy (resulting in menstrual irregularity) and/or structural abnormalities due to androgen excess in utero or suboptimal surgical reconstruction. In women with simple virilizing and salt-losing CAH, respective fertility rates of up to 80% and up to 60% may be achieved with treatment.

In *males*, high levels of adrenal androgens (if poorly controlled) suppress gonadotrophins and therefore testicular function and spermatogenesis. Boys or young men may develop testicular masses composed of ectopic adrenal tissue ('adrenal rests') that is stimulated by the increased ACTH. They are more common in the salt-losing form as they tend to have poorer control and higher ACTH levels.

They are benign but may lead to obstruction of the seminiferous tubules, gonadal dysfunction and infertility.

Stature

Exposure to high levels of sex hormones leads to accelerated growth in childhood but induces premature epiphyseal closure, resulting in a short final adult stature. Excess glucocorticoid therapy may also suppress growth and contribute to adult short stature.

Non-classic CAH (late-onset)

Non-classic or late-onset CAH may present as hirsutism, acne and menstrual irregularity in young women, and early pubarche or sexual precocity in school-age children, or there may be no symptoms.

Rarer forms of CAH

11β-Hydroxylase deficiency

Increased deoxycorticosterone (Fig. 9.1) (which has mineralocorticoid activity) results in hypertension and frequently hypokalaemia. Increased androgens result in the virilization of female foetuses, causing ambiguous genitalia (female pseudohermaphrodism).

3β-Hydroxysteroid dehydrogenase deficiency

Mineralocorticoid (Fig. 9.1) deficiency results in salt wasting and hyperkalaemia. Reduced androgens in men result in ambiguous genitalia (male pseudohermaphrodism) ranging from hypospadias to nearly normal female external genitalia. Increased dehydroepiandrosterone (DHEA) in women may result in a mild virilization of the external genitalia.

17α-Hydroxylase deficiency

Increased mineralocorticoids (Fig. 9.1) result in hypertension and frequently hypokalaemia.

Reduced adrenal and gonadal sex steroids result in ambiguous genitalia in men (male pseudohermaphrodism), with a blind vagina, no uterus or fallopian tubes, intra-abdominal testes and absent puberty/primary amenorrhoea in females.

Investigations

Classic CAH

Most patients with classic CAH are diagnosed in infancy. An elevated level of *17-hydroxyprogesterone* indicates 21-hydroxylase deficiency. 17-Hydroxyprogesterone is a precursor steroid that accumulates upstream of the enzyme defect (see 'Aetiology'). However, the test should be repeated (along with 11-deoxycortisol measurement) after 48 hours of age to distinguish CAH from the physiological hormonal surge in the first 2 days of life. Hyponatraemia and hyperkalaemia indicate a salt-losing crisis. Plasma renin level is useful in confirming salt wasting.

Genetic analysis may be performed to identify specific *CYP21* mutations.

In infants with ambiguous genitalia, *karyotyping* and *gender assignment* should be done urgently. The initial evaluation should include ultrasonography of the internal genitalia (uterus).

Because of the high prevalence of testicular adrenal rests and their association with infertility in male patients, they should be monitored by testicular ultrasonography in adolescence or early adulthood.

Men who desire future fertility should be evaluated with serum testosterone level, semen analysis and testicular ultrasound.

Non-classic CAH

17-Hydroxyprogesterone should be measured at 9 a.m. (because of the diurnal variation in adrenal hormone secretion) and in the follicular phase of the menstrual cycle. False-positive results may occur if 17-hydroxyprogesterone is measured in the luteal phase, as it is also produced by the corpus luteum.

17-Hydroxyprogesterone levels of less than 5 nmol/L are normal, and 17-hydroxyprogesterone levels of over 15 nmol/L are consistent with CAH. However, in patients with 17-hydroxyprogesterone levels of between 5 and 15 nmol/L, an ACTH stimulation test should be done. 17-Hydroxyprogesterone is measured 60 minutes after 250 µg of tetracosactrin (synthetic ACTH) is given intramuscularly or intravenously. In patients with CAH, 17-hydroxyprogesterone values at 60 minutes are typically 43 nmol/L or more, and range between 30 and 300 nmol/L. 17-Hydroxyprogesterone levels of less than 30 nmol/L exclude the diagnosis. Cortisol response to ACTH is usually low normal.

Other tests

Serum testosterone and androstenedione levels are elevated. There is a great overlap with levels in polycystic ovary syndrome, and therefore serum androgen levels cannot distinguish between the two disorders.

A proportion of women with non-classic CAH may have mildly raised plasma renin levels.

Treatment

Salt-losing form

Infants/children

Infants are initially treated with intravenous saline and hydrocortisone. Thereafter, *glucocorticoid* and *mineralocorticoid* replacement are given as oral hydrocortisone and fludrocortisone.

Older adolescents/adults

It is important to plan for the transition from paediatric to adult care.

Glucocorticoids

Dexamethasone (0.25–0.75 mg) is given at bedtime in older adolescents and adults. Once-daily dosing improves compliance. The aim is to suppress the early morning peak of ACTH and thus androgen secretion. Alternatively, some endocrinologists give prednisolone (at a total of 5–7.5 mg per day: two-thirds of the dose at bedtime and one third on waking) or a single or split dosing of hydrocortisone (median 30 mg per day). As with other forms of adrenal insufficiency, glucocorticoid doses should be doubled during illness.

Mineralocorticoids

The usual adult dose of fludrocortisone is 100–200 µg per day, but some patients require more.

Simple virilizing form

Adult women with the simple virilizing form require glucocorticoids. Men require glucocorticoids if they have testicular masses ('adrenal rests') or oligospermia. Testicular masses ('adrenal rests') usually regress with glucocorticoid therapy.

Females with ambiguous genitalia

In children with ambiguous genitalia, karyotyping and gender assignment should be done urgently. The gender assignment in a patient with a 46XX karyotyping and elevated 17-hydroxyprogesterone is female even if the external genitalia are male-like in appearance. Careful evaluation by an experienced team of paediatric endocrinologists, geneticists and paediatric surgeons, as well as sophisticated psychosocial support, is essential. Parents should be offered counselling as soon as the diagnosis is established.

The surgical management of girls with ambiguous genitalia is complex and includes reconstructive surgery (usually clitoroplasty and vaginoplasty). Surgery should be done in a centre with substantial experience at age 2–6 months because it is technically easier than at a later age. Occasionally revisional vaginoplasty may be required at adolescence or young adulthood.

Men who desire future fertility

Men with both forms of classic CAH (salt-losing and simple virilizing) who desire future fertility should be evaluated with serum testosterone, semen analysis and testicular ultrasound.

Non-classic CAH

Female patients with non-classic CAH who are not pursuing fertility are treated with oral contraceptives or cyproterone acetate (an antiandrogen) for acne and hirsutism. Spironolactone should be avoided because of the potential risk of salt wasting and hyper-reninaemia. Oral contraceptives are also recommended for menstrual cycle abnormalities.

Women with non-classic CAH with anovulatory cycles who desire fertility should receive glucocorticoids (dexamethasone 0.25–0.75 mg) as initial therapy for ovulation induction. Those who do not ovulate with glucocorticoid therapy alone should receive additional clomiphene citrate. Patients with non-classic CAH do not require higher glucocorticoid doses during stress.

Males do not usually require treatment unless they have testicular masses (testicular adrenal rest tumours) or oligospermia (in a man desiring fertility). Glucocorticoid therapy may be recommended in these men. Treatment may be discontinued when an adult male no longer seeks fertility.

CAH in pregnancy

For the management of patients with CAH during pregnancy, see Chapter 31.

Follow-up and monitoring

The aims of treatment of CAH in adulthood are:
• to give sufficient glucocorticoids to ensure normal cortisol replacement and to reduce the excessive secretion of ACTH and hyperandrogenaemia
• to avoid glucocorticoid over-replacement, which is associated with an increased risk of osteopenia, obesity and other clinical manifestations of Cushing's syndrome. The lowest dose that ameliorates symptoms should be used.
• to give sufficient mineralocorticoid (in patients with the salt-losing form) to restore blood pressure, serum electrolyte concentrations and extracellular fluid volume to normal.

Classic CAH in adults

Annual follow-up is usually adequate in adults.

Clinical assessment should look for evidence of hyperandrogenism, glucocorticoid overtreatment (Cushingoid appearance), mineralocorticoid undertreatment (postural hypotension) and overtreatment (e.g. dependent oedema). Amenorrhoea in females suggests inadequate treatment.

Serum *17-hydroxyprogesterone* levels should be monitored in women and men receiving glucocorticoid therapy. The aim is to lower serum levels to slightly above the normal range. Normal 17-hydroxyprogesterone levels suggest that the patient is on supraphysiological doses of glucocorticoids, which may result in complications associated with glucocorticoid excess.

Serum *androgen* levels (DHEA sulphate, androstenedione and testosterone) should be monitored in women and men receiving glucocorticoid therapy. The goal is to lower DHEA sulphate, androstenedione and testosterone levels in women, and DHEA sulphate and androstenedione levels in men, to slightly above the upper normal limits. Testosterone levels are measured in men to assess testicular function. Subnormal values should prompt additional evaluation.

Plasma *renin* activity and serum electrolytes should be monitored in patients on mineralocorticoid therapy. The aim is a plasma renin activity in the mid- to upper-normal range. Plasma renin activity is markedly raised in those who are inadequately treated, and is suppressed in those who are overtreated.

Non-classic CAH

Patients should be assessed for an improvement in symptoms (e.g. acne, hirsutism) and features of glucocorticoid excess (Cushingoid appearance).

Serum concentrations of 17-hydroxyprogesterone and androgens (DHEA sulphate, androstenedione, testosterone) should be measured in women with the goal of normalizing testosterone levels. In men, a reduction of serum 17-hydroxyprogesterone levels to slightly above normal is a good index of therapeutic efficacy. Periodic DXA scans should be performed to look for bone loss.

Key points:

- The most common form of CAH is due to 21-hydroxylase deficiency ('classic CAH'), which results in reduced aldosterone and reduced cortisol production causing increased ACTH secretion, which in turn stimulates an increased production of adrenal androgens.
- In patients with 21-hydroxylase deficiency, three main clinical phenotypes have been described: classic salt-losing, classic simple virilizing and non-classic (late onset).
- Patients with the salt-losing form of classic CAH present as infants with failure to thrive, dehydration, hyponatraemia and hyperkalaemia due to aldosterone deficiency.
- Girls with both forms of classic CAH present with ambiguous genitalia caused by the effects of androgen excess on the development of the external genitalia in utero.
- Non-classic or late-onset CAH may present as hirsutism, acne and menstrual irregularity in young women, and early pubarche or sexual precocity in school-age children, or there may be no symptoms.
- Patients with 21-hydroxylase deficiency have elevated 17-hydroxyprogesterone levels.
- Infants with the salt-losing form are treated with glucocorticoids and mineralocorticoids.
- Female patients with non-classic CAH who are not pursuing fertility are treated with oral contraceptives. Those who desire fertility should receive glucocorticoids.

Chapter 10

Adrenal incidentalomas

An adrenal incidentaloma is an adrenal mass greater than 1 cm in diameter that is incidentally discovered when an abdominal computed tomography (CT) or magnetic resonance imaging (MRI) is done for other reasons (Fig. 10.1).

Adrenal incidentalomas may be found in 0.4% of CT scans. Abdominal imaging may also reveal unilateral or bilateral enlarged or unusually shaped adrenals. Although the importance of these changes is not known, the possibility of adrenal disease should be considered.

Following the discovery of an adrenal incidentaloma, close examination of the radiological characteristics, clinical and biochemical assessments should be performed to answer two important questions:

- Is the adrenal incidentaloma *benign* or *malignant*? Malignant incidentalomas include metastases from other cancers (e.g. lung) or, less commonly, primary adrenal carcinomas.
- Is the adrenal incidentaloma *functioning* or *nonfunctioning*? Up to 15% are functioning (about 9% are cortisol secreting, 4–5% are phaeochromocytomas, 1–2% are aldosterone secreting).

Adrenal cysts, adrenal haemorrhage and myelolipoma are usually easily identified as they have distinctive imaging characteristics.

Lecture Notes: Endocrinology and Diabetes. By A. Sam and K. Meeran. Published 2009 by Blackwell Publishing. ISBN 978-1-4051-5345-4.

Radiological evaluation

The size and imaging characteristics ('*imaging phenotype*') of the incidentaloma are important determinants of whether the adrenal mass is benign or malignant. CT scanning is the primary modality of adrenal imaging. The imaging characteristics of adrenal carcinomas, metastases and phaeochromocytomas include:

- size greater than 4 cm in diameter (93% sensitivity but limited specificity; 76% may actually be benign)
- inhomogeneous density (central tumour necrosis resulting in low attenuation)
- irregular border
- attenuation greater than 20 Hounsfield units on unenhanced CT (unlike benign adenomas, which have low attenuation due to a high lipid content)
- less than 50% contrast wash-out at 10 minutes.

Clinical assessment

All patients should be assessed clinically for the possibility of adrenal hormonal hyperfunction and malignancy. A thorough history should be taken to look for features of malignancy and phaeochromocytoma (headache, sweating, palpitations). Physical examination may reveal signs of malignancy, hypertension or features of Cushing's syndrome. However, the absence of signs and

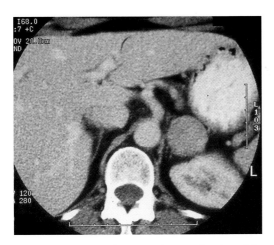

Figure 10.1 Computed tomography scan showing a left-sided adrenal mass.

symptoms does not exclude a phaeochromocytoma, cortisol- or aldosterone-secreting tumour.

Biochemical assessment

Twenty-four-hour *urinary catecholamines* and *fractionated metanephrines* (i.e. metanephrine and normetanephrine measured separately) should be quantified to exclude phaeochromocytoma (see Chapter 8). If the pre-test probability of phaeochromocytoma is high (e.g. a vascular mass with high-attenuation pre-contrast/delayed contrast wash-out, pallor spells or a known germline mutation), plasma free metanephrine and normetanephrine should be measured as this test has a sensitivity of 97–99%. However, it is not very specific (85–89%).

An overnight *dexamethasone suppression test* (1 mg) should be performed to detect autonomous cortisol secretion. If it is abnormal (i.e. an 8–9 a.m. serum cortisol >50 nmol/L after overnight dexamethasone), baseline serum ACTH and a 2-day high-dose dexamethasone suppression test are indicated to confirm the autonomy (see Chapter 16).

If the patient is hypertensive, plasma potassium concentration and plasma *aldosterone-to-renin activity ratio* should be measured to screen for primary hyperaldosteronism. Note that patients with primary hyperaldosteronism may not be hypokalaemic. Patients need to be off spironolactone (for 6 weeks) and off angiotensin-converting enzyme inhibitors and angiotensin receptor blockers (for 2 weeks) prior to this test (see Chapter 7).

Treatment

Indications for surgery

Surgery for an adrenal incidentaloma is recommended in patients with:
- adrenal masses greater than 4 cm in diameter or with a suspicious imaging phenotype
- phaeochromocytoma
- a unilateral aldosterone-secreting mass
- Cushing's syndrome.

Surgery for subclinical Cushing's syndrome (i.e. patients who demonstrate a lack of cortisol suppression after the high-dose dexamethasone suppression test but who do not have any discernible clinical signs) is controversial. Adrenalectomy may be considered in younger patients and those with disorders potentially attributable to the autonomous cortisol secretion (e.g. recent onset of hypertension, diabetes, obesity, osteoporosis). All patients should receive perioperative hydrocortisone because of the risk of adrenal insufficiency.

If there is evidence that the mass is a secondary deposit, a diagnostic CT-guided fine needle aspiration biopsy may be indicated (only after excluding phaeochromocytomas with biochemical testing).

Adjuvant mitotane is recommended for all patients who have undergone surgical resection of an adrenocortical carcinoma as it may prolong recurrence-free survival. Hydrocortisone replacement is necessary because mitotane's adrenolytic activity will result in adrenal insufficiency. Mitotane can also cause aldosterone deficiency.

Laparoscopic adrenalectomy is preferred in most cases as it is an effective, safe and less expensive procedure than open adrenalectomy. However, open adrenalectomy should be performed when adrenocortical cancer is suspected.

Follow-up

Those patients who have non-functioning tumours that are less than 4 cm in size and have a benign imaging phenotype may be followed with scans at

3–6 months and thereafter annually for several years. Any tumour that enlarges during the follow-up period should be removed. Unfortunately, surgical cure of even small carcinomas is not common (42% in one report).

Bilateral adrenal masses

Incidentalomas may be bilateral in 10–15% of cases (Fig. 10.2). In some patients with bilateral masses, one of the adrenal masses may be a non-functioning adenoma and the other may be hormone secreting.

Box 10.1 summarizes the causes of bilateral adrenal masses.

> **Box 10.1 Causes of bilateral adrenal masses**
>
> Cortical adenomas
> Congenital adrenal hyperplasia
> Bilateral macronodular hyperplasia
> Adrenocorticotrophic hormone-dependent
>   Cushing's disease
> Malignancy: phaeochromocytoma, metastases,
>   lymphoma
> Infection, e.g. tuberculosis, fungal
> Infiltration: amyloidosis
> Haemorrhage

> **Key points:**
>
> • An adrenal incidentaloma is an adrenal mass greater than 1 cm in diameter that is incidentally discovered when an abdominal CT or MRI is done for other reasons.
> • Close examination of the imaging characteristics and clinical and biochemical assessments should be performed to determine whether the incidentaloma is benign or malignant, and whether it is functioning (cortisol secreting, phaeochromocytoma or aldosterone secreting).
> • The imaging phenotype (characteristics) of adrenal carcinoma, metastases and phaeochromocytomas includes size greater than 4 cm in diameter, inhomogeneous density, irregular border and high attenuation on unenhanced CT scanning.
> • Patients with non-functioning tumours that are less than 4 cm in size and have a benign imaging phenotype may be followed with scans at 3–6 months and thereafter annually for several years.

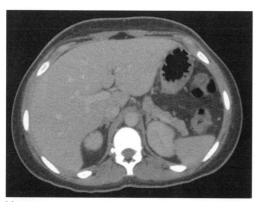

(a)

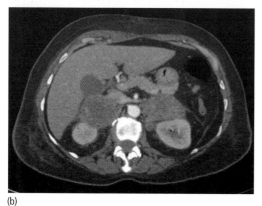

(b)

Figure 10.2 (a) Computed tomography (CT) scan showing normal adrenals for comparison. (b) CT scan showing bilateral adrenal metastases.

Chapter 11

Pituitary anatomy and physiology

The pituitary gland (also called hypophysis) sits in the pituitary fossa (sella turcica) in the sphenoid bone and is anatomically close to some critically important structures (Fig. 11.1). It is connected to the hypothalamus via the pituitary stalk.

Branches of the superior hypophyseal artery form a capillary plexus in the median eminence and upper part of the pituitary stalk (Fig. 11.2). This capillary plexus gives rise to the hypophyseal *portal vessels*, which transmit hypothalamic releasing and inhibitory hormones to the anterior pituitary gland. The posterior pituitary gland is supplied directly by the inferior hypophyseal artery.

Venous blood from the pituitary gland drains by a number of veins into the adjacent cavernous sinuses.

The pituitary gland is divided into anterior pituitary and posterior pituitary:
- The *anterior pituitary* (adenohypophysis) is derived from an upward growth of the ectoderm of the roof of the oropharynx (Rathke's pouch), which becomes pinched off (Fig. 11.3).
- The *posterior pituitary* (neurohypophysis) is derived from a downgrowth of neuroectoderm of the floor of the third ventricle (diencephalon).

Lecture Notes: Endocrinology and Diabetes. By A. Sam and K. Meeran. Published 2009 by Blackwell Publishing. ISBN 978-1-4051-5345-4.

Anterior pituitary hormones

The anterior pituitary secretes at least six different peptide hormones. Each hormone is secreted by a specific group of cells:
- *Growth hormone* (GH) is secreted by somatotrophs (50% of cells).
- *Prolactin* is secreted by lactotrophs (10–30% of cells).
- *Adrenocorticotrophic hormone* (ACTH) is secreted by corticotrophs (20% of cells).
- *Thyroid-stimulating hormone* (TSH) is secreted by thyrotrophs (5% of cells).
- *Luteinizing hormone* (LH) and *follicle-stimulating hormone* (FSH) are secreted by gonadotrophs (15% of cells).

Growth hormone

GH is the most abundant anterior pituitary hormone. It is a protein with 191 amino acids, two disulphide bridges and a molecular weight of 22 kDa.

Effects

GH stimulates the hepatic synthesis and secretion of insulin-like growth factor-1 (IGF-1; a potent growth and differentiation factor). GH stimulates epiphyseal prechondrocyte differentiation and

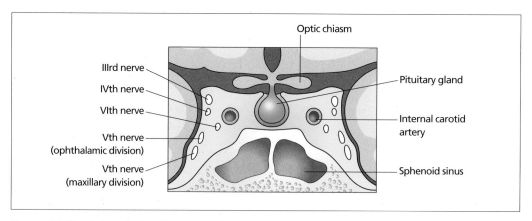

Figure 11.1 The pituitary gland and its anatomical relation to the cavernous sinus and optic chiasm.

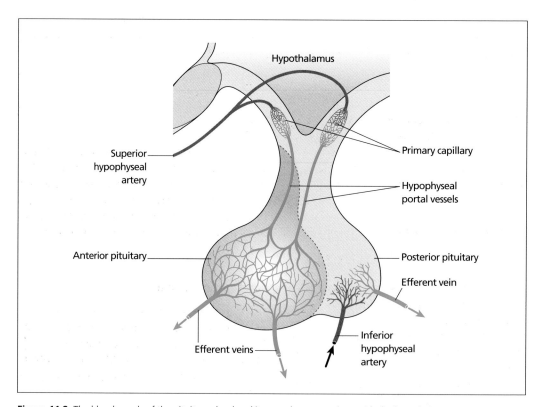

Figure 11.2 The blood supply of the pituitary gland and its vascular connections with the hypothalamus.

linear bone growth in children, stimulates lipolysis, increases protein synthesis, antagonizes insulin action and stimulates phosphate, water and sodium retention.

Mechanism of action

Binding of GH to its plasma membrane receptor (mostly in the liver) leads to receptor dimerization.

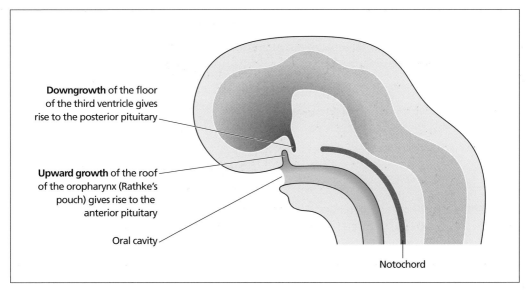

Downgrowth of the floor of the third ventricle gives rise to the posterior pituitary

Upward growth of the roof of the oropharynx (Rathke's pouch) gives rise to the anterior pituitary

Oral cavity

Notochord

Figure 11.3 The embryological origin of the two parts of the pituitary gland.

This is followed by a phosphorylation cascade mediated by Janus kinase (JAK) and components of the signal transduction and activators of transcription (STAT) family, which translocate to the nucleus and regulate target gene expression.

Regulation of secretion

GH secretion is stimulated by hypothalamic GH-releasing hormone, which acts via a G-protein-coupled receptor and increases cyclic AMP levels. Other factors that may stimulate GH release include stress, exercise, sleep, prolonged fasting and ghrelin (a gastric derived peptide). GH secretion is inhibited by IGF-1 (negative feedback) and hypothalamic somatostatin. GH secretion is pulsatile (6–10 pulses separated by long periods during which GH may be undetectable).

Prolactin

Prolactin is a protein with 198 amino acids, three disulphide bonds and a molecular weight of about 22 kDa.

Effects

Prolactin stimulates the proliferation of the breast lobulo-alveolar epithelium and lactation. It also decreases reproductive function by suppressing gonadotrophin-releasing hormone (GnRH) and pituitary gonadotrophin secretion, and by impairing gonadal steroidogenesis in both males and females.

Mechanism of action

Binding of prolactin to its plasma membrane receptor leads to receptor dimerization. This is followed by a phosphorylation cascade mediated by JAK and components of the STAT family, which translocate to the nucleus and regulate target gene expression.

Regulation of secretion

Prolactin secretion is inhibited by hypothalamic dopamine binding to D_2 receptors. Prolactin secretion is stimulated by hypothalamic thyrotrophin-releasing hormone (TRH) and other factors including oestrogen, opiates, serotonin and acetyl-choline. Prolactin levels may be higher in stress, during sleep and following a suckling stimulus, exercise, meals, sexual intercourse and an epileptic fit.

Prolactin secretion is pulsatile, with the highest secretory peaks occurring during rapid eye movement sleep. Peak serum levels occur between 4 and 6 a.m.

ACTH

ACTH is a peptide with 39 amino acids and a molecular weight of 4.5 kDa. ACTH, melanocyte-stimulating hormone and endorphins are products of the same gene: *POMC* (proopiomelanocortin).

Effects

ACTH stimulates the conversion of cholesterol to pregnenolone in the zona fasciculata and reticularis, and therefore stimulates the production of cortisol and adrenal androgens.

Mechanism of action

Binding of ACTH to its plasma membrane receptor in the zona fasciculata of the adrenal gland results in the activation of adenylate cyclase and increased cyclic AMP production. This leads to the stimulation of steroidogenic acute regulatory protein (StAR), which mediates the transport of cholesterol through the cytosol to the inner mitochondrial membrane, where it is converted to pregnenolone. This is the rate-limiting step in cortisol synthesis. The activation of adenylate cyclase also results in the upregulated gene expression of other enzymes involved in steroid synthesis.

Regulation of secretion

ACTH is stimulated by hypothalamic corticotrophin-releasing hormone (CRH) as well as other factors, including stress (e.g. acute inflammatory insults), and is inhibited by cortisol (negative feedback). ACTH secretion is pulsatile and exhibits a characteristic circadian rhythm with a peak at about 8 a.m. and a nadir about midnight.

TSH

TSH is a glycoprotein with two non-covalently bound chains (alpha and beta subunits). The alpha subunit is the same as that of LH, FSH and human chorionic gonadotrophin. However, the beta-subunit is unique to TSH. TSH has a molecular weight of about 30 kDa.

Mechanism of action

Binding of TSH to its plasma membrane receptor results in the activation of adenylate cyclase and increased cyclic AMP production. TSH also stimulates phospholipase C activity.

Effects

TSH stimulates every step in thyroid hormone synthesis and secretion. It also stimulates the expression of many genes in thyroid tissue and causes thyroid hyperplasia and hypertrophy.

Regulation of secretion

TSH secretion is stimulated by hypothalamic TRH. TSH synthesis and release is inhibited by thyroxine (T_4) and triiodothyronine (T_3) directly (via inhibition of transcription of the TSH subunit genes), and indirectly (via inhibition of TRH release). Other factors that may reduce TSH secretion include dopamine, somatostatin, acute non-thyroidal illness and increased human chorionic gonadotrophin (e.g. in early pregnancy).

Gonadotrophins in males

LH and FSH are glycoproteins with two non-covalently bound chains (alpha and beta subunits). They have a molecular weight of about 30 kDa.

Effects

LH stimulates the production of testosterone by Leydig cells in the testes. FSH stimulates spermatogenesis (along with testosterone).

Mechanism of action

Binding of LH and FSH to their plasma membrane receptors results in a stimulation of adenylate cyclase and increased cAMP production. LH stimulates testosterone synthesis by acting on the StAR protein, which delivers cholesterol to the inner mitochondrial membrane, where it is converted to pregnenolone (the rate-limiting reaction in testosterone synthesis).

Regulation of secretion

LH and FSH secretion are stimulated by a pulsatile release of hypothalamic GnRH. Testosterone inhibits hypothalamic GnRH and pituitary LH production (negative feedback). Inhibin B (a glycoprotein consisting of two subunits produced by germ cells) inhibits FSH production. In addition, several other hormones, neurotransmitters and cytokines modulate GnRH secretion.

Gonadotrophins in females

LH and FSH are glycoproteins with two non-covalently bound chains (alpha and beta subunits). They have a molecular weight of about 30 kDa.

Effects

LH stimulates the early steps in steroidogenesis and the production of androgens in ovarian theca cells. The 'LH surge' induces ovulation and thereafter maintains the secretory functions of the corpus luteum. FSH stimulates the recruitment and growth of ovarian follicles and their secretion of oestradiol (by stimulating the aromatase enzyme that locally converts androgens to oestrogens within the ovary mainly in the granulosa cells).

Mechanism of action

Binding of LH and FSH to their plasma membrane receptors activates adenylate cyclase and increases cyclic AMP production. LH stimulates the StAR protein (which transports cholesterol to the inner mitochondrial membrane) and the cholesterol side chain cleavage enzyme (which converts cholesterol to pregnenolone). FSH stimulates the aromatase enzyme that converts androgens to oestrogens.

Regulation of secretion

Gonadotrophin (LH and FSH) secretion is stimulated by pulsatile GnRH secretion from the hypothalamus. The secretion of FSH and LH is fundamentally under negative feedback control by ovarian steroids (particularly oestradiol) and by inhibin (which suppresses FSH). The negative feedback effect of oestradiol on LH secretion changes to a positive feedback effect as oestradiol levels peak before the ovulation (i.e. the oestrogen peak causes the LH surge).

Posterior pituitary hormones

The posterior pituitary stores and secretes *oxytocin* and *vasopressin*, also known as antidiuretic hormone. Vasopressin and oxytocin precursors are synthesized and packaged in granules in the cell bodies of specific magnocellular neurones in the supraoptic and paraventricular nuclei of the hypothalamus. The hormone precursors are transported down the axons in the pituitary stalk to the posterior pituitary. During this transport, they are enzymatically cleaved in the granules to give rise to oxytocin or vasopressin and neurophysin. Neurophysins act as carrier proteins for oxytocin and vasopressin during axonal migration.

Vasopressin

Vasopressin (the nonapeptide also known as antidiuretic hormone) binds to VR_2 membrane receptors on the distal renal tubular cells (in the collecting duct) and causes the activation of adenylate cyclase, the generation of cyclic AMP and the activation of intracellular protein kinases. This results in the insertion of water channel proteins (aquaporin-2) into the tubular membrane, allowing a flow of solute-free water from the hypotonic luminal fluid into the hypertonic renal interstitium. This results in the concentration of urine. At higher concentrations, vasopressin binds to VR_1 receptors on vascular smooth muscle and causes vasoconstriction.

Vasopressin is also secreted into the portal circulation and, together with CRH, stimulates ACTH release from the anterior pituitary.

Vasopressin secretion is stimulated by an increase in serum osmolality (mediated by hypothalamic osmoreceptors), decreased extracellular volume and blood pressure (mediated by baroreceptors in the carotids, atria and aorta) and stress. Vasopressin secretion is inhibited by alcohol and cold.

Oxytocin

Oxytocin release is stimulated by vaginal stimulation caused by the fetus during parturition (the Fergusson reflex), sexual intercourse in both sexes and by nipple stimulation by suckling during lactation. Oxytocin release is inhibited by stress.

Oxytocin stimulates contractions of the uterine muscle, which helps delivery of the fetus and the placenta. It may also help sperm transport in the uterus during sex. Another function of oxytocin is to stimulate the contraction of the myoepithelial cells that surround the alveoli in the breast to aid milk ejection.

Key points:

- The pituitary gland sits in the sella turcica in the sphenoid bone and has close anatomical relations to the optic chiasm and the cavernous sinus.
- Hypophyseal portal vessels transmit hypothalamic releasing and inhibitory hormones to the anterior pituitary gland.
- The anterior pituitary secretes at least six peptide hormones: GH, prolactin, ACTH, TSH, LH and FSH.
- GH is secreted by somatotrophs (stimulated by GH-releasing hormone), prolactin is secreted by lactotrophs (inhibited by dopamine), ACTH is secreted by corticotrophs (stimulated by CRH), TSH is secreted by thyrotrophs (stimulated by TRH), and LH and FSH are secreted by gonadotrophs (stimulated by pulsatile GnRH).
- The posterior pituitary secretes oxytocin and vasopressin (also known as antidiuretic hormone).
- Vasopressin secretion is stimulated by an increase in serum osmolality and decreased extracellular volume and blood pressure.

Chapter 12

Pituitary tumours and other sellar disorders

Pituitary tumours

Pituitary tumours (adenomas) account for about 10% of all intracranial tumours. Pituitary adenomas may be classified according to their size:

- *Macroadenomas*: ≥1 cm
- *Microadenomas*: <1 cm.

'Functioning' pituitary tumours are associated with excess anterior pituitary hormone secretion. Clinical syndromes caused by the hypersecretion of adrenocorticotrophic hormone (ACTH; Cushing's disease), growth hormone (GH; acromegaly), prolactin and thyroid-stimulating hormone (TSH) are described in later chapters.

'Non-functioning' pituitary tumours (adenomas) are not associated with excess anterior pituitary hormone secretion.

Pituitary adenomas can arise from any type of cell in the anterior pituitary gland (Box 12.1).

Epidemiology

The incidence of pituitary tumours is 25 per million per year, peaking at around 30–60 years. Female patients usually present earlier than males. Pituitary tumours are almost always benign. However, up to 0.2% are malignant and spread locally.

Lecture Notes: Endocrinology and Diabetes. By A. Sam and K. Meeran. Published 2009 by Blackwell Publishing. ISBN 978-1-4051-5345-4.

Box 12.1 Pituitary adenomas

Lactotroph adenoma (prolactin secreting): 26%
Corticotroph adenoma (adrenocorticotrophin-secreting or non-functioning): 15%
Somatotroph adenoma (growth hormone-secreting): 14%
Gonadotroph adenoma (usually non-functioning): 8%
Thyrotroph adenoma (thyroid-stimulating hormone-secreting): 1%
Null cell adenomas (non-functioning): 23%
Plurihormonal cell adenoma (particularly prolactin and growth hormone co-secreting): 13%

Lactotroph adenomas (prolactinomas) account for approximately 30–40% of all clinically recognized pituitary adenomas. Non-functioning pituitary adenomas account for 25–30% and are the most common pituitary macroadenoma. Non-functioning pituitary adenomas affect males and females equally and usually present in patients over the age of 50 years.

Aetiology

The mechanism of pituitary tumorigenesis is largely unexplained. Pituitary adenomas are monoclonal in origin and are true neoplasms. Mutations in the following genes may play a role in the development of pituitary adenomas:

- Activating mutations of the alpha subunit of the stimulatory G protein (which links the somatotroph cell membrane GH-releasing hormone receptor to adenylate cyclase) are seen in up to 40% of somatotroph adenomas.

- *PTTG* (the pituitary tumour-transforming gene) is overexpressed in most pituitary adenomas.
- A truncated form of the receptor for fibroblast growth factor-4 has been identified in some pituitary adenomas.
- Loss of function mutations of *MEN1* (a tumour suppressor gene) are responsible for tumours that occur in multiple endocrine neoplasia type 1 syndrome.

Physiological and pathological hyperplasia of the pituitary gland should be distinguished from pituitary adenoma. Examples include lactotroph hyperplasia in pregnancy and lactation, thyrotroph hyperplasia in primary hypothyroidism, gonadotroph hyperplasia in primary hypogonadism, and somatotroph and corticotroph hyperplasia due to ectopic GH-releasing hormone and corticotrophin-releasing hormone hypersecretion respectively.

Clinical presentations

The onset of symptoms and signs of pituitary tumours is often insidious, particularly with non-functioning adenomas. Patients tend to present late, and there is usually a delay in diagnosis. Patients with pituitary tumours may present with features of:
- *hypersecretion* of pituitary hormone(s) in functioning adenomas
- *hypopituitarism*
- *headache*
- *compression* of the surrounding structures such as the optic chiasm.

Hypersecretion of pituitary hormones

- *Prolactin*-secreting adenomas may present with galactorrhoea, oligo/amenorrhoea, infertility and impotence.
- *ACTH*-secreting adenomas cause Cushing's disease (see Chapter 16). ACTH-expressing tumours may also be non-functioning.
- *GH*-secreting adenomas cause acromegaly (see Chapter 15).

- *Luteinizing hormone* (LH) and *follicle-stimulating hormone* (FSH) secretion in LH and/or FSH synthesizing tumours is uncommon and they are usually non-functioning, but they may rarely present with hypogonadism (due to biologically inactive gonadotrophins).
- *TSH*-secreting adenomas (TSHomas) present with secondary hyperthyroidism with or without a goitre.

Hypopituitarism

A pituitary tumour (usually non-functioning) in the anterior pituitary may result in a decreased secretion of anterior pituitary hormones due to compression or destruction of the surrounding normal pituitary cells. Involvement of the posterior pituitary resulting in diabetes insipidus is less common. The order in which hormone deficiencies develop is GH first, followed by gonadotrophins, ACTH and finally TSH. Signs and symptoms resulting from various pituitary hormone deficiencies are summarized below.

GH deficiency

GH deficiency may present with fatigue, impaired psychological well-being, reduced energy, muscle strength and exercise capacity, and increased abdominal adiposity (fat mass).

LH and FSH deficiency

- LH and FSH deficiency in *males* may present with reduced libido, impotence, infertility, loss of body hair, fine perioral wrinkles and flushes.
- LH and FSH deficiency in *females* may present with oligomenorrhoea, amenorrhoea, infertility, dyspareunia, breast atrophy and flushes.

TSH deficiency

Deficiency may present with fatigue, apathy, muscle weakness, cold intolerance, constipation, weight gain and dry skin.

ACTH deficiency

ACTH deficiency may present with fatigue, weakness, nausea, vomiting, weight loss, hypoglycaemia and loss of pubic and axillary hair in females.

Antidiuretic hormone (vasopressin) deficiency

Antidiuretic hormone (ADH, vasopressin) deficiency may present with polyuria, nocturia and polydipsia.

Headache

Headaches are caused by stretching or invasion of the dura. Large tumours with suprasellar extension may occasionally cause obstructive hydrocephalus.

Compression of surrounding structures

Suprasellar extension of the tumour may result in involvement of the optic chiasm, causing bitemporal visual field loss. Superior quadrants are initially affected, and this gradually progresses to a *bitemporal hemianopia* that is characteristically asymmetrical (Fig. 12.1). Other rarer presentations

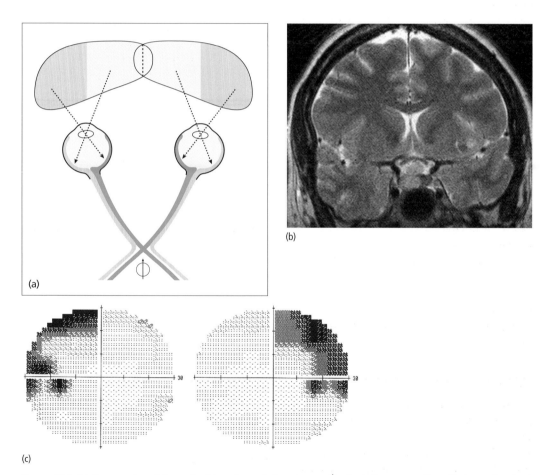

(a)

(b)

(c)

Figure 12.1 (a) Compression of the optic chiasm by a pituitary tumour ⏀ affects those nerve fibres that carry the visual impulse from the nasal retina (dark blue), resulting in an inability to view the temporal fields (dark blue areas). (b) Pituitary MRI showing a non-functioning adenoma compressing the optic chiasm. (c) Humphrey visual field revealing bilateral (mostly superior) temporal field defects.

include hemi-field slide and post-fixational blindness.

Stalk compression causes hyperprolactinaemia, which may cause hypogonadism. Other less common complications include third ventricle obstruction (causing hydrocephalus, vomiting, papilloedema, reduced consciousness level) and hypothalamic damage associated with diabetes insipidus and changes in food intake, temperature regulation or behaviour.

Lateral extension and *cavernous sinus invasion* may cause cranial nerve (IIIrd, IVth, VIth) palsies and diplopia. *Inferior extension* may result in cerebrospinal fluid (CSF) rhinorrhoea due to erosion of the sphenoid sinus.

Pituitary incidentalomas

Pituitary incidentalomas are mass lesions (usually adenomas) that are detected following radiological imaging of the skull base or brain for another clinical reason.

Management depends on pituitary function and whether the optic chiasm is involved. Microadenomas that are intrasellar and non-functioning may be followed up with an annual magnetic resonance imaging (MRI) scan to monitor their size. Macroadenomas that are non-functioning, have not caused hypopituitarism and do not involve the optic chiasm may also be followed up with an annual MRI.

Investigations

Investigations in patients with suspected pituitary tumours include basal and dynamic *pituitary function tests*, *pituitary MRI* and formal *visual field assessment*. In addition, patients with suspected syndromes of pituitary hormone hypersecretion such as Cushing's disease and acromegaly should undergo specific investigations for these disorders. These are described in detail in separate chapters.

Basal pituitary function tests

Basal anterior pituitary function tests are summarized in Box 12.2.

> **Box 12.2 Basal anterior pituitary function tests**
>
> Prolactin
> Insulin-like growth factor-1
> Luteinizing hormone, follicle-stimulating hormone, testosterone in men and oestradiol in women
> Thyroid-stimulating hormone and free thyroxine
> 9 a.m. cortisol

Prolactin

Prolactin levels can be elevated in non-functioning adenomas due to stalk compression, resulting in a reduction of the inhibitory effect of dopamine on prolactin secretion ('disconnection' hyperprolactinaemia). However, prolactin levels of more than 4000 mU/L are usually due to prolactin hypersecretion from a lactotroph adenoma (prolactinoma).

When measuring prolactin levels, it is important to be aware of two laboratory pitfalls:
- The '*hook effect*' occurs when the assay uses antibodies that recognize two different sites on the prolactin molecule. The prolactin molecule is 'sandwiched' between these two antibodies: one capturing it and the other labelling it (Fig. 12.2a). Very high prolactin levels may be artefactually reported as normal or only modestly elevated. This is because the very high serum prolactin saturates both the capture and labelling antibodies and prevents the binding of the two in a 'sandwich' (Fig. 12.2b). This can be avoided by repeating the assay using a dilution of serum (e.g. 1:100).
- Hyperprolactinaemia may be due to decreased clearance of a complex of prolactin with immunoglobulin G ('macroprolactin'). This condition is referred to as *macroprolactinaemia*. Macroprolactin is not biologically active but does get measured in routine assays, thereby causing falsely elevated results. The percentage of macroprolactin should be identified and, if significant, the prolactin result should be amended accordingly. Misdiagnosis can be avoided by pretreating the serum with polyethylene glycol to precipitate the macroprolactin before the immunoassay for prolactin.

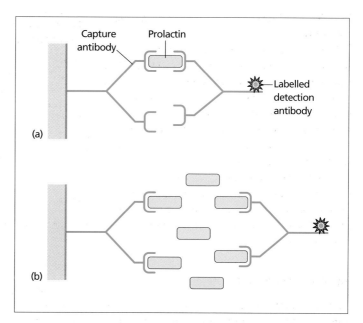

Figure 12.2 (a) A two-site immunometric assay for the measurement of serum prolactin uses two antibodies that are specific for different epitopes of prolactin. Prolactin is sandwiched between a 'capture' antibody attached to a solid-phase matrix and a labelled detection antibody. (b) The hook effect: very high serum prolactin levels simultaneously saturate both the capture and detection antibodies, preventing sandwich formation and the detection of prolactin.

Insulin-like growth factor-1

Insulin-like growth factor-1 (IGF-1) is a peptide that is synthesized and secreted by the liver under the control of GH. IGF-1 adjusted for sex and age is low in patients with GH deficiency. GH levels are affected by a number of factors including stress, and therefore GH deficiency can only be proven by failure to respond to stimulation in dynamic tests (see below). IGF-1 levels are high in patients with GH-secreting pituitary tumours, causing acromegaly.

LH, FSH, testosterone in men and oestradiol in women

- *Women* with secondary hypogonadism have reduced oestradiol with reduced or inappropriately normal LH and FSH.
- *Men* with secondary hypogonadism have reduced testosterone with reduced or inappropriately normal LH and FSH.

TSH and free thyroxine

In secondary hypothyroidism, free thyroxine is low and TSH is either low or inappropriately normal.

8–9 a.m. cortisol and ACTH

In secondary adrenal insufficiency, 8–9 a.m. cortisol levels are low, and ACTH levels are either reduced or inappropriately normal. However, cortisol levels, like GH, are affected by stress, and deficiencies can be proved only by a failure to respond to stimulation in dynamic tests (see below).

ADH (vasopressin) deficiency

Tests of posterior pituitary function include measurement of serum and urine osmolality and sodium concentrations, and the water deprivation test (see Chapter 17).

Dynamic pituitary function tests

Insulin tolerance test

Insulin-induced hypoglycaemia (glucose <2.2 mmol/L) stimulates GH (to >20 mU/L or 6 µg/L) and cortisol (to >500 nmol/L) in normal individuals. Patients with a basal cortisol below 80 nmol/L are very unlikely to have a normal response and may therefore not need the test.

The *insulin tolerance test* (ITT) is contraindicated in patients with a history of epilepsy or ischaemic heart disease. All patients should have a normal ECG before the test. Untreated hypothyroidism impairs the GH and cortisol response.

Insulin is injected intravenously at a dose of 0.10 U/kg (0.2–0.3 U/kg in acromegaly and Cushing's disease). Blood samples are taken for GH, cortisol and glucose, and blood glucose is also checked with a glucometer before insulin injection and after 30, 60, 90 and 120 minutes. A further insulin dose may be given if the patient does not become hypoglycaemic by 30 minutes. Once blood glucose is less than 2.2 mmol/L and blood specimens have been taken, patients do not need to remain hypoglycaemic. The false-positive rate is about 5%.

Glucagon test

The glucagon test may be done when an ITT is contraindicated. This test is slightly less reliable than an ITT. In adults, 1 mg of intramuscular glucagon is given. Blood samples are taken for glucose, cortisol and GH prior to glucagon injection and at 90, 120, 150 and 180 minutes. The criteria for adequate cortisol and GH response are the same as those for ITT. The false-positive rate is about 8%. The false-negative rate for cortisol response is 30%.

Metyrapone test

Some endocrinologists prefer to test the ACTH reserve using the metyrapone test. Metyrapone blocks the conversion of 11-deoxycortisol to cortisol. Thus in normal individuals, metyrapone (750 mg given orally every 4 hours for 24 hours) causes a fall in serum cortisol (8 a.m. cortisol <172 nmol/L after 24 hours of metyrapone) and stimulates ACTH secretion. The increase in ACTH leads to an increase in adrenal steroid synthesis up to and including 11-deoxycortisol (8 a.m. 11-deoxycortisol ≥289 nmol/L). In patients with ACTH deficiency, 8 a.m. 11-deoxycortisol after 24 hours of metyrapone is <289 nmol/L.

The metyrapone-induced cortisol deficiency should be reversed by 100 mg of hydrocortisone administered intravenously at the end of the 24 hours (after the 8 a.m. blood sample is taken). The main disadvantage of this test is that the patient must be observed in an inpatient setting. Lying and standing blood pressure and pulse must be measured before each metyrapone dose. If postural hypotension occurs, the test should be terminated and 100 mg of hydrocortisone should be given intravenously.

Pituitary imaging

MRI is the preferred imaging modality for the pituitary gland. It can effectively characterize soft tissues, and demonstrates the size of the adenoma and whether it extends outside the sella turcica. Patients are not exposed to ionizing radiation. The renal function must be checked before MRI with gadolinium since some patients with impaired renal function have been reported to develop nephrogenic systemic fibrosis as a side-effect of the contrast agent.

On T1-weighted MRI images (Fig. 12.3), the anterior pituitary is isointense with white matter. The posterior pituitary exhibits a higher signal intensity (due to an accumulation of neurosecretory granules consisting of an ADH–neurophysin complex packaged within phospholipid membranes). Following gadolinium administration, the pituitary gland and stalk enhance brightly.

In patients with suspected microadenomas, both coronal and sagittal sections are required. Pituitary microadenomas are usually hypointense relative to the surrounding normal pituitary tissue. This can be further clarified following enhancement with gadolinium as microadenomas take longer to enhance.

In patients with macroadenomas, pituitary MRI can detect involvement of the surrounding structures (i.e. optic chiasm, cavernous sinus, carotid arteries, sphenoid sinus, orbit and temporal lobe) and the presence of haemorrhage.

A computed tomography (CT) scan may be done when an MRI is contraindicated (cardiac pacemakers, metallic clips on aneurysms—except for newer titanium clips—and any metallic foreign body in the eye, spinal canal or close to a major blood vessel). Artefacts from the skull base and metallic

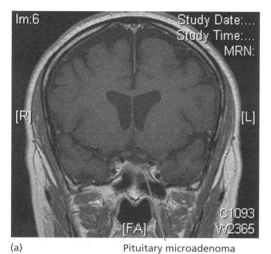

(a)   Pituitary microadenoma

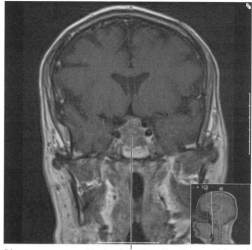

(b)   Pituitary macroadenoma

Figure 12.3 (a) Coronal magnetic resonance imaging (MRI) scan showing a pituitary microadenoma (note that the microadenoma is hypointense relative to the surrounding normal pituitary tissue). Coronal (b) and sagittal (c) MRI scans showing a pituitary macroadenoma.

(c)   Pituitary macroadenoma

dental materials can obscure and compromise the characterization of soft tissues.

Treatment

The aims of treatment for patients with pituitary tumours include:
- the treatment of pituitary hormone hypersecretion: see the specific chapters on Cushing's disease, acromegaly and prolactinomas
- the treatment of hypopituitarism (see Chapter 13)
- the treatment of space-occupying (local compression) effects of the tumour.

The space-occupying effects of pituitary tumours are treated with *pituitary surgery*. In some cases, pituitary surgery may be followed with *radiotherapy*.

Pituitary surgery

The indications for pituitary surgery include:
- reducing local compression effects such as worsening visual fields (Fig. 12.4). Surgery may also be

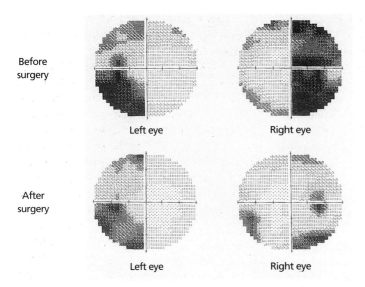

Before surgery

Left eye · Right eye

After surgery

Left eye · Right eye

Figure 12.4 Improvement in temporal visual field defects before and after trans-sphenoidal surgery.

indicated to prevent future compressive effects if the pituitary is shown to be growing over time on serial scans and likely to cause problems before the patient dies of natural causes.

• reducing excess hormone secretion (e.g. Cushing's disease, acromegaly, TSHomas and prolactinomas not responding to medical treatment).

When surgery is indicated, the *trans-sphenoidal* approach is the first-line surgery for almost every case. Patients must be informed of the possible complications of trans-sphenoidal pituitary surgery (Box 12.3). Patients should be aware of the need for lifelong follow-up.

Secondary adrenal insufficiency should be treated with hydrocortisone (see Chapter 13).

> **Box 12.3 Complications of trans-sphenoidal surgery**
>
> **A**nterior pituitary hormone deficiencies (about 10% for macroadenomas, uncommon with microadenomas)
> **B**leeding, carotid artery injury (rare)
> **C**erebrospinal fluid leakage/rhinorrhoea, meningitis
> **D**iabetes insipidus (transient 5%, permanent 0.1%)
> **E**yes: visual deterioration, cranial (e.g. IIIrd) nerve damage
> **F**ailure of the surgery
> **G**eneral anaesthetic complications
> **H**yponatraemia

Treatment of secondary hypothyroidism should be commenced only after excluding or treating adrenal insufficiency. Secondary hypothyroidism is treated with thyroxine if surgery is not imminent, and with triiodothyronine (20 µg three times a day) for 4 days preoperatively if the surgery is urgent.

For the management of patients with prolactinomas, acromegaly and Cushing's disease, see the specific chapters. In patients with Cushing's disease, metyrapone or ketoconazole may be given for at least 6 weeks prior to surgery. These inhibit adrenal steroid hormone synthesis, correcting the hypercortisolaemia, which allows for an improvement in healing and in the general state of the patient.

Craniotomy may be required for craniopharyngiomas, parasellar tumours (e.g. meningiomas) and very large tumours with extensive suprasellar extension and lateral invasion where trans-sphenoidal surgery is unlikely to achieve removal of a significant portion of the tumour.

Perioperative measures

Some centres advocate prophylactic perioperative antibiotics, which may reduce the risk of meningitis.

Perioperative *hydrocortisone* must be given to patients with Cushing's disease and those with a deficient or unknown steroid reserve. Hydrocortisone 50 mg intramuscularly is started with premedication on the day of surgery and is continued 6-hourly. This may be converted to oral hydrocortisone (20 mg, 10 mg, 10 mg) when the patient starts eating and drinking. Oral hydrocortisone may then be temporarily stopped and 9 a.m. cortisol checked (i.e. after stopping hydrocortisone the night before and on the morning of the test).

In those without Cushing's disease:
• If 9 a.m. cortisol >350 nmol/L, the patient can stay off hydrocortisone.
• If 9 a.m. cortisol <300 nmol/L, the patient is sent home on regular oral hydrocortisone (10 mg, 5 mg, 5 mg) until further assessment. Patients must be provided with advice regarding sick day rules (doubling the dose during illness), intramuscular preparation of hydrocortisone for emergencies, a steroid warning card and a MedicAlert bracelet.
• If 9 a.m. cortisol is 300–350 nmol/L, the patient should be supplied with oral (and intramuscular preparation of) hydrocortisone and written advice about starting hydrocortisone if he or she becomes unwell.

In those with Cushing's disease, 9 a.m. cortisol below 50 nmol/L is suggestive of remission, and regular hydrocortisone replacement should be started. This is because prolonged elevation of circulating cortisol levels has suppressed the hypothalamic–pituitary axis and, following cure, patients may become steroid deficient. Some endocrinologists recommend hydrocortisone replacement (for approximately 4–6 weeks) until further assessment for all patients with Cushing's disease regardless of the immediate postoperative cortisol levels due to the risk of delayed remission.

Visual fields should be formally assessed 3–5 days postoperatively.

Fluid balance must be very closely monitored postoperatively to watch for the possible development of *diabetes insipidus*, which may occur due to manipulation of the pituitary and its stalk during surgery. Diabetes insipidus presents with polyuria. Postoperatively, the patient's urine must be checked regularly for specific gravity (SG) on the ward. This is much more practical and quicker than sending urine to the laboratory for measurement of osmolality.

The SG of dilute urine is below 1.005. If the patient becomes polyuric (i.e. passes 200–300 mL per hour for three or more consecutive hours), it is important to distinguish psychogenic polydipsia (i.e. the patient drinking water because of mouth-breathing as the nose is packed) from true diabetes insipidus. Both result in dilute urine, but in true diabetes insipidus the plasma osmolality is high. In some centres, it is easier to measure plasma sodium rather than plasma osmolality, and it gives the same information. If the serum osmolality is low, the patient may be overdrinking. A low urine SG (<1.005) or osmolality is appropriate in this case.

Diabetes insipidus is confirmed if the plasma osmolality is high (>295 mosm/L) or plasma sodium is over 145 mmol/L in the presence of an inappropriately low urine osmolality/SG (SG <1.005). Patients must be encouraged to drink more. However, if they cannot keep up with the diuresis and plasma osomolality rises to more than 299 mosm/L or sodium increases to over 147 mmol/L, desmopressin is given (1 µg subcutaneously). If polyuria recurs up to 4 days postoperatively, regular desmopressin should be considered.

Serum sodium must be checked 7–10 days postoperatively as there is a risk of *hyponatraemia*. Hyponatraemia occurring 5–10 days postoperatively may be due to the syndrome of inappropriate ADH (SIADH) or rarely cerebral salt wasting (CSW). SIADH is probably due to excess ADH released from degenerating ADH-producing neurones whose axons were damaged during the surgery. CSW is associated with large amounts of urinary salt loss and hypovolaemia. This should be differentiated from SIADH by assessing fluid status and central venous pressure which show hypovolaemia in CSW and euvolaemia in SIADH. CSW is treated using saline administration, whereas SIADH is treated with fluid restriction.

Pituitary radiotherapy

Conventional radiotherapy delivers repeated small doses (fractions) of radiation (e.g. over 35 days).

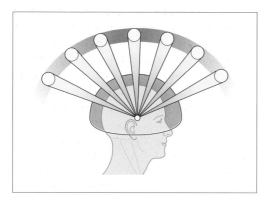

Figure 12.5 The gamma knife delivers convergent radiation beams from an array of [60]cobalt sources.

Stereotactic radiosurgery delivers a single, relatively large dose of radiation to a precisely defined target. A 'gamma knife' delivers convergent radiation beams from an array of [60]cobalt sources (Fig. 12.5). A linear accelerator delivers the radiation beam via a gantry that rotates around the patient.

The indications for radiotherapy following pituitary surgery are to shrink residual or recurrent tumour, to reduce the likelihood of regrowth and to treat persistent hormone hypersecretion.

Short-term complications include nausea, headache and hair loss. Long-term complications include hypopituitarism (due to the effect of radiotherapy on the hypothalamus) and visual impairment (which may occur within 3 years of radiotherapy and is possibly due to damage to the vascular supply of the optic chiasm).

Radiotherapy is also associated with a small increased risk of second intracranial tumours, for example astrocytoma, meningioma and meningeal sarcoma (a 1.9% cumulative risk over 20 years) and stroke.

Follow-up and monitoring

Patients should be evaluated 4–6 weeks after the surgery with a formal assessment of *visual acuity and fields*, and *pituitary function testing*, including 8–9 a.m. serum cortisol (12–24 hours after discontinuation of hydrocortisone), free thyroxine, TSH, LH, FSH, testosterone in men or oestradiol in pre-menopausal women. Hydrocortisone should be resumed after the test until the results are known.

If the 8–9 a.m. serum cortisol is over 550 nmol/L, hydrocortisone can be stopped. If not, the patient should be assessed with an ITT. Patients on hydrocortisone replacement should be offered an ITT 1–2 years after surgery as there is a chance of recovery of normal corticotroph function.

If the patient has polyuria, a 24-hour urine collection should be made, and a water deprivation test should be done if the urine output is above 3 L per day.

Pituitary MRI is best repeated 3 months after the surgery so that the immediate inflammatory postoperative changes will not influence the results.

Long-term monitoring should include clinical assessment, visual field assessment and repeat MRI. The optimal protocol for imaging follow-up is not known. An accepted practice is to do a pituitary MRI 3 months after surgery, then annually for 5 years and then every 2 years thereafter.

Visual fields should be assessed annually, and a pituitary MRI should be done if any deterioration is noted.

Following postoperative radiotherapy, loss of any pituitary hormone can occur from a few months to at least 10 years after radiation. Therefore pituitary function tests should be repeated 6 months after radiotherapy and then annually.

Other pituitary and sellar disorders

Pituitary apoplexy

Pituitary apoplexy is acute haemorrhagic infarction of a pituitary tumour (usually large) resulting in gland destruction and compression of surrounding structures by the oedematous enlarged pituitary tumour. Hypertension may be an important predisposing factor. It presents with acute headache, meningism, visual impairment, ophthalmoplegia and sometimes altered consciousness. Patients may also have postural hypotension due to acute cortisol deficiency. Silent bleeds into a pituitary adenoma are much more common.

Investigations include pituitary MRI and pituitary function tests. In the first 3–5 days, haemorrhage within the sella is isointense on T1-weighted images and hypointense on T2-weighted sequences.

Initial treatment should include hydrocortisone replacement. It has been suggested that surgery within 8 days provides the optimal chance of neurological recovery. However, patients with no significant visual or other neurological loss may be managed conservatively. Long-term follow-up is required initially, with an annual MRI.

Sheehan's syndrome

Sheehan's syndrome refers to pituitary gland necrosis caused by hypotension due to postpartum haemorrhage. Patients may present after delivery with failure of lactation, failure to resume menses as well as signs of other pituitary hormone deficiencies, for example fatigue, anorexia and weight loss.

Empty sella syndrome

Empty sella syndrome (Fig. 12.6) is characterized by an enlarged sella filled with CSF.

'Primary' empty sella syndrome may be due to a defective and enlarged diaphragma sella opening. It may be caused by a developmental anomaly or increased intracranial pressure, and can result in compression and posterior displacement of the anterior pituitary. It is more common in middle-aged women and is usually incidental with no clinical significance. Hyperprolactinaemia (due to the stalk effect) and intrasellar prolapse of the optic chiasm may occasionally occur. The latter is usually asymptomatic.

'Secondary' empty sella syndrome may be due to infarction, surgery or radiotherapy of a pituitary adenoma/sella mass. Visual impairment may occur due to fibrosis and ischaemia of the prolapsed optic chiasm.

Other sellar and parasellar disorders

In addition to pituitary adenomas, a number of other disorders can also occur in or near the sella turcica and suprasellar cistern (Box 12.4). These lesions can have similar presentations to pituitary adenomas, with headaches, visual impairment, hypopituitarism and hydrocephalus depending on their size, location and the extent of their impingement on the local tissues. Diabetes insipidus is more common in patients with non-pituitary lesions than those with pituitary adenomas.

The diagnosis is dependent on careful clinical and radiological assessment of these lesions.

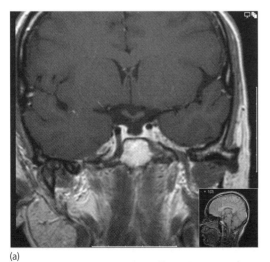

(a)

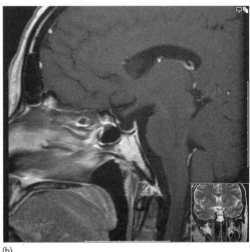

(b)

Figure 12.6 Coronal (a) and sagittal (b) magnetic resonance imaging scans showing an empty sella.

Box 12.4 Sellar and parasellar disorders

Pituitary adenoma, carcinoma (very rare)
Cysts: Rathke's cleft, arachnoid, dermoid
Craniopharyngioma
Meningiomas
Malignant tumours: germ cell tumour, sarcoma, chordoma, lymphoma, metastases (lung, breast)
Infection: abscesses (bacterial, tuberculosis, fungal, parasitic)
Inflammation/infiltration: lymphocytic hypophysitis, sarcoidosis, haemochromatosis, Langerhans cell histiocytosis
Vascular: aneurysms
Trauma

Craniopharyngiomas are benign tumours that arise from squamous epithelial remnants of Rathke's pouch. Around 50% present during childhood and adolescence. Most are suprasellar, and only 20% originate in the sella. Craniopharyngiomas can be cystic and/or solid. Histology may be either 'adamantinous' with cyst formation and calcification, or 'papillary' (with generally a better prognosis).

Craniopharyngiomas commonly cause diabetes insipidus. The major presenting symptoms are growth retardation in children and visual abnormalities in adults.

Total excision of craniopharyngiomas may be associated with considerable morbidity, operative mortality, recurrence and long-term neurological and endocrine complications. Therefore many centres recommend less aggressive surgery followed by external beam irradiation.

Craniopharyngioma is a locally aggressive tumour and has a high recurrence rate. Further surgical removal may be indicated when symptoms are caused by increased tumour size.

Meningiomas are usually benign tumors arising from the meninges. Some arise near the sella, causing visual impairment and hormonal deficiencies. On MRI they are isointense with grey matter, and following gadolinium contrast they become hyperintense.

Germ cell tumours are usually associated with simultaneous lesions in the pineal gland, and patients may have a paralysis of upward conjugate gaze (Parinaud's syndrome). Human chorionic gonadotrophin-beta is detected in the serum or CSF. These tumours are very radiosensitive. Fifty per cent are malignant and metastasize.

Abscesses in the pituitary may result from local spread, for example from sphenoid sinusitis, or may be secondary to septicaemia. Tuberculosis may present with hypopituitarism and basilar meningitis. Some but not all patients have fever, leukocytosis and meningism. Imaging studies may be unable to distinguish between pituitary abscess and pituitary adenoma, and most patients are diagnosed at the time of surgical exploration.

Lymphocytic hypophysitis is characterized by lymphocytic infiltration of the anterior pituitary followed by fibrosis. It is associated with other autoimmune endocrine conditions and possibly has an autoimmune origin. It almost always affects women, most commonly during pregnancy or the postpartum period. It is characterized by headaches of an intensity out of proportion to the size of the lesion and hypopituitarism, in which adrenal insufficiency is unusually prominent.

Sarcoidosis is an inflammatory granulomatous multisystem disorder that may affect multiple organs such as the eyes (anterior uveitis), skin (erythema nodosum, papules), lungs (e.g. hilar lymphadenopathy, pulmonary fibrosis), joints and central nervous system (with a predilection for the base of the brain). It may affect the pituitary stalk or hypothalamus.

Hereditary haemochromatosis is an inherited disorder characterized by increased intestinal iron absorption and iron deposition in various organs (e.g. liver, heart, pituitary gland) due to mutations in the *HFE* gene. Gonadotrophin deficiency is the most common endocrine abnormality. Iron studies should be performed if there is an appropriate family history or if the patient has other suggestive manifestations such as bronzed skin, diabetes mellitus or otherwise unexplained heart or liver disease. Repeated phlebotomy to remove iron may reverse the gonadotrophin deficiency.

Langerhans cell histiocytosis may present with diabetes insipidus. The lesions are eosinophilic granulomata and affect multiple organs such as bones (e.g. radiolucent lesions in the skull, marrow involvement), skin (histiocytomas), central nervous system (particularly the hypothalamic–pituitary axis), ear (otitis externa, discharge), lungs (obstructive and restrictive defects), lymph nodes, liver and spleen (enlargement).

Cysts: Rathke's cleft, arachnoid and dermoid cysts can produce sellar enlargement and may cause visual impairment, hypopituitarism and hydrocephalus. Rathke's cleft cysts (like craniopharyngiomas) are derived from the remnants of Rathke's pouch. They are lined by ciliated cuboidal/columnar epithelium (compared with squamous epithelium in craniopharyngiomas). Symptomatic patients are treated by decompression. Recurrence after treatment is rare.

Aneurysms are best diagnosed with magnetic resonance angiography.

Traumatic brain injury may result in hypopituitarism. In the acute phase, patients may show evidence of deficiency of gonadotrophins (80%), GH (18%), ACTH (16%) and ADH abnormalities (40%) causing diabetes insipidus or SIADH. Some of the early abnormalities are transient. However, new endocrine dysfunctions may become apparent in the post-acute phase. About 25% of the long-term survivors have one or more pituitary hormone deficiencies. This is a higher frequency than previously thought and suggests that most cases of post-traumatic hypopituitarism remain undiagnosed.

Key points:

- Pituitary tumours are classified according to size (microadenoma <1 cm, macroadenoma ≥1 cm) and whether they are functioning (secreting one or more anterior pituitary hormones) or non-functioning.
- Tumours may present with hormone hypersecretion syndromes, hypopituitarism or mass effects due to tumour impingement on surrounding structures.
- Work-up includes basal and dynamic pituitary function testing, visual field assessment and pituitary MRI.
- Pituitary surgery is indicated for certain hypersecretion syndromes, to relieve pressure effects or where medical therapy has failed.
- The trans-sphenoidal approach is favoured where possible. Patients should be cared for by a multidisciplinary team including a specialist pituitary neurosurgeon and endocrinologists.
- Postoperative complications include hypopituitarism, cerebral infection and diabetes insipidus.
- Radiotherapy may be considered for large postoperative tumour remnants, to reduce the risk of tumour regrowth or for persistent hormone hypersecretion. Subsequent hypopituitarism may ensue, often after a long latency, so long-term endocrine follow-up is mandatory.
- Pituitary apoplexy is acute haemorrhagic infarction of a pituitary tumour presenting with acute headache, meningism, visual impairment, ophthalmoplegia and sometimes altered consciousness. Initial life-saving treatment is with intravenous hydrocortisone. All cases, particularly those with neurological complications, should be discussed with a neurosurgeon.
- Other sellar and parasellar pathologies that may present with hypopituitarism or mass effects include cysts, tumours of surrounding structures, infiltrative disorders, infection and vascular abnormalities. These are more likely to cause posterior pituitary dysfunction compared with pituitary adenomas.

Chapter 13

Hypopituitarism

Hypopituitarism refers to the reduced secretion of pituitary hormones, which can result from diseases of either the pituitary gland or the hypothalamus (causing a decreased secretion of hypothalamic releasing hormones that stimulate anterior pituitary hormone release).

A total of 76% of cases of hypopituitarism are due to pituitary tumours or their treatment. Another 13% may be due to extrapituitary tumours (e.g. craniopharyngioma). The cause of hypopituitarism in up to 8% of patients may remain unknown.

Box 13.1 summarizes major causes of hypopituitarism. Pituitary adenomas and other sellar and parasellar disorders were discussed in Chapter 12.

Genetic causes of hypopituitarism may be due to mutations in the genes encoding the transcription factors necessary for the differentiation of anterior pituitary cells. Mutations in the *PROP1* gene are the most common cause of both familial and sporadic congenital combined pituitary hormone deficiency. Mutations in *PROP1* result in deficiencies in growth hormone (GH), prolactin, thyroid-stimulating hormone (TSH), luteinizing hormone (LH) and follicle-stimulating hormone (FSH).

Mutations in *HESX1*, *LHX3* and *LHX4* also cause deficiencies of GH, prolactin, TSH, LH and FSH. Mutations of the gene that encodes *PIT1* (which

---

Lecture Notes: Endocrinology and Diabetes. By A. Sam and K. Meeran. Published 2009 by Blackwell Publishing. ISBN 978-1-4051-5345-4.

> **Box 13.1 Causes of hypopituitarism**
>
> **Pituitary adenomas**
>
> **Other tumours/cysts**
> Craniopharyngiomas, meningiomas, malignant tumours (germ cell tumours, chordoma, sarcoma), pituitary metastases (e.g. lung, breast), cysts (e.g. Rathke's cleft)
>
> **Pituitary/hypothalamic surgery**
>
> **Trauma** (basal skull fracture)
>
> **Pituitary/hypothalamic radiation**
>
> **Infarction**
> Apoplexy, Sheehan's syndrome
>
> **Inflammation/infiltration/infection**
> Lymphocytic hypophysitis, sarcoidosis, haemochromatosis, Langerhans cell histiocytosis, tuberculous meningitis
>
> **Genetic**
> e.g. *PROP1* or *PIT1* mutations

acts temporally just after *PROP1*) lead to congenital deficiencies of GH, prolactin and sometimes TSH. Mutations in *TPIT* cause adrenocorticotrophic hormone (ACTH) deficiency, and result in neonatal death if not detected early.

Clinical presentations

Signs and symptoms resulting from various pituitary hormone deficiencies are summarized below.

GH deficiency

GH deficiency can result in fatigue, impaired psychological well-being, reduced energy, muscle strength and exercise capacity, and increased abdominal adiposity (fat mass).

LH and FSH deficiency

- LH/FSH deficiency in *men* results in secondary hypogonadism: reduced libido, oligospermia and infertility, loss of body hair, fine perioral wrinkles, flushes and osteoporosis (see Chapter 19).
- LH/FSH deficiency in *women* results in secondary hypogonadism: oligomenorrhoea/amenorrhoea, infertility, dyspareunia, breast atrophy, hot flushes and osteoporosis (see Chapter 21).

ACTH deficiency

ACTH deficiency results in secondary adrenal insufficiency: fatigue, weakness, nausea, vomiting, weight loss, hypoglycaemia and loss of pubic and axillary hair in females (see Chapter 6).

TSH deficiency

TSH deficiency results in secondary hypothyroidism: fatigue, apathy, muscle weakness, cold intolerance, constipation, weight gain and dry skin (see Chapter 2).

Antidiuretic hormone deficiency

Antidiuretic hormone (ADH) deficiency results in diabetes insipidus: polyuria, nocturia and polydipsia (see Chapter 17).

Prolactin deficiency

The only known presentation of prolactin deficiency is the inability to lactate after delivery.

Investigations

Pituitary function tests and pituitary imaging are discussed in Chapter 12.

Treatment and monitoring

ACTH deficiency

Hydrocortisone is the logical option for glucocorticoid replacement because it is the glucocorticoid normally made by the adrenals. A daily regimen of 10 mg in the morning, 5 mg at noon and 5 mg in the evening is probably the 'best-guess' starting dose. Cortisol has a plasma half-life of less than 2 hours. The traditional hydrocortisone regimen of 20 mg in the morning and 10 mg in the evening is suboptimal for two reasons. First, it may result in low cortisol levels and low quality of life scores in late afternoon. Second, hydrocortisone production rates in normal individuals are lower than previously believed. Chronic over-replacement (>20 mg per day) may result in Cushing's syndrome.

It is essential that patients are provided with:
- information regarding doubling of hydrocortisone dose at times of intercurrent illness
- an emergency intramuscular hydrocortisone supply (to be given at times of vomiting on their way to hospital)
- a steroid card and MedicAlert bracelet.

Glucocorticoid replacement may unmask underlying central diabetes insipidus, leading to marked polyuria.

These patients usually do not require mineralocorticoid replacement therapy (unlike patients with primary adrenal failure) because aldosterone release is under the control of the renin–angiotensin system and is not ACTH driven.

Follow-up and monitoring

Under-replacement results in a persistence (or recurrence) of the symptoms of cortisol deficiency, whereas over-replacement may result in symptoms of cortisol excess and bone loss. The adequacy of treatment is monitored by:
- asking about symptoms
- measurement of lying and standing blood pressure (to exclude postural hypotension)
- hydrocortisone day curves.

Many endocrinologists use hydrocortisone day curves to adjust the dose and timing of hydrocortisone replacement therapy. All oestrogens therapy should be discontinued 6 weeks prior to the test as they increase cortisol-binding globulin levels and result in misleadingly high measured total cortisol levels. Blood is taken in the morning, before and 1 hour after the lunchtime and evening doses. Aim for adequate cortisol levels throughout the day (peak <900 nmol/L, trough >50–100 nmol/L). Once adequate levels have been achieved, this process rarely needs to be repeated.

TSH deficiency

Levothyroxine is started at a dose of 100 µg per day in young patients without cardiac disease. In the elderly or those with cardiac disease, levothyroxine is started at a dose of 25–50 µg per day. Levothyroxine must only be started *after* hydrocortisone replacement as it may increase the clearance of the little cortisol that is produced, and may precipitate an Addisonian crisis.

Follow-up and monitoring

Serum TSH cannot be used to monitor treatment in central (secondary) hypothyroidism. The treatment aim should be a serum thyroxine in the middle of the normal range. Long-term over-replacement increases the risk of osteoporosis and atrial fibrillation.

LH and FSH deficiency in women

- Women who *do not desire fertility* should receive oestrogen–progestin replacement therapy for the prevention of osteoporosis, for symptomatic control (vasomotor symptoms, vaginal dryness) and possibly for the prevention of coronary heart disease (see Chapter 21).
- Those who *do wish to become fertile* may be treated with pulsatile gonadotrophin-releasing hormone (GnRH) or gonadotrophins (daily FSH to stimulate follicle development followed by human chorionic gonadotrophin (hCG) to induce ovulation when the ovarian follicles are mature).

Gonadotrophin replacement

FSH is given according to a step-up or step-down protocol. The step-down protocol mimics the physiology of normal cycles more closely. FSH is started at a dose of 150 IU per day shortly after progesterone-induced bleeding and is continued until a dominant follicle (>10 mm) is seen on transvaginal ultrasonography. The dose is then reduced to 112.5 IU per day followed by a further reduction to 75 IU per day after 3 days, which is continued until hCG is administered. The ovarian response to FSH therapy is monitored using transvaginal ultrasonography and serum oestradiol.

hCG is given on the day that at least one follicle appears to be mature (a follicle diameter of 18 mm and a serum oestradiol of 734 pmol/L per dominant follicle). If three or more follicles bigger than 15 mm are present, stimulation should be stopped to prevent multiple pregnancies and ovarian hyperstimulation.

Pulsatile GnRH is more likely than gonadotrophins to result in the development and ovulation of a single follicle, thereby reducing the risk of ovarian hyperstimulation and multiple gestations. However, in more than 50% of women with organic pituitary disease, residual gonadotrophin function may be insufficient to allow pulsatile GnRH therapy.

LH and FSH deficiency in men

- Men with secondary hypogonadism who *do not desire fertility* should receive testosterone replacement therapy if there are no contraindications. For the treatment and monitoring of patients on testosterone replacement therapy, see Chapter 19.
- Men with secondary hypogonadism who *do desire fertility* can be treated with gonadotrophin replacement therapy or pulsatile GnRH. Both regimens may take up to 2 years to achieve adequate spermatogenesis.

Gonadotrophin replacement

Initially, hCG injections are administered (1000–2000 IU intramuscularly or subcutaneously, three times a week). hCG has the biological activity of LH but a longer half-life in the circulation. It stimulates the Leydig cells to secrete testosterone. Serum testosterone is measured every 1–2 months and is used to adjust the hCG dose. The response to therapy is measured on semen analysis (every 4 weeks).

Most patients who eventually reach a normal sperm count (>20 million/mL or 40 million/ejaculate) do so within 6 months. If adequate spermatogenesis is not achieved within 6–12 months, human menopausal gonadotrophin or recombinant FSH is added (37.5–75 IU three times a week). Human menopausal gonadotrophin is purified from the urine of postmenopausal women and contains FSH. It may take 12 months or more for a response to be seen.

Pulsatile GnRH may be given subcutaneously via a catheter attached to a mini-pump. This regimen is suitable in men with a hypothalamic defect with normal pituitary gonadotrophin function.

GH deficiency

Adult-onset GH deficiency is associated with unfavourable serum lipid profiles, increased body fat, decreased muscle mass and bone mineral density, and a lower sense of well-being and overall quality of life.

In the USA, many endocrinologists replace GH in patients with adult-onset GH deficiency if they meet at least two criteria for GH therapy: a poor GH response to at least two standard stimuli, and hypopituitarism due to pituitary or hypothalamic damage.

In the UK, GH replacement in adults is considered only in GH-deficient patients with a severely impaired quality of life, reflected by a score of at least 11 (range 0–25) in the Quality of Life Assessment of GH Deficiency in Adults (QoL-AGHDA) questionnaire. GH therapy should be discontinued after 9 months if the QoL-AGHDA score improves by fewer than 7 points. The 9-month period allows a dose titration interval of 3 months followed by a 6-month therapeutic trial period.

GH may be started at a low dose (0.15–0.3 mg per day) given once daily subcutaneously. The dose may be increased every 4–6 weeks based on the clinical response and insulin-like growth factor-1 (IGF-1) levels until a steady replacement dose is reached (maximum 1 mg daily).

GH treatment results in:

- decreased fat mass and increased muscle mass (following 12 months' therapy)
- increased bone mineral density (over 24 months of GH replacement)
- an improved sense of well-being, and overall quality of life in some patients
- reduced serum total cholesterol, low-density lipoprotein and triglyceride levels. However, a complicating factor is the apparent increase in lipoprotein (a) (a lipoprotein associated with an increased risk of coronary heart disease) seen in some studies.

Follow-up and monitoring

Monitoring includes:
- assessment of quality of life
- measurement of weight, waist-to-hip ratio and blood pressure
- measurement of lipid profile, glycated haemoglobin and IGF-1.

ADH deficiency

For details of ADH replacement therapy see Chapter 17.

Prolactin deficiency

The only known presentation of prolactin deficiency is the inability to lactate after delivery. There is currently no treatment available for this.

> **Key points:**
>
> - Hypopituitarism refers to a reduced secretion of pituitary hormones.
> - Hypopituitarism may be caused by sellar/parasellar tumours, surgery, trauma, radiation, infarction, inflammation/infiltration or mutations in the genes involved in the differentiation of anterior pituitary cells.
> - Patients with hypopituitarism may present with features of GH deficiency, hypogonadism, secondary adrenal insufficiency, hypothyroidism and occasionally diabetes insipidus. Depending on the specific pituitary hormone deficiency, patients may require replacement therapy with hydrocortisone, levothyroxine, sex steroids and GH. Pulsatile GnRH or gonadotrophins may be given if the patient desires fertility.

Chapter 14

Hyperprolactinaemia

Hyperprolactinaemia is the presence of abnormally high circulating prolactin levels secreted by the lactotroph cells in the anterior pituitary. The causes of hyperprolactinaemia are summarized in Box 14.1.

Prolactin gene expression and synthesis is upregulated by *oestrogen*. This explains the higher prolactin levels in premenopausal women than in men, and the higher prolactin levels (up to 10-fold) seen during pregnancy and lactation.

Prolactin secretion is inhibited by dopamine (via activation of D_2 receptors). Therefore hyperprolactinaemia may be caused by:

- reduced dopamine secretion
- reduced dopamine delivery to the anterior pituitary via the portal vessels (due to pituitary stalk compression by a sellar/parasellar lesion or stalk section caused by trauma)
- dopamine (D_2) receptor antagonists (e.g. antipsychotics and some antiemetics).

Prolactin levels are also higher following exercise, meals and sexual intercourse, during physical or psychological stress, and following an epileptic fit.

In some patients, the underlying cause of the hyperprolactinaemia is not found ('idiopathic hyperprolactinaemia'). Many of these patients may have microadenomas not visible on magnetic resonance imaging (MRI).

Lecture Notes: Endocrinology and Diabetes. By A. Sam and K. Meeran. Published 2009 by Blackwell Publishing. ISBN 978-1-4051-5345-4.

Box 14.1 Causes of hyperprolactinaemia

Physiological
Pregnancy
Lactation
Stress

Drugs
Antipsychotics: phenothiazines, butyrophenones, flupenthixol, risperidone
Antidepressants: tricyclic antidepressants, selective serotonin reuptake inhibitors, monoamine oxidase inhibitors
Metoclopramide, domperidone
Oestrogens
Opiates
Others: omeprazole, H_2 antagonists, verapamil, methyldopa, bezafibrate, protease inhibitors

Pituitary tumours and other sellar/parasellar lesions
Prolactinomas
Mixed growth hormone/prolactin-secreting tumours
Sellar and parasellar lesions causing stalk compression ('disconnection hyperprolactinaemia')

Primary hypothyroidism (thyrotrophin-releasing hormone stimulates prolactin release)

Chronic renal failure (reduced clearance of prolactin)

Severe liver disease (disordered hypothalamic regulation)

Polycystic ovary syndrome

Epidemiology

Prolactinomas are the most common functioning pituitary tumour. Lactotroph adenomas (prolactinomas) account for approximately 30–40% of all clinically recognized pituitary adenomas. Microprolactinomas (<1 cm) are more common than macroprolactinomas (>1 cm). Women with microprolactinomas present earlier (with menstrual irregularities) than men.

Clinical presentations

The main action of prolactin is to stimulate lactation. Excess prolactin can result in an inhibition of gonadotrophin-releasing hormone (GnRH) and pituitary gonadotrophin release, and an impairment of gonadal steroidogenesis. Therefore patients with hyperprolactinaemia may present with *galactorrhoea* and symptoms of *hypogonadism*.

Women present with galactorrhoea (30–80%) and menstrual irregularities (oligomenorrhoea or amenorrhoea) or delayed menarche. Mild hyperprolactinaemia can cause infertility even when there is no abnormality of the menstrual cycle. These women account for about 20% of those evaluated for infertility. Galactorrhoea is less common in those with longstanding oestrogen deficiency.

Men present with reduced libido, impotence or infertility. They rarely present with galactorrhoea.

In addition to the symptoms of hyperprolactinaemia, patients with pituitary tumours may present with local mass affects, i.e. *headache* and *visual field defects*, and cranial nerve palsies (due to cavernous sinus invasion) or symptoms of *hypopituitarism* (e.g. adrenal insufficiency, hypothyroidism). Longstanding hyperprolactinaemia may result in low bone mineral density and osteoporosis. Most prolactinomas in females are small at the time of diagnosis.

Evaluation

It must be remembered that stress, sleep, exercise, intercourse and meals can cause a transient rise in serum prolactin levels. Thus borderline results should be repeated.

As mentioned above, prolactin levels can be elevated in patients with non-functioning adenomas due to pituitary stalk compression resulting in a reduction of the inhibitory effect of dopamine on prolactin secretion ('disconnection' hyperprolactinaemia). In non-functioning adenomas, elevated prolactin levels due to pituitary stalk compression rarely exceed 2000 mU/L and are almost never more than 4000 mU/L. Prolactin levels of more than 4000 mU/L are usually due to prolactin hypersecretion from a lactotroph adenoma (prolactinoma).

When measuring prolactin levels, it is important to be aware of the following two laboratory pitfalls (Fig. 14.1).

Macroprolactinaemia

Hyperprolactinaemia may be due to a decreased clearance of '*macroprolactin*', which is a complex of the normal 22 kDa prolactin with immunoglobulin G (Fig. 14.1b). In macroprolactinaemia, the free prolactin concentration may be normal. The most extensively used method to detect macroprolactin is to pretreat the serum with polyethylene glycol to precipitate the macroprolactin before the immunoassay for prolactin. Most laboratories now perform an automatic screen for macroprolactin on samples with an elevated result. The laboratory will report either the percentage of macroprolactin or the corrected monomeric prolactin estimation. Macroprolactin is present in 1.5% of the normal population and is biologically inactive.

The hook effect

The '*hook effect*' occurs when the assay uses antibodies that recognize two ends of the molecule (one capturing it and the other labelling it). Very high prolactin levels may be artefactually reported as normal or modestly elevated. This is because the very high serum prolactin saturates both the capture and labelling antibodies and prevents the binding of the two in a 'sandwich' (Fig. 14.1c). This can be avoided by repeating the assay using a 1:100 dilution of serum. This has clinical significance in the case of large prolactinomas, which may be

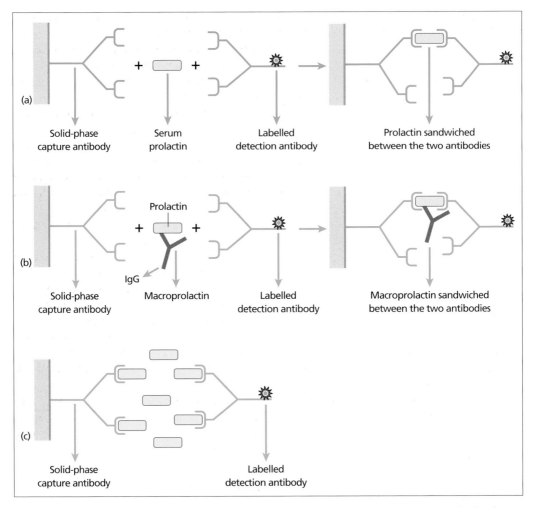

Figure 14.1 (a) A two-site immunometric assay for the measurement of serum prolactin uses two antibodies that are specific for different epitopes of prolactin. Prolactin is sandwiched between a capture antibody attached to a solid-phase matrix and a labelled detection antibody. (b) Circulating macroprolactin (complexes of immunoglobulin G [IgG] and prolactin) is detected but it is not bioactive. Thus the result is a false positive and clinically misleading. (c) The 'hook effect': very high serum prolactin levels simultaneously saturate both the capture and detection antibodies, preventing 'sandwich formation' and the detection of prolactin. This will result in a falsely low measurement.

misdiagnosed as non-functioning tumours if the hook effect is not taken into account, resulting in the patient undergoing unnecessary surgery.

The cause of hyperprolactinaemia (Box 14.1) can usually be identified by taking a history (with particular attention to drug history), examining the patient, performing a pregnancy test and measuring thyroid, renal and liver function.

Once physiological causes, drugs and metabolic causes (primary hypothyroidism, chronic renal failure, severe liver disease) have been excluded, a gadolinium-enhanced *pituitary MRI* should be performed. Prolactinomas can be divided into *macroadenomas* (>1 cm) and *microadenomas* (<1 cm) based on MRI measurement of the tumour size.

Patients with macroadenomas should have formal *visual field testing* and *pituitary function tests* to look for hypopituitarism.

Dual-energy X-ray absorptiometry scans should be done to assess the bone mineral density in patients with longstanding hyperprolactinaemia.

Treatment

Indications for treatment of hyperprolactinaemia include:
• existing or impending neurological symptoms due to local compression by a macroprolactinoma
• a desire for fertility
• the presence of symptoms: oligomenorrhoea/amenorrhoea, galactorrhoea, loss of libido
• bone density maintenance.

Dopamine agonists

Dopamine agonists reduce prolactin secretion and the size of prolactinomas. Prolactinomas (micro- and macroadenomas) are treated first line with dopamine (D_2) receptor agonists (cabergoline or bromocriptine) regardless of the size of the adenoma and the severity of the neurological sequelae.

Cabergoline

Cabergoline is a long-acting D_2 receptor agonist and is the initial choice of dopamine agonist. It is preferred to bromocriptine because it is:
• better tolerated (fewer and milder side-effects) for a similar drop in prolactin
• more effective in reducing prolactin levels (90% vs 59%)
• more effective in restoring ovulatory cycles (85% vs 52%).

Cabergoline can reduce the size of macroadenomas in 90% of patients. The initial dose in adults is 250 μg twice weekly. The dose may be increased by 250 μg twice weekly at 4-weekly intervals to a maximum of 4.5 mg weekly (usually 1.5 mg three times a week). However, prolactin levels are usually normalized with a dose of 250 μg twice weekly.

It has recently been reported that patients with Parkinson's disease treated with doses of cabergo-line much higher than that used in the treatment of hyperprolactinaemia (e.g. >20 mg per week) have an increased risk of valvular heart disease. It has therefore been recommended to use the lowest possible dose of cabergoline necessary to normalize prolactin levels.

If the prolactin level and pituitary size have been normal for 2 or more years, a trial of withdrawal should be attempted and prolactin should be monitored. If prolactin levels have normalized on dopamine agonist therapy but a small tumour remains on imaging, many endocrinologists still attempt weaning off drug treatment after a few years with monitoring of prolactin levels, since many patients will remain in remission.

In women, the menopause is often associated with a spontaneous resolution of prolactinomas. Moreover, at this stage in life, hypogonadism does not usually need to be treated. Most endocrinologists advocate treating until the age of 50 and then withdrawing cabergoline and monitoring prolactin levels. Re-initiation of treatment is reserved for the patients who undergo tumour expansion.

If a patient does not tolerate one dopamine agonist or fails to respond to it—in terms of prolactin levels and adenoma size—an alternative dopamine agonist should be tried.

Bromocriptine

Bromocriptine may be started at a dose of 1.25 mg once at night to minimize the side-effects, such as nausea, postural hypotension and depression. The bromocriptine dose can be increased by 1.25 mg per week (i.e. 1.25 mg twice a day after the first week). A dose of 5–7.5 mg of bromocriptine is usually needed to normalize prolactin levels and restore normal menstrual cycles.

For a woman who wishes to conceive, bromocriptine is used by most endocrinologists as first choice, as there is more extensive experience with bromocriptine (used since 1974) and greater certainty that it has no teratogenic effects. However, cabergoline (used since 1994) has not been shown to be unsafe in early pregnancy and is used by some endocrinologists.

Pregnancy

For the management of prolactinomas in pregnancy, see Chapter 31.

Treatment in those who cannot tolerate or do not respond to dopamine agonists

- In premenopausal women with microadenomas who wish to conceive, ovulation induction with clomiphene citrate or pulsatile GnRH therapy should be considered.
- In premenopausal women with microadenomas who do not wish to conceive, oestrogen and progesterone replacement therapy may be given to prevent osteoporosis.
- Trans-sphenoidal surgery is reserved for patients in whom dopamine agonists have failed to lower the serum prolactin level or size of the macroadenoma, and in whom symptoms or signs due to hyperprolactinaemia or adenoma size (e.g. visual field defect) persist during treatment.

Radiotherapy may be considered in patients with large macroadenomas following transsphenoidal surgery to prevent regrowth of the residual tumour.

Treatment of other causes of hyperprolactinaemia

Hyperprolactinaemia due to causes other than prolactinoma should be treated if it results in hypogonadism. In patients with hyperprolactinaemia and hypogonadism secondary to antipsychotic drugs, withdrawal of the antipsychotic drug may not be possible. These patients should receive gonadal steroid replacement (oestrogen–progesterone in women, testosterone in men). Antipsychotics such as quetiapine, which are relatively 'prolactin-sparing', should be considered.

Prognosis

In a prospective study of 200 patients treated with cabergoline for hyperprolactinaemia (105 with microadenomas, 70 with macroadenomas, 25 with idiopathic hyperprolactinaemia), dopamine agonist withdrawal was attempted when serum prolactin levels normalized and MRI showed no adenoma or a greater than 50% reduction with no cavernous sinus invasion and more than 5 mm distance from the optic chiasm. After 2–5 years of observation, hyperprolactinaemia recurred in 24%, 31% and 36% of patients with idiopathic hyperprolactinaemia, microadenomas and macroadenomas respectively. Adenoma regrowth was not seen in any patient. Hyperprolactinaemia was more likely to recur if an adenoma remnant was seen on MRI when treatment was stopped (78 vs 33% for macroadenomas, 42 vs 26% for microadenomas).

Giant adenomas (>3 cm) may behave more aggressively, as shown by case reports of rapid, significant regrowth within weeks of withdrawal of treatment.

Key points:

- Causes of hyperprolactinaemia include physiological (pregnancy, lactation), drugs (e.g. antipsychotics), pituitary tumours (prolactinomas or due to stalk compression), primary hypothyroidism, chronic renal failure and severe liver disease.
- Prolactinomas are the most common functioning pituitary tumour.
- Women present with galactorrhoea and oligomenorrhoea/amenorrhoea. Men present with reduced libido, impotence and infertility. Patients with macroadenomas may present with local mass affects (headache and visual field defects).
- Once physiological causes, drugs and metabolic causes have been excluded, a gadolinium-enhanced pituitary MRI should be performed.
- Prolactinomas are treated medically with dopamine agonists (cabergoline or bromocriptine).
- Indications for treatment include existing or impending neurological symptoms due to local compression by the prolactinoma, symptoms (oligomenorrhoea/amenorrhoea, galactorrhoea, loss of libido), a desire for fertility and bone density maintenance.

Chapter 15

Acromegaly

Acromegaly is a clinical condition caused by chronic excessive circulating levels of *growth hormone* (GH) in adults. Excessive GH secretion before epiphyseal fusion results in gigantism.

Epidemiology

The incidence of acromegaly is 5 per million per year, and the prevalence is 50 per million. Males and females are equally affected. Patients with acromegaly are mostly diagnosed at age 40–60 years. Pituitary gigantism is less common than acromegaly.

Aetiology

Around 99% of cases are caused by a GH-secreting pituitary adenoma. Macroadenomas (i.e. >1 cm) are more common than microadenomas. Prolactin is co-secreted by 30% of tumours.

An ectopic secretion of GH-releasing hormone from a carcinoid tumour (e.g. lung, pancreas) or hypothalamus is a much rarer cause. Ectopic secretion of GH (from a pancreatic islet cell tumour) is extremely rare. An activating mutation of the gene

Lecture Notes: Endocrinology and Diabetes. By A. Sam and K. Meeran. Published 2009 by Blackwell Publishing. ISBN 978-1-4051-5345-4.

encoding the alpha subunit of the stimulatory G protein, resulting in a constitutive activation of adenylyl cyclase, is seen in about 40% of GH-secreting pituitary adenomas.

Familial cases may be seen as part of multiple endocrine neoplasia type 1 (see Chapter 32) and Carney's complex (see Chapter 16).

Clinical presentations

Acromegaly is an insidious disease, and the average time from the onset of symptoms to diagnosis may be 5–10 years or longer. Acromegaly in older patients usually presents with a smaller tumour and lower GH levels. Patients may present with:
- symptoms and signs of acromegaly due to *excess GH* or *insulin-like growth factor-1* (IGF-1) secretion (summarized in Box 15.1)
- *local compression* of the optic apparatus resulting in visual field defects (often initially bitemporal superior quadrantanopia progressing to bitemporal hemianopia)
- *hypopituitarism* (symptoms of other anterior pituitary hormone deficiencies).

Pituitary gigantism is suspected when increased growth velocity is seen without manifestations of premature puberty. An arm span larger than standing height suggests an onset of disease before fusion of the epiphyses.

Box 15.1 Clinical presentations of acromegaly due to excess growth hormone/insulin-like growth factor-1

General
Increased sweating (>80%), headache, fatigue/lethargy

Face
Coarse features, frontal bossing, enlarged nose, deep nasolabial furrows, prognathism, increased interdental separation, macroglossia

Hands/feet
Enlarged (change in ring/shoe size; Fig. 15.1), carpal tunnel syndrome (40%)

Cutaneous
Oily skin, skin tags

Cardiovascular
Coronary artery disease probably related to an increased incidence of hypertension, impaired glucose tolerance (40%) and type 2 diabetes (20%), cardiac failure

Respiratory
Obstructive sleep apnoea

Gastrointestinal
Colonic polyps (9–39%)

Musculoskeletal
Osteoarthritis, arthralgia

Other
Goitre, deep voice, oligomenorrhoea/amenorrhoea, hypercalcaemia and hypercalciuria (growth hormone stimulates the renal 1α-hydroxylation of vitamin D)

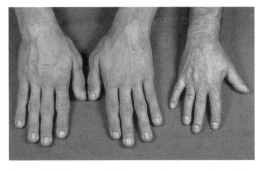

Figure 15.1 Acromegalic hands and a normal hand for comparison.

Investigations

Measurement of random GH has little value in the diagnosis of acromegaly. This is because GH secretion is pulsatile and the pulses are separated by long periods during which GH may be undetectable. In addition, GH secretion may be stimulated by a variety of factors such as short-term fasting, exercise, stress and sleep.

IGF-1 levels do not fluctuate widely throughout the day and are almost always raised in patients with acromegaly, except in severe intercurrent illness. A patient with a normal serum IGF-1 is unlikely to have acromegaly. However, IGF-1 levels may be decreased by malnutrition and liver disease (as the liver is the source of 75% of plasma IGF-1).

Like IGF-1, serum IGF-binding protein-3 (IGFBP-3) secretion is GH dependent, and IGFBP-3 levels are elevated in acromegaly. However, there is considerable overlap of IGBP-3 values between those with acromegaly and normal persons.

If serum IGF-1 concentration is high (or equivocal), serum GH should be measured after a 75 g *oral glucose tolerance test* (OGTT). In normal individuals, GH levels fall following oral glucose. Acromegaly is diagnosed when there is a failure of GH suppression to less than 1 µg/L. False-positive results may be seen in anorexia nervosa or malnutrition, adolescence, chronic liver and renal failure, diabetes mellitus and opiate addiction.

When acromegaly is biochemically confirmed, a *pituitary MRI* should be performed to determine the presence of a pituitary adenoma and whether there is suprasellar extension or invasion of the cavernous sinus by the tumour.

If the pituitary MRI is normal, a chest and abdominal computed tomography scan and serum GH-releasing hormone measurements may be performed to look for an extrapituitary cause. However, these are extremely rare.

Once diagnosis is established, patients should have:

• anterior pituitary function tests: prolactin, 9 a.m. cortisol, thyroid-stimulating hormone and free thyroxine, luteinizing hormone, follicle-stimulating hormone, testosterone (in men), oestradiol (in women)

- formal visual field perimetry
- tests to look for any complications: ECG, chest X-ray, echocardiography, sleep study (if obstructive sleep apnoea is suspected), fasting glucose, glycated haemoglobin, serum calcium and large-joint X-rays (if osteoarthritis is suspected).

Treatment

Overview

Patients with acromegaly should be referred to a centre with endocrinologists, dedicated pituitary neurosurgeons and radiotherapists experienced in treating this condition.

- *Trans-sphenoidal surgery* by an experienced neurosurgeon is the first-line treatment of choice for all microadenomas and macroadenomas that are fully resectable or are causing visual impairment.
- *Somatostatin analogues* may be given as primary therapy in those with macroadenomas that are not fully resectable and in patients who are unfit for general anaesthesia or are unwilling to have surgery. Somatostatin analogues are also used to treat patients whose disease remains active after surgery (see below).

- If somatostatin analogues alone are ineffective, other treatments such as *cabergoline* or *pegvisomant* (see below) may be used either alone or in combination.
- If, despite medical therapy, the pituitary adenoma continues to increase in size, *radiotherapy* or repeat surgery should be considered.

Somatostatin analogues

Somatostatin analogues (Table 15.1) such as *octreotide* and *lanreotide* bind to somatostatin receptors-2 and -5 on somatotrophs and inhibit GH secretion. They may lead to normal IGF-1 levels in up to 60% of patients. The long-term response may be predicted before starting treatment by measuring hourly GH levels for 6 hours after a subcutaneous injection of $100\,\mu g$ of octreotide.

Short-acting octreotide is useful in patients with 'acromegaly headache'. Side-effects include nausea, diarrhoea and gallstones.

Cabergoline

Cabergoline is a dopamine agonist and binds to D_2 receptors on somatotrophs. It may be particularly

Table 15.1 Somatostatin analogues

	Route	Initial dose and dose adjustment
Short-acting octreotide	Subcutaneous	$50\,\mu g$ three times a day Adjust the dose every 2 weeks based on levels of insulin-like growth factor-1 Maximum: $500\,\mu g$ three times a day
Long-acting octreotide Lar	Intramuscular	20 mg every 4 weeks Adjust at 3 months Maximum: 40 mg every 4 weeks
Lanreotide LA	Intramuscular	30 mg every 2 weeks Increase frequency according to response Maximum: 30 mg every 7 days
Lanreotide Autogel	Deep subcutaneous	60 mg every 4 weeks Adjust at 3 months Maximum: 120 mg every 4 weeks

helpful in patients with adenomas that co-secrete prolactin. Significant tumour shrinkage may occasionally be seen in these cases. Side-effects include nausea, constipation and mood changes, particularly irritability. Cabergoline may lead to normal IGF-1 in 20% of patients. Cabergoline is started at a dose of 250μg twice a week and may be increased as required to maximum 1.5mg three times weekly.

Pegvisomant

Pegvisomant binds to GH receptors and blocks receptor dimerization and activation. It may result in a normalization of IGF-1 in about 97% of patients. However, more data on the effect on tumour size are needed. Serum GH increases with pegvisomant, and only IGF-1 is used to monitor the response. Serious side-effects include hepatitis in about 1% of patients.

Radiotherapy

The number of patients treated with radiotherapy has declined as medical treatment is now mostly used for patients who are not cured by surgery. However, radiotherapy is an important treatment option for large and invasive tumours.

Two techniques are available: external beam radiation (usually given in several fractions over several weeks) or a single dose of highly focused sterotactic radiotherapy. Both techniques result in hypopituitarism. It may take about 4–6 years to achieve 'safe' GH levels following radiotherapy. Those who have had radiotherapy and are on medical treatment with somatostatin analogues should have a withdrawal period every year to assess disease activity.

'Safe' GH levels

It is difficult ever to say that a patient with acromegaly is 'cured'. The aim of treatment is to reduce the GH level to one that will no longer present the risks of acromegaly in terms of morbidity or mortality (a 'safe' GH level). The actual 'safe' level of GH is, however, controversial.

A normal serum IGF-1 concentration (for age and gender), a serum GH concentration less than 1μg/L after an OGTT and a mean GH of less than 1.9μg/L during a GH day curve (involving GH measurement at five points during the day) have been used as markers of remission.

Follow-up and monitoring

- Pituitary function tests and an OGTT are repeated about 4–6 weeks after pituitary surgery (see Chapter 12).
- Patients are monitored during treatment with clinical examination, serum IGF-1 levels and OGTTs. Some endocrinologists use GH day curves (see above). Medical treatment may then be titrated up or down accordingly.
- Pituitary function tests should be performed annually.
- Formal visual field assessment should be performed annually.
- The MRI should be repeated yearly for the first few years after initial treatment, and less often thereafter.
- *Colonoscopy* should be done every 3 years in patients over 50 years old and in those with more than three skin tags for the early detection and treatment of premalignant colonic polyps. Patients with polyps should have annual colonoscopy.

Prognosis

Life expectancy in untreated individuals is reduced by approximately 10 years. Mortality in untreated patients is twice that of the normal population. Cardiovascular disease is the major cause of mortality in these patients. The early remission rate following surgery is 80–90% for microadenomas and 40–50% for macroadenomas. Bony abnormalities generally do not regress, and joint symptoms persist after treatment.

Key points:

- Acromegaly is caused by chronic excessive circulating levels of GH in adults.
- Patients may present with symptoms and signs due to excess GH/IGF-1, local compression (e.g. visual field defects) or hypopituitarism.
- A patient with a normal serum IGF-1 is unlikely to have acromegaly.
- If the serum IGF-1 concentration is high or equivocal, an OGTT should be performed. Acromegaly is diagnosed when there is failure of suppression of GH following a glucose load.
- Patients who have a biochemical diagnosis of acromegaly should have formal visual field perimetry, anterior pituitary function tests and a pituitary MRI.
- Trans-sphenoidal surgery by an experienced neurosurgeon is the first-line treatment of choice for all microadenomas and macroadenomas that are fully resectable or are causing visual impairment.
- Somatostatin analogues may be given in those who are unfit for or unwilling to have surgery.
- Follow-up should include measurement of serum IGF-1, an OGTT or GH day curve, pituitary function tests, visual field assessment, pituitary MRI and colonoscopy (for the early detection of premalignant colonic polyps).

Chapter 16

Cushing's syndrome

Cushing's syndrome comprises a collection of signs and symptoms caused by a chronic inappropriate elevation of free circulating cortisol.

Aetiology

The most common cause of Cushing's syndrome is iatrogenic from excess exogenous glucocorticoids (oral, inhaled, topical, rectal, injected).

The aetiology of endogenous Cushing's syndrome can be divided into:

- adrenocorticotrophic hormone (ACTH) dependent (80%):
  — excess ACTH secreted from a pituitary adenoma, which is referred to as *Cushing's disease* (80%)
  — ACTH secreted from an ectopic source, mostly tumours arising from neuroendocrine cells, for example small-cell lung carcinomas, pulmonary, pancreas and thymic carcinoid tumours (20%)
- ACTH-independent (20%):
  — excess cortisol secreted from a benign adrenal adenoma (60%)
  — excess cortisol secreted from an adrenal carcinoma (40%).

Rarer causes of Cushing's syndrome include a corticotrophin-releasing hormone (CRH) secreting tumour and excess cortisol secretion by ACTH-independent macronodular or micronodular adrenal hyperplasia (Box 16.1).

Several disorders other than Cushing's syndrome (Box 16.2) can be associated with hypercortisolism and some of the clinical features of Cushing's syndrome ('pseudo-Cushing's syndrome'). The abnormal cortisol secretion presumably results from hypothalamic–pituitary–adrenal axis hyperactivity. In these conditions, hypercortisolism

---

Box 16.1 Causes of Cushing's syndrome

Excess exogenous glucocorticoids
ACTH-secreting pituitary adenoma
Ectopic ACTH-secreting tumours
Adrenal adenoma
Adrenal carcinoma

Rare causes
ACTH-independent micronodular adrenal hyperplasia
ACTH-independent macronodular adrenal hyperplasia
Ectopic corticotrophin-releasing hormone

Box 16.2 Physiological causes of hypercortisolism

Stress: physical or psychological
Depression or other psychiatric disorders
Chronic alcoholism
Severe obesity
Poorly controlled diabetes mellitus
Pregnancy

Lecture Notes: Endocrinology and Diabetes. By A. Sam and K. Meeran. Published 2009 by Blackwell Publishing. ISBN 978-1-4051-5345-4.

disappears after reversal of the underlying cause (e.g. abstinence with chronic alcoholism).

Epidemiology

Traditionally, the incidence of Cushing's syndrome was reported as 2–4 per million per year. However, Cushing's syndrome may be more common than previously thought. An unexpectedly high incidence of unrecognized Cushing's syndrome has been demonstrated in high-risk populations, for example 0.5–1% of hypertensive patients, 2–3% of patients with poorly controlled diabetes mellitus and 3–5% of obese, hypertensive patients with type 2 diabetes. Endogenous Cushing's syndrome is more common in females.

Clinical presentations

Many features of Cushing's syndrome, such as weight gain, fatigue, depression, hirsutism, acne and menstrual abnormalities, are also common in the general population, and the spectrum of clinical presentation is broad. Therefore confirmation of the diagnosis may be delayed until 1–2 years after the onset of the symptoms. A review of old photographs of the patient may be useful as those with Cushing's syndrome usually have progressive clinical features.

Some features of Cushing's syndrome that are common in the general population are more likely to be due to Cushing's syndrome if the onset is at a younger age. These include:
- type 2 diabetes mellitus
- hypertension
- osteoporosis
- thin skin.

Signs that are more discriminatory (although not unique to Cushing's syndrome) include:
- easy bruising
- proximal muscle weakness
- facial plethora
- reddish-purple striae on the abdomen, breast or thighs more than 1 cm wide (Fig. 16.1)
- weight gain with decreasing growth velocity in children.

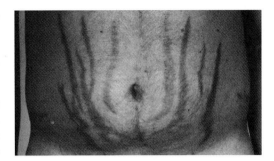

Figure 16.1 Abdominal striae in a patient with Cushing's syndrome.

Patients with pseudo-Cushing's syndrome seldom have easy bruising, thin skin or proximal muscle weakness.

Other features seen in Cushing's syndrome that may have other causes include:
- reduced concentration, impaired memory, psychosis
- reduced libido
- unusual infections
- poor skin healing
- pigmentation (in ACTH-dependent cases)
- hypokalaemia (usually in ACTH-dependent ectopic cases).

Investigations

A thorough history should be taken to exclude exogenous glucocorticoid use causing iatrogenic Cushing's syndrome before performing any biochemical tests.

Endogenous Cushing's syndrome is rare, and conditions such as obesity, depression, diabetes and hypertension are common. Thus the risk of false-positive results following biochemical tests is high. The rate of false-positive cases may be reduced if tests are performed only in patients with a *high pre-test probability* of having Cushing's syndrome, i.e. patients with:
- unusual features for their age (see above)
- multiple and progressive signs and symptoms, especially those which best discriminate Cushing's syndrome (see above)
- adrenal incidentalomas (2–20% prevalence of Cushing's syndrome)

- children with increasing weight and reducing height percentile.

Initial high-sensitivity tests

The following tests have a sensitivity of more than 90%, and any one of them may be used as the initial test depending on their suitability (some tests are preferred over others in certain situations; see the sections on pitfalls below).

24-Hour urinary free cortisol

Two or three 24-hour urinary free cortisol (UFC) measurements should be made. Urinary creatinine and volume should also be measured to ensure adequate urine collection over 24 hours.

Pitfalls

UFC measurement is not recommended in patients with renal failure as levels may be falsely low due to reduced glomerular filtration. A high fluid intake (≥5 L per day) may result in false-positive results.

Overnight dexamethasone and low-dose dexamethasone suppression tests

In the *overnight test*, 1 mg dexamethasone is taken at midnight. If the serum cortisol measured next morning between 8 and 9 a.m. is over 50 nmol/L (failure of suppression), the test is considered abnormal.

In the *low-dose dexamethasone suppression test* (LDDST), 0.5 mg is taken at intervals of exactly 6 hours for 48 hours (i.e. at 9 a.m., 3 p.m., 9 p.m. and 3 a.m.). If serum cortisol measured at 9 a.m. on day three (48 hours after the first dose of dexamethasone) is over 50 nmol/L (a failure of suppression), the test is considered abnormal.

Pitfalls

Assays used for serum cortisol in dexamethasone suppression tests measure total cortisol (free and bound to cortisol-binding protein). Oestrogens increase cortisol-binding protein levels and therefore increase total cortisol levels (but not free cortisol levels). They should be stopped for 6 weeks prior to the test as they may result in false-positive results.

Dexamethasone metabolism and clearance may be increased by some drugs (e.g. phenytoin, carbamazepine, rifampicin). Dexamethasone clearance is decreased in patients with renal or liver failure. Thus simultaneous measurement of cortisol and dexamethasone (if available) in these circumstances is helpful.

Late-night salivary cortisol measurements (if available)

In normal individuals, cortisol falls to very low levels at midnight. In Cushing's syndrome, there is a loss of normal circadian rhythm. Saliva is collected either into a plastic tube by passive drooling or by placing a cotton pledget (Salivette) in the mouth and chewing for 1–2 minutes. The sample should be collected at home (in a stress-free environment).

Pitfalls

Circadian rhythm may also be blunted in shift-workers. Cigarette smoking should be avoided prior to the collection of salivary cortisol as tobacco contains an inhibitor of 11β-hydroxysteroid dehydrogenase type 2, an enzyme that metabolizes cortisol.

In patients with normal test results, Cushing's syndrome is unlikely. However, if signs or symptoms progress, tests may be repeated in 6 months' time. If any one of the above tests is abnormal, another one or two of the above high-sensitivity tests should be performed.

As mentioned above, some conditions, such as depression, anxiety, obesity, alcoholism and poorly controlled diabetes, may be associated with hypercortisolism. These conditions may cause abnormal results on UFC measurement or the overnight dexamethasone suppression test. In these cases, the results should be treated with caution.

Hypokalaemia occurs more commonly in patients with ectopic ACTH secretion, but it may also be seen in up to 10% of patients with Cushing's disease. This is because these patients have higher levels of cortisol, which saturate the cortisol metabolizing enzyme 11β-hydroxysteroid dehydrogenase type 2. This results in excess cortisol acting as a mineralocorticoid in the kidney, causing potassium loss.

Determining the cause

Patients with positive results on the initial screening tests should have further tests to determine the cause of Cushing's syndrome.

Plasma ACTH

Samples should be cold-centrifuged immediately after venesection and flash-frozen before storage, as ACTH is degraded quickly and falsely low results may be measured.

- ACTH levels of less than 5 pg/mL are seen in patients with adrenal causes of Cushing's syndrome.
- ACTH levels of more than 15 pg/mL can be attributed to ACTH-dependent causes of Cushing's syndrome.
- Plasma levels of between 5 and 15 pg/mL should be repeated and interpreted with caution.

High-dose dexamethasone suppression test

The high-dose dexamethasone suppression test (HDDST) test was previously used to differentiate between excess ACTH secretion from a pituitary adenoma and from an ectopic source. The HDDST is based on the observation that hypercortisolaemia caused by pituitary ACTH-secreting tumours is more sensitive to suppression by dexamethasone than hypercortisolaemia caused by ectopic ACTH-secreting tumours.

The HDDST involves giving 2 mg of dexamethasone at 6-hourly intervals. Serum cortisol is measured before the first dexamethasone dose and 48 hours after the first dose. Cortisol is suppressed to less than 50% in about 80% of patients with Cushing's disease (i.e. a sensitivity of around 80%). The test has a specificity of about 80% (i.e. cortisol suppression is also seen in some patients with ectopic ACTH secretion).

The HDDST has now been largely abandoned in centres where inferior petrosal sinus sampling is available (see below).

Imaging

Pituitary magnetic resonance imaging (MRI) scans should be performed if the biochemical tests have indicated the presence of an ACTH-secreting corticotroph adenoma (Cushing's disease). Initial biochemical confirmation is important as pituitary incidentalomas may be seen in up to 10% of normal people, and 40% of corticotroph adenomas may be missed on MRI. Corticotroph adenomas may be seen as hypointense lesions on pituitary MRIs that do not enhance with gadolinium.

A low plasma ACTH concentration (<5 pg/mL or <1.1 pmol/L) should be followed by thin section computed tomography (CT) or MR imaging of the adrenal glands.

Those with a suspected ectopic source of ACTH should have further imaging (a radio-labelled octreotide scan and MR/CT imaging) to look for ectopic ACTH-secreting tumours. High-resolution chest CT may identify the most common sites of ectopic ACTH secretion, i.e. small cell lung cancer and bronchial carcinoid tumours. Radiolabelled octreotide scans are also used to detect carcinoid tumours as they express somatostatin receptors.

Inferior petrosal sinus sampling

This is the most reliable test for differentiating pituitary and non-pituitary sources of ACTH.

The inferior petrosal sinuses receive venous drainage from the cavernous sinus (which in turn receives blood from the pituitary gland) and drain into the sigmoid sinuses. Femoral catheters can be advanced bilaterally up to the internal jugular vein, sigmoid sinuses and finally into the inferior petrosal sinuses to collect 'central' blood. Blood is also collected from a peripheral vein.

Patients with Cushing's disease show a basal central-to-peripheral ACTH ratio of more than 2:1 or a central-to-peripheral ACTH gradient of over 3:1 after CRH administration.

Treatment

The treatment of Cushing's syndrome due to exogenous glucocorticoid therapy is to reduce the glucocorticoid dose and discontinue it if possible. This should be done gradually as most patients will have developed hypothalamic–pituitary–adrenal suppression and insufficiency following chronic glucocorticoid treatment.

ACTH-secreting pituitary adenomas (Cushing's disease)

The treatment of choice for Cushing's disease is *trans-sphenoidal surgery* by an experienced neurosurgeon.
• If a clearly circumscribed microadenoma is identified by the neurosurgeon, trans-sphenoidal microadenectomy is the treatment of choice.
• If no clearly circumscribed microadenoma is identified and future fertility is not an issue, subtotal (85–90%) anterior pituitary resection may be performed.
• If no clearly circumscribed microadenoma is identified by the neurosurgeon and future fertility is an important concern, radiotherapy may be used.

Patients with post trans-sphenoidal surgery cortisol levels of less than 50 nmol/L are more likely to have prolonged remission. Patients with evidence of remission (cortisol <50 nmol/L) following surgery should have hydrocortisone replacement. This is because prolonged exposure to high cortisol levels in these patients has resulted in suppression of the hypothalamic–pituitary–adrenal axis.

Medical treatment with *adrenal enzyme inhibitors* (ketoconazole, metyrapone) may be given before surgery to control hypercortisolism and stabilize the patient. The dose is titrated to achieve a mean serum cortisol of 150–300 nmol/L.

Metyrapone inhibits 11β-hydroxylase and blocks the final step in cortisol biosynthesis. It can exacerbate hirsutism due to increased adrenal androgen production. Hypertension can also occur as a result of increased production of deoxycorticosterone (see the steroid synthesis pathway in Chapter 5). Metyrapone may be started at a dose of 250 mg twice a day and may be increased every 3 days up to 1 g four times a day.

Ketoconazole inhibits the first step in cortisol biosynthesis (side chain cleavage) and to a lesser extent the conversion of 11-deoxycortisol to cortisol. It also inhibits ACTH secretion by impairing corticotroph adenylate cyclase activation. Ketoconazole may be started at a dose of 200 mg twice a day and is increased at 2–3-weekly intervals. Doses higher than 400 mg three times a day are seldom effective.

Liver function tests should be monitored weekly initially as ketoconazole can cause hepatitis. Other side-effects of ketoconazole include headache, sedation, nausea, vomiting, gynaecomastia, impotence and decreased libido (due to inhibition of testosterone production).

Hypertension and diabetes mellitus should be treated as normal. Patients with marked bone loss should receive oral bisphosphonate therapy, calcium and vitamin D supplementation.

Radiotherapy may be used in those who are not cured and have persistent hypercortisolaemia after trans-sphenoidal resection of the tumour. Pituitary irradiation is as likely to cure children as is surgery and may therefore be considered as the initial therapy. Stereotactic radiotherapy provides less irradiation to the surrounding tissues (see Chapter 12).

Pituitary irradiation using a linear accelerator may correct hypercortisolism in about 45% of adults and 85% of children. The maximal benefits do not occur for at least 9–12 months and occasionally as long as 2 years in adults. Children usually respond within 3 months. During this time, adrenal enzyme inhibitors should be used to control the hypercortisolism.

The major side-effect of radiotherapy is *progressive hypopituitarism*. Nearly all patients will have growth hormone deficiency 10 years post radiotherapy, and luteinizing hormone/follicle-stimulating hormone deficiency may be seen in up to 15%.

In refractory cases where surgery and radiotherapy fail to normalize cortisol secretion, surgical bilateral total adrenalectomy or medical adrenalectomy with mitotane with lifelong glucocorticoid and mineralocorticoid replacement is the final definitive cure. Monitoring of mitotane levels and dose adjustment is frequently advocated.

In patients who cannot be treated with adrenalectomy, adrenal enzyme inhibitors may be used long term to ameliorate the hypercortisolism.

Bilateral adrenalectomy may rarely be complicated by development of *Nelson's syndrome*. This was originally characterized by a locally aggressive pituitary tumour causing skin pigmentation due to excessive ACTH secretion. With the advent of pituitary imaging with CT/MR, corticotroph tumour progression can be detected very early and therefore Nelson's syndrome is rarely seen. The corticotroph adenoma may require surgery and radiotherapy. Pituitary radiotherapy at the time of adrenalectomy is effective in preventing Nelson's syndrome.

Ectopic ACTH-secreting tumours

In patients with ACTH-secreting ectopic tumours, complete excision often results in remission.

However, in patients who are not cured after surgical resection of the tumour, adrenal enzyme inhibitors may be used to control hypercortisolism.

Adrenal tumours

In patients with an isolated cortisol-secreting adenoma, unilateral adrenalectomy has a good prognosis. In patients with adrenocortical carcinoma, mitotane is used as adjuvant therapy following surgery. Adrenal enzyme inhibitors may be used when surgery is contraindicated or if the tumour is metastatic or occult.

Prognosis

In the past, Cushing's disease had a 5-year survival rate of 50% when not treated. However, with modern treatments, the standard mortality ratio following normalization of cortisol is similar to that of an age-matched population. In patients with persistent hypercortisolism after treatment, the standard mortality ratio may be increased to 4–5 times that of the general population. Most deaths are due to cardiovascular, thromboembolic

or hypertensive complications, or bacterial/fungal infections.

The initial remission rate with an experienced neurosurgeon is about 70–80%. However, permanent cure rate is about 60–70% due to late recurrence.

The symptoms and signs of patients with Cushing's syndrome gradually resolve in the year following surgery. Impaired glucose tolerance, hypertension and osteoporosis improve but may not disappear. Impaired health-related quality of life resolves partially but not completely after trans-sphenoidal surgery. It may remain below that of age- and gender-matched subjects for up to 15 years. Depression usually persists for many years following successful treatment.

In children, bone density and growth rate both increase after treatment, but neither returns to normal.

Patients with ectopic ACTH secretion or an adrenocortical carcinoma may have a poor prognosis associated with the underlying tumour. The prognosis for adrenocortical carcinomas is poor. They almost invariably recur and usually do not respond to irradiation or chemotherapy.

Follow-up and monitoring

The follow-up of patients after pituitary surgery is discussed in Chapter 12.

Patients should be followed up clinically for recurrence of features of Cushing's syndrome, and dexamethasone suppression tests should be performed when recurrence is clinically suspected. In patients in whom remission is achieved with surgery and who are taking hydrocortisone replacement, an insulin tolerance test should be done 1–2 years after surgery to look for the recovery of normal corticotroph function.

Rare causes of ACTH-independent Cushing's syndrome

Micronodular adrenal hyperplasia

Micronodular adrenal hyperplasia, also known as primary pigmented nodular adrenocortical disease

(PPNAD), is characterized by multiple small pigmented, autonomously functioning adrenocortical nodules. It may be sporadic or familial (isolated or as part of Carney's complex).

Carney's complex is an autosomal dominantly inherited syndrome characterized by spotty skin pigmentation (café-au-lait spots), endocrine tumours (most commonly PPNAD) and non-endocrine tumours (such as myxomas of the skin, heart, breast and other sites). Three responsible genes have so far been identified: *PRKAR1A*, *PDE11A* and *MYH8*.

Macronodular adrenal hyperplasia

Macronodular adrenal hyperplasia is characterized by adrenal glands that contain multiple non-pigmented nodules larger than 5 mm in diameter. An ectopic adrenal expression of some G-protein-coupled receptors (gastric inhibitory polypeptide, beta-adrenergic, luteinizing hormone/human chorionic gonadotrophin, serotonin receptors) or an increased expression/activity of some eutopic receptors (e.g. V_1 vasopressin receptors) may mediate the increase in cortisol secretion.

These patients have increased serum and urinary cortisol, and undetectable plasma ACTH in the basal state and after administration of CRH. Cortisol production is suppressed minimally, if at all, by high-dose dexamethasone.

Cushing's syndrome associated with McCune–Albright syndrome is a rare variant of ACTH-independent macronodular adrenal hyperplasia. McCune–Albright syndrome is a sporadic disease caused by activating mutations of the gene coding for the alpha subunit of stimulatory G protein, which results in constitutive activation of the cyclic AMP pathway in the nodules and excess cortisol secretion. McCune–Albright syndrome is characterized by café-au-lait spots, polyostotic fibrous dysplasia, precocious puberty and other endocrine disorders.

Surgical bilateral adrenalectomy is used in patients with micronodular adrenal hyperplasia and most patients with macronodular adrenal hyperplasia.

Key points:

- Cushing's syndrome comprises a collection of signs and symptoms caused by a chronic inappropriate elevation of free circulating cortisol.
- Cushing's syndrome may be caused by excess exogenous glucocorticoids, an ACTH-secreting pituitary adenoma, an ectopic ACTH-secreting tumour, an adrenal adenoma or an adrenal carcinoma.
- Biochemical tests should only be performed in patients with a high pre-test probability of having Cushing's syndrome (e.g. patients with unusual features for their age or multiple and progressive features that best discriminate Cushing's syndrome).
- Initial high-sensitivity tests for Cushing's syndrome include 24-hour UFC measurements, an overnight dexamethasone suppression test, low-dose dexamethasone suppression test and a late-night salivary cortisol measurement (if available).
- Investigations to determine the underlying cause of Cushing's syndrome include plasma ACTH, pituitary or adrenal imaging (depending on the plasma ACTH result) and inferior petrosal sinus sampling.
- The treatment of choice for Cushing's disease is trans-sphenoidal surgery by an experienced neurosurgeon.
- The treatment of Cushing's syndrome due to an adrenal adenoma is unilateral adrenalectomy.

Chapter 17

Diabetes insipidus

Diabetes insipidus (DI) is characterized by hypotonic polyuria (i.e. urine output of more than 3 L per day with osmolality <300 mosmol/kg).

DI is classified into:
- *central DI*: due to a deficiency of the posterior pituitary hormone antidiuretic hormone (ADH) which is also known as arginine vasopressin (AVP)
- *nephrogenic DI*: due to renal resistance to ADH
- *dipsogenic DI* (more commonly known as *primary polydipsia*): due to excessive drinking.

Epidemiology

DI is a rare condition. Males and female are affected equally, and most cases present in adults. However, familial cases mostly present in childhood. The prevalence of central DI is about 4 per 100 000. The prevalence of nephrogenic DI and primary polydipsia is not clear.

Aetiology

Central DI

Causes of central DI include:
- Idiopathic: 33% of cases (possibly due to autoimmune injury to the ADH-secreting neurones)
- head trauma/neurosurgery

Lecture Notes: Endocrinology and Diabetes. By A. Sam and K. Meeran. Published 2009 by Blackwell Publishing. ISBN 978-1-4051-5345-4.

- pituitary tumours (primary or metastases)
- granulomatous diseases (e.g. sarcoidosis, histiocytosis X).

Less common causes include vascular, for example Sheehan's syndrome (see Chapter 12), central nervous system infections, hypoxic encephalopathy (cardiopulmonary arrest or shock), the mutations of genes involved in ADH production and DIDMOAD (Wolfram's syndrome, characterized by DI, diabetes mellitus, optic atrophy and deafness).

Wolfram's syndrome is inherited as an autosomal recessive trait with incomplete penetrance. It is caused by at least two different genes: *WFS1* and *ZCD2*. Wolframin, the product of *WFS1*, is a transmembrane protein expressed in pancreatic beta cells and neurones.

Nephrogenic DI

Nephrogenic DI is due to resistance to the action of ADH and may be secondary to:
- X-linked mutations in the gene encoding the ADH receptor V_2, or autosomal dominant mutations in the gene encoding aquaporin-2 (ADH-sensitive water channel)
- persistent hypercalcaemia (>2.75 mmol/L)
- severe hypokalaemia (<3.0 mmol/L)
- drugs: lithium (may cause irreversible DI), demeclocycline, antifungals and antineoplastic agents.

Gestational DI is an unusual condition due to increased placental vasopressinase activity and degradation of vasopressin. Gestational DI resolves after delivery.

Primary polydipsia

Primary polydipsia is due to excess fluid intake resulting in an inhibition of ADH release. These patients often have a history of a psychiatric condition. Thirst may be affected by the psychiatric condition or the drugs used in the treatment.

Diagnosis

Initial tests

A urine volume of over 3 L per day with a urinary osmolality of 300 mosmol/kg or less is suggestive of DI. DI can be diagnosed if plasma osmolality is more than 295 mosmol/kg, plasma sodium is more than 145 mmol/L and urine osmolality is less than 300 mosmol/kg. In equivocal cases, a water deprivation test should be done (see below).

Serum *sodium* is usually normal or only slightly elevated in DI as long as water is available. Serum sodium is usually low in primary polydipsia because of water overload.

In all patients presenting with polyuria, *glucose*-induced osmotic diuresis due to uncontrolled diabetes mellitus should be excluded first.

Serum *potassium* and *calcium* should be measured to exclude nephrogenic DI caused by hypercalcaemia or hypokalaemia.

Water deprivation test

Water deprivation tests may be used to differentiate between cranial DI, nephrogenic DI and primary polydipsia. In the first stage of the test, no fluid is allowed for 8 hours (e.g. between 8.30 a.m. and 4.30 p.m.). Plasma and urine osmolality are checked at intervals. It is essential to weigh the patient hourly; the test must be terminated if there is more than 3% weight loss (the test then being considered positive).

In the second stage of the test (i.e. after 8 hours), desmopressin is given (20 µg intranasally or 2 µg intramuscularly) to patients who have not concentrated their urine adequately (i.e. to more than

750 mosmol/kg), and hourly urine volumes and osmolality are measured for 4 hours. Patients may drink freely during the second stage.

Plasma samples should also be collected at baseline and after 8 hours (i.e. prior to the administration of desmopressin) for measurement of ADH if necessary (i.e. in cases where the history and water deprivation test provide equivocal results).

Interfering medication such as diuretics should be stopped before the test. Cortisol and thyroxine deficiencies should be corrected before the test as their deficiency impairs water excretion.

Interpretation

In normal individuals, water deprivation stimulates ADH release. Urine is therefore concentrated to greater than 750 mosmol/kg, and plasma osmolality remains below 300 mosmol/kg.

In patients with central/nephrogenic DI, reduced ADH release/action inhibits urine concentration (urine osmolality remains less than 300 mosmol/kg), and plasma osmolality may rise above 300 mosmol/kg.

After desmopressin administration, patients with cranial DI (a deficiency of ADH) can concentrate their urine (osmolality >750 mosmol/kg). However, those with nephrogenic DI (resistance to the action of ADH) cannot concentrate their urine.

In patients with primary polydipsia, urine is concentrated to a lesser degree than in healthy individuals (between 300 and 750 mosmol/kg). This is because chronic polyuria washes out the medullary interstitial solutes (and the osmotic gradient) and impairs the urine-concentrating ability. In addition, chronic overhydration in primary polydipsia causes a suppression of ADH release. In these patients, plasma osmolality may initially be low but rises to normal with water deprivation.

There is, however, a potential error with the water deprivation test. Patients with primary polydipsia may have a water deprivation test result similar to those with partial central DI. Patients with partial central DI are hyper-responsive to a submaximal rise in ADH following the water deprivation test (possibly due to receptor upregulation) and may concentrate their urine to some extent.

The history may provide important clues: for example, a gradual onset and a history of psychiatric illness favour primary polydipsia. A therapeutic trial of desmopressin with careful in-hospital monitoring of fluid balance and plasma sodium may occasionally be used to differentiate between primary polydipsia and partial central DI. In patients with partial central DI, an improvement in polydipsia and polyuria may be seen. In patients with primary polydipsia, polyuria is decreased but polydipsia persists. These patients may develop acute hyponatraemia (hence the need for close monitoring). In patients with nephrogenic DI, no effect is seen.

In patients with cranial DI diagnosed on water deprivation testing, the hypothalamic–pituitary anatomy should be assessed with a *magnetic resonance imaging* (MRI) scan.

Treatment

Central DI

Desmopressin is a synthetic modification of ADH or AVP with prolonged antidiuretic effects and no vasopressive activity.

- *Intranasal administration.* An initial dose of 5 µg is usually given at bedtime to control nocturia. The dose can be titrated up according to night-time and daytime symptoms to a maintenance dose of about 10–20 µg once or twice daily. Some endocrinologists recommend starting with the intranasal preparation to ensure that the patient understands what a good antidiuretic response is. The therapy can then be changed to tablets.
- *Oral administration.* Only about 5% is absorbed from the gut. The initial dose is 100 µg at bedtime and can then be titrated up to 100–400 µg three times a day according to symptoms. The absorption of desmopressin may be decreased by up to 50% when taken with meals.
- *Subcutaneous administration* is occasionally used. The usual dose is 1 µg twice a day.

Desmopressin is safe during pregnancy for both mother and fetus.

Plasma sodium and osmolality and clinical response should be monitored, and the desmopressin dose should be modified if necessary to ensure that patients are not becoming hyponatraemic (due to water intoxication). Physicians should be aware of interactions of desmopressin with other drugs (e.g. carbamazepine, indapamide) that may increase its action.

Nephrogenic DI

The underlying cause (e.g. hypokalaemia or hypercalcaemia) should be treated if possible and the causative drug stopped. Treatment includes a low-sodium diet, thiazides and non-steroidal anti-inflammatory drugs (NSAIDs). Thiazides act by inducing mild volume depletion, resulting in increased proximal tubular sodium and water reabsorption. This leads to decreased water delivery to the collecting tubules (where ADH normally acts) and reduces urine output.

NSAIDs inhibit renal prostaglandin synthesis and augment ADH action. In patients who cannot be treated with NSAIDs or who have persistent symptomatic polyuria after the addition of NSAIDs, a trial of desmopressin may be given.

Primary polydipsia

The underlying psychiatric disorder should be treated.

Key points:

- DI is characterized by hypotonic polyuria (a urine output of >3 L per day with osmolality <300 mosmol/kg).
- DI may be central (due to deficiency of ADH produced in the posterior pituitary), nephrogenic (due to renal resistance to the action of ADH) or dipsogenic, also known as primary polydipsia (due to excessive drinking).
- In all patients presenting with polyuria, glucose-induced osmotic diuresis should be excluded first.
- A water deprivation test is used to differentiate between cranial DI, nephrogenic DI and primary polydipsia.
- In patients with central DI, the hypothalamic–pituitary anatomy should be assessed with an MRI scan.
- Patients with central DI are treated with desmopressin. Plasma sodium and osmolality and clinical response should be monitored.

Chapter 18

Hyponatraemia and syndrome of inappropriate ADH secretion

Hyponatraemia is commonly defined as a serum sodium concentration of less than 135 mmol/L.

Epidemiology

Hyponatraemia is the most common electrolyte disorder in hospitalized patients. Mild hyponatraemia is seen in 15–20% of hospitalized patients.

Aetiology

Causes of hyponatraemia are summarized in Box 18.1. Hyponatraemia may be associated with low, normal or high plasma osmolality. The majority of causes of hyponatraemia are associated with low plasma osmolality and increased antidiuretic hormone (ADH) levels (see below). Assessing the volume status of the patient is essential in determining the aetiology of hyponatraemia. The possibility of artifactually low sodium concerntration in blood taken proximal to an intravenous infusion should always be excluded.

Hyponatraemia with low plasma osmolality

Most cases of hyponatraemia are caused by an increase in extracellular water relative to extracellular sodium. This is usually due to an impairment of renal water excretion capacity and water retention caused by increased plasma ADH levels.

Increased plasma ADH levels in hypovolaemic patients

Increased secretion of ADH in patients with volume depletion (e.g. secondary to urinary, gastrointestinal or third-space fluid losses) is mediated by the carotid sinus baroreceptors, which sense the reduced pressure.

Thiazide diuretics are the most common cause of hyponatraemia in adults. Patients with hyponatraemia caused by thiazides may be either hypovolaemic or euvolaemic, depending on the magnitude of the sodium loss and water retention. Hyponatraemia is less common with loop diuretics, as the inhibition of sodium chloride transport in the loop of Henle prevents the generation of the countercurrent gradient and limits the ability of ADH to cause water retention.

Cerebral salt wasting is a rare syndrome described in patients with cerebral disease, particularly subarachnoid haemorrhage. Salt wasting is the primary defect and is possibly due to the release of brain natriuretic peptide and/or reduced central sympathetic activity. The ensuing volume depletion causes a rise in ADH release.

Lecture Notes: Endocrinology and Diabetes. By A. Sam and K. Meeran. Published 2009 by Blackwell Publishing. ISBN 978-1-4051-5345-4.

Box 18.1 Causes of hyponatraemia

Hyponatraemia with low plasma osmolality

Increased plasma ADH in hypovolaemic patients
Renal fluid and sodium loss: thiazide diuretics, salt-losing nephropathy, cerebral salt wasting
Extrarenal fluid and sodium loss: diarrhoea, vomiting, third-space losses (burns, pancreatitis, bowel obstruction)

Increased plasma ADH in euvolaemic patients
Adrenal insufficiency
Hypothyroidism
Syndrome of inappropriate ADH secretion
Pregnancy

Increased plasma ADH in hypervolaemic patients
Cardiac failure
Cirrhosis
Nephrotic syndrome

Excessive water intake
Primary polydipsia
Ecstasy
Marathon runners (excessive water intake combined with sodium loss due to sweating)

Decreased solute intake
Beer drinkers

Hyponatraemia with normal plasma osmolality
Pseudohyponatraemia
Hyperlipidaemia
Paraproteinaemia

Renal failure
Sodium-free isosmotic irrigant solutions (used in laparoscopy, hysteroscopy and transurethral resection of the prostate)

Hyponatraemia with high plasma osmolality
Hyperglycaemia
Rarer causes: administration and retention of mannitol or maltose (e.g. intravenous immunoglobulin in 10% maltose)

Box 18.2 Causes of syndrome of inappropriate antidiuretic hormone secretion

Central nervous system pathology
Vascular (infarction, haemorrhage, cerebral venous thrombosis), infection (meningitis, encephalitis), inflammatory conditions (e.g. systemic lupus erythematosus, demyelination), trauma, tumours

Pulmonary pathology
Infection (pneumonias, abscess, tuberculosis, aspergillosis), bronchiectasis, carcinoma, mesothelioma, mechanical ventilation

Malignancy
Small cell lung carcinomas, mesothelioma, oropharynx, stomach, duodenum, pancreas, ovaries, bladder, prostate, endometrium, thymoma, lymphoma, sarcoma, olfactory neuroblastoma

Drugs
Selective serotonin reuptake inhibitors, tricyclic antidepressants, antipsychotics, clofibrate, carbamazepine, nicotine, opiates, vincristine, cyclophosphamide, desmopressin

Miscellaneous
Acute intermittent porphyria, postoperative state, pain, severe nausea, AIDS

Idiopathic

Increased plasma ADH levels in hypervolaemic patients

The increased secretion of ADH in patients with cardiac failure and cirrhosis is mediated by the carotid sinus baroreceptors, which sense the reduced pressure due to reduced cardiac output and peripheral vasodilatation respectively in these conditions.

Increased plasma ADH levels in euvolaemic patients

• *Hypothyroidism*: increased plasma ADH levels may be caused by reduced cardiac output and activation of the carotid sinus baroreceptors.
• *Adrenal insufficiency*: increased plasma ADH levels may be caused by reduced systemic blood pressure and cardiac output (due to a lack of cortisol), by hypovolaemia (due to aldosterone deficiency) or from removal of the inhibitory effect of cortisol on corticotrophin-releasing hormone and ADH.
• *Syndrome of inappropriate ADH secretion (SIADH)*: this may be due to central nervous system pathology, pulmonary pathology, malignancy (ADH secreted by the tumour), drugs or a number of other causes (Box 18.2). Increased ADH results in

reduced water excretion. The elevated level of fluid is detected by the renal juxtaglomerular cells and causes a reduction in renin and aldosterone levels. This results in increased sodium excretion, which prevents fluid overload but perpetuates hyponatraemia.

Cases of 'nephrogenic syndrome of inappropriate antidiuresis' due to activating mutations of the V_2 receptor in the renal collecting ducts have been reported.

Excessive water intake

Excessive water intake (more than 10L per day) may occasionally be seen in psychiatric patients with polydipsia, following ecstasy (MDMA) or in marathon runners. If the excessive water intake exceeds the water excretion capacity of the kidneys, water retention and hyponatraemia ensue.

Decreased intake of solutes

A decreased intake of solutes in beer drinkers or other malnourished patients may also result in hyponatraemia. Beer contains little or no sodium, potassium or protein. The fall in daily solute excretion results in a reduction in water excretory capacity.

Hyponatraemia with normal plasma osmolality

In patients with marked hyperlipidaemia (e.g. uncontrolled diabetes) or hyperproteinaemia (e.g. multiple myeloma), the aqueous fraction of the plasma volume is reduced. This results in a decrease in the sodium concentration if it is measured in the total plasma volume using flame photometry. However, this is a measurement artefact since the sodium concentration in the aqueous fraction of plasma is unchanged ('*pseudohyponatraemia*'). This artefact may be avoided with the use of ion-selective electrodes that directly measure the sodium concentration in the aqueous fraction of the plasma.

In *renal failure*, water retention can lead to hyponatraemia with normal plasma osmolality, as the decrease in osmolality due to low sodium is offset by the increased urea. (Remember that osmolality = $2 \times [Na^+ + K^+]$ + urea + glucose.) Although plasma osmolality is normal, plasma tonicity (the contribution to osmolality by effective osmoles) is low since urea is an ineffective osmole (i.e. it can freely cross cell membranes and does not induce water movement out of the cell).

Hyponatraemia with normal serum osmolality may occasionally be seen in patients who have received and absorbed large volumes of isosmotic, sodium-free irrigant solutions (containing glycine or sorbitol) during laparoscopic surgery or transurethral prostatectomy.

Hyponatraemia with high plasma osmolality

Hyponatraemia with high plasma osmolality may be seen in patients with *hyperglycaemia*. The rise in plasma glucose pulls water out of the cells and results in a reduction in plasma sodium concentration by dilution ('translocational' hyponatraemia). An increase of 2.3mmol/L in blood glucose decreases serum sodium concentration by about 1.0mmol/L.

Hyponatraemia with increased plasma osmolality may also occur with the administration and subsequent retention of hypertonic mannitol or with maltose (e.g. when intravenous immune globulin is given in a 10% maltose solution).

Clinical presentations

Most patients with a serum sodium concentration of more than 125mmol/L are asymptomatic.

The clinical manifestations of hypotonic hyponatraemia (Box 18.3) are more prominent when the

---

Box 18.3 Clinical presentations of hyponatraemia

Headache
Anorexia, nausea, vomiting
Lethargy
Muscle cramps
Depressed reflexes
Confusion, restlessness, disorientation
Seizures
Coma, death

decrease in the serum sodium concentration is large or has occurred rapidly within a period of hours.

Hypotonic hyponatraemia causes entry of water into the brain, resulting in cerebral oedema and intracranial hypertension. A process of adaptation starts within a few hours as solutes leave the brain tissues, resulting in a reduction of brain swelling.

Hypovolaemic patients may have tachycardia, postural hypotension, dry mucous membranes and reduced tissue turgor. Hypervolaemic patients have may have a raised jugular venous pressure and peripheral oedema.

In addition, patients may have features of the underlying cause, for example clubbing and cachexia in malignancy (causing SIADH) or increased pigmentation in Addison's disease. Patients must be thoroughly examined for features of malignancy (including breast examination).

The correction in sodium concentration must not exceed 10 mmol/L in the first 24 hours and 18 mmol/L in the first 48 hours. Rapid correction of hyponatraemia must be avoided as it can result in shrinkage of the brain, which triggers demyelination of the pontine and extrapontine neurones. This 'osmotic demyelination' is known as *cerebral pontine myelinolysis*. Patients can present one to several days after aggressive treatment of hyponatraemia with quadriplegia, pseudobulbar palsy, seizures, coma and death. The risk of this complication is higher in patients with alcoholism, malnutrition, liver failure and potassium depletion.

Investigations

Serum lipids and protein should be measured to rule out pseudohyponatraemia. Blood glucose must be measured as hyperglycaemia causes translocational hyponatraemia (see above).

Hypothyroidism and adrenal insufficiency must be excluded by measuring thyroid-stimulating hormone, free thyroxine and 9 a.m. cortisol. If 9 a.m. cortisol is less than 550 nmol/L a short Synacthen test must be done.

Hypovolaemic patients with a renal cause of fluid and sodium loss (e.g. thiazide diuretics) have a high spot urinary sodium (>20 mmol/L), whereas those with an extrarenal cause of fluid and sodium loss (e.g. diarrhoea or vomiting) have a low spot urinary sodium (<20 mmol/L).

SIADH should be considered in euvolaemic patients (who have been off diuretics for 2 weeks) in whom hypothyroidism and adrenal insufficiency has been excluded. The key tests are *paired plasma osmolality and urine osmolality* and *sodium concentration*. Patients with SIADH have low plasma osmolality, and high urine osmolality (>100 mosmol/kg) and sodium levels (>20 mmol/L).

It is important to remember that SIADH is not a diagnosis. Once it has been confirmed, the underlying cause must be diagnosed. Patients should be investigated by brain imaging (computed tomography [CT] scan with contrast, or magnetic resonance imaging) and chest CT. Patients with normal brain and lung imaging should have further imaging to look for malignancy elsewhere (e.g. with CT of the abdomen/pelvis).

Treatment

The treatment of hyponatraemia should include correction of the underlying cause, such as stopping the causative drug or the administration of hydrocortisone and mineralocorticoids to patients with adrenal insufficiency and thyroxine to hypothyroid patients.

Hypovolaemic patients

Hypovolaemic patients must be rehydrated with isotonic (0.9%) saline. The administration of isotonic saline to patients with volume depletion removes the hypovolaemic stimulus to ADH release and allows excretion of the excess water.

Hypervolaemic patients

Hypervolaemic patients (e.g. those with cardiac failure or cirrhosis) are treated with fluid restriction. Their drugs should be reviewed.

Euvolaemic patients with SIADH

Mild-to-moderate hyponatraemia

Patients with chronic mild-to-moderate hyponatraemia (a serum sodium concentration of 120–

130 mmol/L) are usually asymptomatic. However, recent observations suggest that some of these 'asymptomatic' patients have subtle neurological manifestations (e.g. reduced mental functioning, unsteadiness and falls in elderly patients) that may be improved by raising the serum sodium. They are often treated with fluid restriction (up to 1 L per day). It is important to note that the administration of normal saline may worsen hyponatraemia in SIADH. This is because the administered sodium is excreted in the urine, while some of the water is retained.

If hyponatraemia continues, an increased dietary intake of salt should be encouraged. Patients who do not tolerate fluid restriction may occasionally receive demeclocycline (300–600 mg twice a day). Demeclocycline reduces the responsiveness of the collecting tubule cells to ADH and therefore increases water excretion. It may take 1–2 weeks to see its effect. Renal function should be monitored, since nephrotoxicity can occur with this drug.

Severe hyponatraemia

Patients with severe hyponatraemia (<115 mmol/L) presenting with seizures and a reduced conscious level require hypertonic 3% saline (513 mmol/L) solution. The increase in plasma sodium concentration following hypertonic saline is due to the water loss induced by excretion of the extra sodium. Hypertonic saline must be given with extreme caution as rapid correction can result in central pontine myelinolysis (see above).

The change in sodium concentration must not exceed 10 mmol/L in the first 24 hours, and 18 mmol/L in the first 48 hours. Serum sodium concentration should be increased by 1–2 mmol/L per hour in the first 3 hours. The rate of correction may then be slowed to 0.5 mmol/L per hour. Plasma sodium should be monitored regularly (initially every 2–4 hours).

A loop diuretic (e.g. furosemide 20 mg intravenously) may be beneficial as it inhibits sodium chloride reabsorption in the thick ascending limb of the loop of Henle and interferes with the countercurrent concentrating mechanism.

Calculating the rate of hypertonic saline infusion

If you give (hypothetically) 1 L of 3% saline to a patient, the serum sodium will increase by approximately:

$$(\text{fluid }[Na^+] - \text{serum }[Na^+])/[\text{total body water} + 1]$$

(where '1' denotes the 1 L that has been infused).

Total body water is estimated as lean body weight $\times$ 0.6 for men, and body weight $\times$ 0.5 for women. So, for example, in an 80 kg woman with a serum sodium concentration of 103 mmol/L, 1 L of 3% saline increases the serum sodium concentration by 10 mmol/L: $(513 - 103)/[(0.5 \times 80) + 1]$. Therefore an infusion of 100 mL of 3% saline per hour will increase her serum sodium concentration by 1 mmol/L per hour.

After 3 hours, the hypertonic saline infusion must be stopped and the serum sodium concentration rechecked. Correction of hyponatraemia can then be resumed at a slower rate, such as 0.5 mmol/L per hour, or 50 mL of 3% saline per hour, in this case. The hypertonic saline should be stopped if the serum sodium concentration rises too rapidly, once it is above 120 mmol/L or when the patient's symptoms settle.

A simpler strategy that results in similar correction rates is to infuse 3% saline initially at a rate of 1–2 mL/kg per hour to increase the serum sodium level by 1–2 mmol/L. The rate can then be slowed to 0.5 mL/kg per hour.

Effect of potassium

It is important to remember that giving potassium can raise the plasma sodium concentration in a hyponatraemic subject. This is because most of the given potassium goes into the cells, and to maintain electroneutrality sodium moves out of the cells. In addition, water moves into the cells secondary to a movement of chloride ions into the cells with potassium. This is clinically important in patients with severe diuretic- or vomiting-induced hyponatraemia who are also hypokalaemic.

The increase in sodium concentration caused by concurrent potassium administration should be taken into account to avoid an over-rapid correction of hyponatraemia. Any potassium added to the infused solution should be considered as sodium in the equation above, i.e.:

$$\text{change in } [Na^+] = \{\text{fluid } [Na^+] + \text{fluid } [K^+]\} - \text{serum } [Na^+]/(\text{total body water} + 1).$$

Novel therapies

Vasopressin receptor antagonists cause a selective water diuresis without affecting sodium and potassium excretion. Tolvaptan (an oral selective V_2 receptor antagonist) has been used in clinical trials for the management of patients with euvolaemic hyponatraemia (mostly due to SIADH) and hypervolaemic hyponatraemia (e.g. heart failure, cirrhosis). Vasopressin receptor antagonists are likely to be useful in the management of moderate chronic hyponatraemia if water restriction is insufficient.

Key points:

- Most cases of hyponatraemia are caused by an increase in the extracellular water due to increased plasma ADH levels.
- Assessing the volume status of the patient is essential in determining the aetiology of hyponatraemia.
- The clinical manifestations of hyponatraemia are more prominent when it has occurred acutely (i.e. within a period of hours).
- SIADH is not a diagnosis, and the underlying cause must be investigated.
- Correction of sodium concentration must not exceed 10 mmol/L in the first 24 hours.
- SIADH can be diagnosed in euvolaemic patients in whom hypothyroidism and adrenal insufficiency have been excluded and who have low plasma osmolality and high urine osmolality.
- Treatment of hyponatraemia generally includes correction of the underlying cause, volume replacement in hypovolaemic patients, and fluid restriction in euvolaemic and hypervolaemic patients.

Chapter 19

Male reproductive physiology and hypogonadism

Testicular anatomy and physiology

Anatomy

The testes contain (Fig. 19.1):
• seminiferous tubules composed of *Sertoli cells* and *germ cells*
• an interstitium containing *Leydig cells* that produce testosterone.

Physiology of the hypothalamic–pituitary–testicular axis

Pulsatile gonadotrophin-releasing hormone

Hypothalamic neurones (in the preoptic area) secrete gonadotrophin-releasing hormone (GnRH) in a *pulsatile* fashion into the hypophyseal portal system (see Chapter 11). Pulsatile GnRH in turn stimulates the pulsatile release of *luteinizing hormone* (LH) and *follicle-stimulating hormone* (FSH) from the anterior pituitary (Fig. 19.2).

GnRH binds to receptors on the plasma membrane of pituitary gonadotrophs and stimulates LH and FSH release by a calcium-dependent mechanism that may involve diacylglycerol.

Lecture Notes: Endocrinology and Diabetes. By A. Sam and K. Meeran. Published 2009 by Blackwell Publishing. ISBN 978-1-4051-5345-4.

LH and FSH

LH and FSH are composed of two glycoprotein chains. They interact with cell membrane receptors and stimulate adenylate cyclase. LH stimulates the production of testosterone by Leydig cells. LH stimulates testosterone synthesis by acting on the steroidogenic acute regulatory protein, which delivers cholesterol to the inner mitochondrial membrane, where it is converted to pregnenolone (the rate-limiting reaction). Sperm are produced under stimulation from testosterone and FSH (Fig. 19.2).

LH secretion is inhibited by testosterone, which acts on the hypothalamus (to slow the hypothalamic pulse generator) and directly on the anterior pituitary. Some of the effects of testosterone are mediated by oestradiol (produced from the aromatization of testosterone).

FSH secretion is inhibited by inhibin B (a glycoprotein consisting of two subunits, produced by Sertoli cells) as well as testosterone and oestradiol (produced from the aromatization of testosterone).

In addition, several other hormones, neurotransmitters and cytokines modulate GnRH secretion. Testosterone levels may be reduced in acute and chronic illnesses (due to increasing corticotrophin-releasing hormone and cytokines) and fasting (due to lower levels of leptin, which is required for normal pulse generator activity).

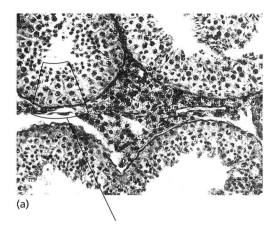

(a)

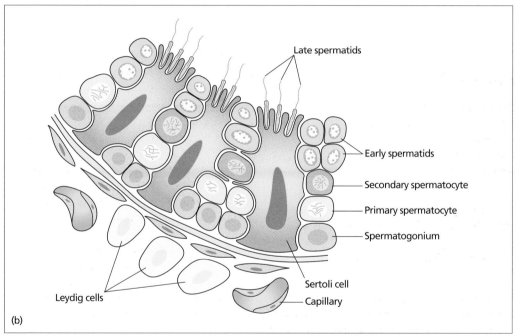

(b)

Figure 19.1 (a) A section of testis showing several seminiferous tubules containing Sertoli and spermatogenic cells. Leydig cells are in the interstitial space between the adjacent seminiferous tubules. (b) Part of a seminiferous tubule and interstitial space as indicated by the boxed area in (a). Spermatogonia differentiate into spermatocytes and spermatids as they move toward the lumen of the seminiferous tubules. Tight junctions between the Sertoli cells separate the tissue into two functional compartments.

Free and total testosterone

Only 2% of plasma testosterone is free (unbound). Of the rest, 44% of testosterone is bound to a hepatic glycoprotein called *sex hormone-binding globulin* (SHBG), and 54% of testosterone is loosely bound to albumin. Almost all of the albumin-bound testosterone is available for tissue uptake. Therefore bioavailable testosterone in plasma is the sum of free (2%) plus albumin-bound hormone (54%).

The serum SHBG levels may be increased and decreased by a number of factors (Box 19.1).

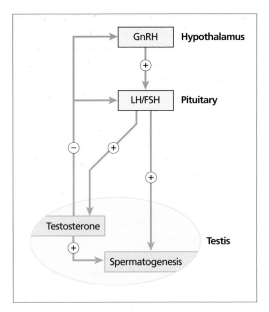

Figure 19.2 Pulsatile gonadotrophin-releasing hormone (GnRH) release from the hypothalamus stimulates luteinizing hormone (LH) and follicle-stimulating hormone (FSH) release from the anterior pituitary. LH stimulates testosterone synthesis by the Leydig cells. Sperm are produced under stimulation by testosterone and FSH. LH secretion is inhibited by testosterone, which acts on the hypothalamus and directly on the anterior pituitary.

Box 19.1 Causes of altered sex hormone-binding globulin (SHBG)

Increased SHBG
Ageing
Antiepileptic agents
Liver disease
Oestrogens
Thyrotoxicosis
Growth hormone deficiency

Decreased SHBG
Diabetes mellitus
Obesity
Corticosteroids, anabolic steroids
Hypothyroidism
Acromegaly

However, changes in the SHBG levels do not affect free androgen levels. This is because the hypothalamic–pituitary system responds to acute changes in the concentrations of bioavailable testosterone (caused by changes in SHBG levels) by altering testosterone synthesis.

Mechanism of action of testosterone

Testosterone is converted to active metabolites *5α-dihydrotestosterone* (by 5α-reductase) and *17β-oestradiol* (by aromatase). Testosterone and its metabolites bind to intracellular receptors, which in turn bind to specific DNA sequences ('response elements') and regulate the transcription of certain genes.

Physiological actions of testosterone

The physiological actions of testosterone are the result of the combined effects of testosterone itself plus its active metabolites. The major functions of androgens in males include:
- the regulation of gonadotrophin secretion from the hypothalamic–pituitary system
- the initiation and maintenance of spermatogenesis
- the formation of the male genital tract during embryogenesis
- the development of male secondary sexual characteristics and sexual potency at puberty, and their maintenance thereafter.

Male hypogonadism

Male hypogonadism is a syndrome of decreased testosterone production, sperm production or both.

Aetiology

Male hypogonadism may result from disease of the testes (*primary hypogonadism*) or disease of the pituitary or hypothalamus (*secondary hypogonadism*).

Known causes of hypogonadism are summarized in Box 19.2. However, many cases of hypogonadism remain unexplained (idiopathic).

Primary hypogonadism

In primary hypogonadism, reduced testosterone levels result in elevated gonadotrophin levels (due to a reduced negative feedback effect of

---

Box 19.2 Causes of male hypogonadism

Primary
Klinefelter's syndrome and other chromosomal
  abnormalities
Cryptorchidism
Infections (e.g. mumps orchitis)
Testicular trauma or torsion
Drugs, e.g. chemotherapy, ketoconazole, sulfasalazine,
  excess alcohol
Radiotherapy
Autoimmune damage
Chronic illnesses
Rare causes: mutations in genes encoding enzymes
  necessary for testosterone synthesis, mutations in
  the gene encoding the follicle-stimulating hormone
  receptor, myotonic dystrophy

Secondary
GnRH deficiency
Kallmann's syndrome (associated with anosmia),
  idiopathic

Pituitary or hypothalamic disease
Pituitary adenomas, cysts, craniopharyngiomas, other
  tumours, surgery, head trauma, infections, infarction,
  infiltrative disorders, e.g. haemochromatosis

Suppression of gonadotrophins
Chronic systemic illness, diabetes mellitus, hyperprolactinaemia, androgen excess (e.g. anabolic steroids),
  cortisol excess (exogenous or Cushing's syndrome),
  oestrogen excess (e.g. produced by a testicular
  tumour), gonadotrophin-releasing hormone analogues, opiates
Rare causes: Laurence–Moon–Biedl syndrome, Prader–
  Willi syndrome, mutations in the genes encoding
  GPR54 (the kisspeptin receptor), gonadotrophin-
  releasing hormone receptor, luteinizing hormone,
  follicle-stimulating hormone, leptin, leptin receptor,
  DAX1 (associated with congenital adrenal hypoplasia),
  LHX3, LHX4, HESX1 and PROP1 (transcription factors
  necessary for early differentiation of the pituitary).

---

testosterone on the hypothalamus and pituitary).
Thus primary hypogonadism is also known
as hypergonadotrophic hypogonadism. Primary
hypogonadism may be congenital or acquired.

Congenital causes
Congenital primary hypogonadism may be due to
Klinefelter's syndrome, other chromosomal abnor-
malities or cryptorchidism.

Klinefelter's syndrome is the most common congenital cause of primary hypogonadism and occurs
in about 1 in 500–1000 live male births. It is caused
by one or more extra X chromosomes in men,
resulting in damaged seminiferous tubules and
Leydig cells. The greater the number of extra X
chromosomes, the greater the phenotypic consequences. The most common genotype is 47XXY.
The 47XXY genotype results from non-disjunction
of the sex chromosomes of either parent during
meiotic division. 46XY/47XXY mosaicism probably results from non-disjunction during mitotic
division after conception.

In addition to features of hypogonadism,
patients may have:
- intellectual dysfunction and behavioural
abnormalities that cause difficulty in social
interactions
- a predisposition to develop chronic bronchitis,
bronchiectasis and emphysema, germ cell tumours
(e.g. involving the mediastinum), breast cancer (a
20-fold increased risk), possibly non-Hodgkin's
lymphoma, varicose veins, leg ulcers and diabetes
mellitus.

A large number of *other chromosomal abnormalities* have been reported that result in testicular
hypofunction. The 46XY/X0 karyotype results in a
syndrome characterized by short stature and features typical of Turner's syndrome (see Chapter
21). Gonadectomy should be performed in a
patient who has both a streak gonad and a dysge-
netic testis, as the risk of gonadoblastoma is about
20%. Up to 20% of men with azoospermia or severe
oligospermia have microdeletions in specific
regions of the long arm of the Y chromosome.

Cryptorchidism refers to unilateral or bilateral
(10%) undescended testes (in the abdominal cavity
or in the inguinal canal) that cannot be manipu-
lated manually into the scrotum by the age of 1
year. The risk of testicular cancer is increased
(3–14-fold).

Acquired causes
Acquired primary hypogonadism may be due to
infections (e.g. mumps orchitis), testicular trauma
or torsion, chemotherapy, radiotherapy, autoimmune damage or chronic illnesses (e.g. chronic

obstructive pulmonary disease, congestive cardiac failure, Crohn's disease, coeliac disease, chronic liver disease, chronic kidney disease, chronic anaemia, rheumatoid arthritis, AIDS).

Secondary hypogonadism

Secondary (or hypogonadotrophic) hypogonadism is due to impaired secretion of hypothalamic GnRH or pituitary gonadotrophins. Secondary hypogonadism may be congenital or acquired.

Congenital GnRH deficiency

Congenital secondary hypogonadism may be associated with anosmia in *Kallmann's syndrome*. The incidence of Kallmann's syndrome is 1 in 10 000 males. Kallmann's syndrome is usually X-linked (although autosomal dominant transmission can also occur). It may be due to sporadic or familial mutations of several genes (e.g. *KAL1* and *FGFR1* [*KAL2*], *PROK2*, *PROKR-2*) encoding the cell surface adhesion molecules or their receptors required for the migration of GnRH-secreting neurones into the hypothalamus. Kallmann's syndrome may also be associated with red–green colour blindness, midline facial abnormalities (e.g. cleft palate), urogenital tract abnormalities, synkinesis (mirror movements of the hands) and hearing loss.

Secondary hypogonadism may very rarely be caused by a number of mutations in the genes involved in the regulation of the hypothalamic–pituitary–gonadal axis (Box 19.2). Congenital secondary hypogonadism may be associated with mental retardation and obesity in Prader–Willi syndrome (caused by deletion of part of paternally derived chromosome 15q) and Laurence–Moon–Biedl syndrome (also associated with polydactyly and retinitis pigmentosa).

Pituitary or hypothalamic disease

Secondary hypogonadism may be caused by any pituitary or hypothalamic disease such as pituitary adenoma, craniopharyngioma, pituitary surgery, infarction, infection and infiltrative disorders such as haemochromatosis, sarcoidosis, histiocytosis, tuberculosis and fungal infections.

Suppression of gonadotrophins

Gonadotrophin secretion may be suppressed by chronic systemic illness, diabetes mellitus, hyperprolactinaemia, androgen excess (e.g. anabolic steroids, congenital adrenal hyperplasia, testicular/adrenal tumours), cortisol excess (exogenous or Cushing's syndrome), oestrogen excess (e.g. produced by a testicular tumour), chronic opiate administration and GnRH analogues.

Clinical presentations

The clinical presentations depend on whether the onset of hypogonadism is before or after puberty.

Hypogonadism occurring before the onset of puberty results in delayed puberty (see Chapter 29). Hypogonadism occurring after the onset of puberty may present with:

- fatigue, reduced energy and lowered physical strength
- low mood, irritability and poor concentration
- reduced libido and/or sexual function, loss of spontaneous morning erections, and infertility
- osteoporosis and fragility fractures.

The major action of testosterone on male sexuality is on libido. Men who present with erectile dysfunction usually have microvascular or macrovascular disease, and testosterone deficiency accounts for fewer than 5% of cases. Erectile responses to erotic stimuli are usually normal in hypogonadal men. However, spontaneous nocturnal or morning erections are testosterone dependent and are reduced in untreated hypogonadal men.

Patients should be asked about the features of the possible causes of hypogonadism (Box 19.2).

The clinical signs of hypogonadism are summarized in Box 19.3.

Primary hypogonadism is more likely to be associated with gynaecomastia, probably due to the stimulation of testicular aromatase activity by the increased serum FSH and LH, resulting in increased conversion of testosterone to oestradiol and also increased testicular secretion of oestradiol relative to testosterone.

Box 19.3 Clinical signs of hypogonadism
Hypogonadism occurring before onset of puberty
Testes <5 mL
Penis <5 cm long
Reduced pubic, axillary and facial hair
Gynaecomastia
Eunuchoid proportions: arm span > height, lower segment > upper segment (due to delayed fusion of the epiphyses and continued growth of the long bones)
Features of the underlying cause, e.g. cryptorchidism, anosmia (Kallmann's syndrome)
Hypogonadism occurring after puberty
Testes soft, <15 mL
Penis normal length (>5 cm) and width (>3 cm)
Reduced pubic, axillary and facial hair
Gynaecomastia
Normal skeletal proportions
Fine perioral wrinkles
Features of the underlying cause, e.g. visual field defects due to a pituitary tumour, signs of systemic/chronic illness

Investigations

The diagnosis of hypogonadism can be confirmed by finding low serum testosterone and/or decreased sperm in the semen.

Serum testosterone levels

Measurement of the serum total (free plus protein-bound) testosterone concentration is usually an accurate reflection of testosterone secretion. Testosterone exhibits a diurnal variation (particularly in young men), with maximum levels at about 8 a.m. and lower levels in the evening. Thus testosterone levels should be measured at 8 a.m. If a single testosterone value is low or borderline low, it should be repeated once or twice.

Measurement of the serum free testosterone concentration by equilibrium dialysis is usually not necessary (unless it is suspected that an abnormality in testosterone binding to SHBG coexists with hypogonadism, e.g. in obesity). However, free and bioavailable testosterone levels (free testosterone plus testosterone bound weakly to albumin) can be calculated from the total testosterone, SHBG and albumin levels.

LH and FSH levels

In a hypogonadal patient (with low serum testosterone and/or a subnormal sperm count):
- high LH and FSH concentrations indicate testicular damage (primary hypogonadism)
- low or inappropriately normal LH and FSH levels suggest pituitary or hypothalamic disease (secondary hypogonadism).

Semen analysis

Semen analysis for sperm number and motility should be performed in men presenting with infertility. (Healthy men produce >40 million sperm per ejaculate; >50% are motile and >50% have normal morphology.) Four or more abnormal analyses over several months are necessary to indicate an abnormality that is likely to be of clinical importance.

Follow-up of initial tests

Men with primary hypogonadism should have a peripheral leukocyte *karyotype* to determine whether Klinefelter's syndrome is present.

Men with secondary hypogonadism should have basal pituitary function tests: 8–9 a.m. cortisol, free thyroxine and thyroid-stimulating hormone, and prolactin. Iron saturation should be done if hereditary haemochromatosis is suspected.

Magnetic resonance imaging (MRI) of the hypothalamic–pituitary area should be performed if the patient has other pituitary hormonal abnormalities, headache or visual field defects. If there is no other evidence of pituitary/hypothalamic disease, MRI is warranted in young men if the confirmed testosterone value is less than 9 nmol/L. However, in elderly men (>65 years), a total testosterone value of below 7 nmol/L is necessary to warrant an MRI as the serum testosterone level decreases with increasing age.

Treatment

Treatment should be directed at any underlying disorders. The aim of therapy is to relieve the symptoms and to preserve bone density.

Boys who have not gone through puberty are started on low doses of testosterone, which are gradually increased (see Chapter 29).

Primary hypogonadism

In symptomatic men with a total testosterone of consistently less than 8 nmol/L, testosterone replacement therapy may be started if there are no contraindications (Box 19.4). Those with testosterone levels of 8–10 nmol/L require careful individual evaluation. The borderline low levels of testosterone commonly seen in ageing men are generally compatible with adequate sexual function.

Testosterone preparations

A number of different preparations are available for testosterone replacement therapy. The choice of preparation depends on local availability and patient preference.

Box 19.4 Testosterone replacement therapy: side-effects and contraindications

Side-effects

Acne on the upper trunk, particularly in younger patients
Prostate: enlargement (obstructive symptoms), stimulation of growth in previously undiagnosed tumours
Polycythaemia
Gynaecomastia (develops during commencement of therapy, resolves with continued use)
Fluid retention (mild)
Sleep apnoea
Other: mood fluctuations and sexually aggressive behaviour with supraphysiological levels
Side-effects of the particular route of administration

Contraindications

Prostate cancer or severe symptomatic benign prostatic hypertrophy
Polycythaemia (haematocrit >0.54)
Breast carcinoma
Sleep apnoea
Conditions in which fluid retention may be harmful, e.g. congestive cardiac failure

---

Testosterone gel (Testogel, Testim, Tostran) is applied on the skin of the shoulder and upper arm. When applied to the skin in doses of 50–100 mg once a day, the serum testosterone levels reach the normal male range within a month and remain steady throughout 24 hours. The gel has several advantages, including self-administration, avoidance of painful injections and stable pharmacokinetics. It dries quickly but could be transferred to the partner through skin contact. Patients should not shower for 6 hours.

Intramuscular testosterone (e.g. Sustanon: mixed testosterone esters) may be given at a dose of 250 mg every 2–3 weeks. Disadvantages include pain at the injection site, fluctuating plasma testosterone levels that may lead to mood swings, and polycythaemia caused by repetitive post-injection supraphysiological testosterone levels. Nebido, a depot preparation (1 g testosterone undecanoate in 4 mL castor oil), maintains stable physiological testosterone levels for about 12 weeks. The second dose is administered after 6 weeks to achieve rapid steady state levels, and thereafter injections are given every 12 weeks.

With *subcutaneous testosterone implants*, three or four 200 mg pellets are implanted under local anaesthesia every 6 months. This preparation requires minor surgery. Complications include infection, bleeding, extrusion (8–10% risk) and scarring. It is useful in patients who wish to avoid frequent treatment.

Buccal testosterone (Striant SR) may be given at a dose of 30 mg every 12 hours. It is delivered via the superior vena cava, and hepatic first-pass metabolism is avoided. Steady-state testosterone concentrations are achieved in 24 hours. Disadvantages include alterations in taste and irritation of gums and oral mucosa.

Other preparations include testosterone patches, which commonly cause local skin irritation, and oral testosterone undecanoate, which has limited efficacy due to poor and variable bioavailability, a short half-life requiring frequent administration, and risk of hepatic injury.

The side-effects of testosterone replacement therapy and its contraindications are summarized in Box 19.4.

Men who desire fertility

Assisted reproductive techniques may be used for men with oligospermia and azoospermia. Intra-uterine insemination may be used in couples with mild male infertility. In vitro fertilization is used for the treatment of male infertility in patients with moderate oligospermia.

Intracytoplasmic sperm injection (ICSI) can be used for men with very severe oligospermia and even azoospermia. A single spermatozoon is directly injected into the cytoplasm of a human oocyte (usually obtained from follicles produced under controlled ovarian hyperstimulation). When the ejaculate does not contain any sperm but there are germ cells in the testes, ICSI may be performed with spermatozoa isolated from testicular biopsies or fine needle aspirates.

In men presenting with infertility, 30–40% of cases are due to primary hypogonadism and 1–2% are due to secondary hypogonadism (see below). A total of 10–20% are secondary to post-testicular defects (disorders of sperm transport), and 40–50% are non-classifiable.

Secondary hypogonadism

The underlying cause should be treated if possible. For example, patients with prolactinomas are treated with dopamine agonists. Normal spermatogenesis takes 3 months. Therefore restoration of a normal sperm count usually does not occur for 3–6 months after the serum prolactin and testosterone levels have normalized.

Men with secondary hypogonadism who do not desire fertility should receive testosterone replacement therapy if there are no contraindications (see above).

Men who desire fertility

Men who have secondary hypogonadism due to hypothalamic or pituitary diseases can be treated with gonadotrophins. However, only men with secondary hypogonadism due to hypothalamic disease can be treated with pulsatile GnRH. Both regimens may take up to 2 years to achieve adequate spermatogenesis. Once they are effective, storing several samples of frozen sperm for any future attempts at pregnancy should be considered.

With *gonadotrophin replacement*, initially human chorionic gonadotrophin (hCG) injections are administered (1000–2000 IU subcutaneously or intramuscularly, three times a week). hCG has the biological activity of LH. The response to therapy is measured on semen analysis and may take 6–12 months. If adequate spermatogenesis is not achieved, human menopausal gonadotrophin or recombinant FSH is added (37.5–75 IU three times a week). It may take 12 months or more for a response to be seen.

Pulsatile GnRH therapy may be given subcutaneously via a catheter attached to a mini-pump. This regimen is suitable in men with a hypothalamic defect with normal pituitary gonadotrophin function.

Follow-up and monitoring

Clinical assessment

Patients should be asked about improvements in symptoms (e.g. libido, erectile/sexual function, energy, stamina, mood and cognition, hair pattern) and symptoms of possible treatment complications—mood swings, features of sleep apnoea (daytime sleepiness and apnoea witnessed during sleep by a partner) and prostate-related symptoms—every 6–12 months.

Patients should be assessed for weight gain, peripheral oedema and gynaecomastia at baseline and yearly during follow-up. In men over 40 years, *digital rectal examination* should be performed at baseline and 3 and 6 months and yearly thereafter to look for prostate enlargement.

For follow-up of patients with secondary hypogonadism due to pituitary disease and hyperprolactinaemia, see Chapters 12 and 14.

Laboratory tests

- *Haemoglobin/haematocrit* should be measured at baseline, after 3 and 6 months, and yearly thereafter to detect polycythaemia.

• *Prostate-specific antigen* (PSA) should be measured at baseline, after 3 and 6 months and yearly thereafter.

• *Liver function tests* and *fasting lipid profile* should be measured before starting therapy and then yearly.

• *Testosterone levels* should be monitored. The timing of testosterone measurement depends on the preparation used. The aim is to maintain testosterone levels in the mid-normal range: (15–20 nmol/L). If it is above 15 nmol/L or below 8 nmol/L, adjust the dosing interval, dose or both.

   — Testosterone gel: levels can be measured at any time after the patient has received treatment for at least 1 week.

   — Testosterone undecanoate injections, implants and buccal testosterone: measure nadir testosterone levels before each administration.

   — Mixed testosterone ester injections: measure testosterone levels mid-way between injections.

Referral to urologists for prostate biopsy should be considered if patients complain of increasing obstructive symptoms, if digital rectal examination is abnormal or if PSA is increased (>4 ng/mL or an increase of ≥1.0 ng/mL within any 12-month period). PSA measurement should be repeated in patients with a PSA increase of 0.7–0.9 ng/mL.

A sleep study should be performed if obstructive sleep apnoea is clinically suspected. For selected men, bone mineral density monitoring during therapy might be helpful to confirm end-organ effects.

Key points:

• LH stimulates testosterone synthesis by the Leydig cells. Sperm are produced under stimulation from testosterone and FSH.

• Male hypogonadism may result from disease of the testes (primary hypogonadism) or disease of the pituitary or hypothalamus (secondary hypogonadism).

• Klinefelter's syndrome is the most common congenital cause of primary hypogonadism. It is caused by one or more extra X chromosomes.

• The clinical presentation depends on whether the onset of hypogonadism is before or after puberty. Hypogonadism occurring before the onset of puberty results in delayed puberty.

• The investigation of patients with hypogonadism should include measurement of serum testosterone, LH and FSH (high in primary hypogonadism and low or inappropriately normal in secondary hypogonadism), semen analysis, karyotyping in primary hypogonadism (to exclude Klinefelter's syndrome), and pituitary function tests and MRI of the hypothalamic–pituitary area in secondary hypogonadism.

• A number of different testosterone preparations are available for testosterone replacement therapy. The choice of preparation depends on local availability and patient preference.

Chapter 20

Gynaecomastia

Gynaecomastia is a benign proliferation of the glandular tissue of the male breast (Fig. 20.1). It is usually bilateral but may be unilateral.

Gynaecomastia must be differentiated from pseudogynaecomastia (due to excessive adipose tissue without glandular proliferation, often seen in obese men) and male breast carcinoma, which is far less common.

Epidemiology

Gynaecomastia is common in infancy, adolescence and elderly men. A total of 60–90% of infants may have transient gynaecomastia (for 2–3 weeks) due to the high oestrogen levels in pregnancy. The second peak of gynaecomastia occurs during puberty and affects about 65% of boys. Almost all cases regress spontaneously. The third peak of gynaecomastia occurs in 25–65% of middle-aged and elderly men, with the highest prevalence at 50–80 years.

Aetiology

Oestrogens stimulate ductal epithelial growth and proliferation of the periductal fibroblasts.

Lecture Notes: Endocrinology and Diabetes. By A. Sam and K. Meeran. Published 2009 by Blackwell Publishing. ISBN 978-1-4051-5345-4.

Conditions (Box 20.1) that cause an increase in the production of oestrogens (and hence their stimulatory effect) and/or a decrease in the production/activity of androgens (and hence their inhibitory effect) result in gynaecomastia.

The factors that define the net oestrogen/androgen balance are:
- the production of oestrogens/androgens or their precursors by the adrenals and testes
- aromatase activity: aromatase is the enzyme that converts androgens to oestrogens in peripheral tissues, for example adipose tissue, liver, skin, muscle, bone and kidney
- sex hormone-binding globulin (SHBG) levels: SHBG has a higher affinity for androgens than for oestrogens. Thus changes in SHBG levels result in an imbalance in unbound oestrogens and androgens
- the responsiveness of the target cells to androgens and oestrogens.

The histological picture of gynaecomastia changes over time, with early proliferation and inflammation, and later fibrosis.

Box 20.1 summarizes the causes of gynaecomastia. During puberty, serum oestradiol rises to adult levels before serum testosterone, and this transient imbalance in oestrogen/testosterone levels may account for pubertal gynaecomastia.

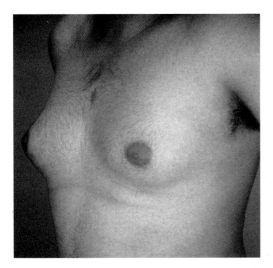

Figure 20.1 Gynaecomastia.

Clinical presentations

Gynaecomastia (enlargement of the glandular tissue) should be differentiated from pseudogynaecomastia (excessive adipose tissue often seen in obese men) and breast cancer.

Ask the patient to lie on his back with his hands behind his head. Place your thumb and forefinger on each side of the breast and slowly bring them together toward the nipple. In gynaecomastia, a rubbery/firm disk of glandular tissue (at least 0.5 cm in diameter) will be felt extending concentrically from the nipple. In pseudogynaecomastia, the fingers will not meet any resistance until they reach the nipple.

Breast cancer tends to be eccentrically positioned (rather than symmetrical to the nipple), tends to be firm to hard in texture, and may be associated with skin dimpling, nipple retraction, discharge and axillary lymphadenopathy.

A careful history and physical examination are essential in detecting the symptoms and signs of the underlying cause of gynaecomastia (Box 20.1). Patients should be asked about any of the drugs that can cause gynaecomastia. Look for symptoms and signs of the possible underlying cause, i.e. hypogonadism, hyperthyroidism, chronic liver or chronic renal disease, thyrotoxicosis and testicular

Box 20.1 Causes of gynaecomastia

Physiological
Puberty, persistent pubertal (25% of cases), elderly

Drugs (10–25%)
Oestrogens, antiandrogens, spironolactone (antiandrogenic effects), cimetidine, nifedipine, herbal products/oils

Hypogonadism (primary 8%, secondary 2%)
Reduced serum testosterone production

Chronic liver disease (8%)
Enhanced aromatization (many patients are also on spironolactone)

Chronic renal failure (1%)
Reduced serum testosterone due to Leydig cell dysfunction

Thyrotoxicosis (1.5%)
Enhanced aromatization

Tumours
Testicular germ cell tumours secrete human chorionic gonadotrophin (hCG) resulting in enhanced aromatization
Testicular Leydig cell tumours secrete increased oestradiol
Other hCG-secreting tumours, e.g. lung, stomach, renal cell and liver
Oestrogen-secreting adrenal tumours

No detectable abnormality (25%)

Rare causes
Aromatase excess syndrome—rare autosomal dominant disorder of increased aromatase activity
Androgen insensitivity syndrome (testicular feminization) due to defective/absent androgen receptor in the target tissues. Thus patients are genotypic males but appear to be phenotypic females

or other (human chorionic gonadotrophin [hCG]- or oestrogen-secreting) tumours.

Investigations

In adolescent boys, gynaecomastia is almost always due to pubertal gynaecomastia and often resolves spontaneously.

Asymptomatic gynaecomastia that is discovered during a physical examination in a patient who

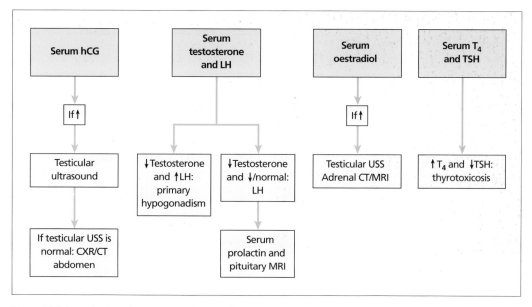

Figure 20.2 Investigation of gynaecomastia. CXR, chest X-ray.

does not have one of the possible causative conditions should be re-evaluated in 6 months.

Serum hCG, luteinizing hormone (LH), testosterone, oestradiol, free thyroxine (T$_4$) and thyroid-stimulating hormone (TSH) should be measured, particularly if the gynaecomastia is of recent onset or painful (Fig. 20.2).

- If *hCG is elevated*, a testicular ultrasound scan should be performed to look for a testicular germ cell tumour. If testicular ultrasound is normal, a chest radiograph and abdominal computed tomography (CT) should be done to look for an hCG-secreting tumour.
- If *testosterone is low and LH levels are increased*, the diagnosis is primary hypogonadism.
- If *testosterone is low and LH levels are low or inappropriately normal*, the diagnosis is secondary hypogonadism. Serum prolactin should be measured and magnetic resonance imaging (MRI) of the pituitary should be performed.
- If *free T$_4$ levels are high and TSH is suppressed*, the diagnosis is thyrotoxicosis.
- If the *oestradiol levels are increased and LH levels are low or normal*, testicular ultrasound should be performed to look for a Leydig or Sertoli cell tumour. If the testicular ultrasound is normal,

adrenal imaging (CT/MRI) should be performed to look for an adrenal tumour. If the imaging is normal, increased extraglandular aromatase activity is likely.

- If all *tests are normal*, the diagnosis is 'idiopathic gynaecomastia'.

Treatment, follow-up and monitoring

The treatment of gynaecomastia depends on its cause, its severity, the presence of tenderness and its duration.

Adolescents

Most adolescents with gynaecomastia should be followed up and re-evaluated every 3–6 months. Gynaecomastia usually resolves spontaneously within 6 months to 2 years.

In boys with severe gynaecomastia causing substantial tenderness and/or embarrassment, a 3-month trial of tamoxifen (10 mg twice a day) may be considered. Patients and parents should be told that these drugs are not approved for this purpose.

Adult male

● *Men with an identifiable cause* should be followed up and re-evaluated after the possible cause has been treated.

● *Men with no identifiable cause and tender gynaecomastia persisting for longer than 3 months* may be treated with a 3–6-month trial of tamoxifen (10 mg twice daily). Patients should be told that tamoxifen is not approved for this purpose.

● *Men with persistent gynaecomastia (>1–2 years) who find it psychologically troubling* should be offered surgery, as the breast tissue has probably become fibrotic and medical therapy is unlikely to be effective.

● *Men with advanced prostate cancer who are on anti-androgens* may be given tamoxifen to reduce the risk of developing gynaecomastia. Prophylactic radiation is also an alternative. Tamoxifen may be also be tried in men who have already developed gynaecomastia on antiandrogen therapy.

Key points:

● Gynaecomastia is a benign proliferation of the glandular tissue of the male breast.

● Gynaecomastia must be differentiated from pseudo-gynaecomastia (excessive adipose tissue without glandular proliferation, often seen in obese men) and male breast carcinoma.

● Physiological gynaecomastia is common in infants, adolescents and elderly men.

● Conditions that cause an increase in the production of oestrogens (and hence their stimulatory effect) and/or a decrease in the production/activity of androgens (and hence their inhibitory effect) result in gynaecomastia.

● Causes of gynaecomastia include hypogonadism, chronic liver disease, chronic kidney disease, thyrotoxicosis, testicular tumours and other hCG- and oestrogen-secreting tumours.

● Blood tests in patients with gynaecomastia include serum hCG, LH, testosterone, oestradiol, free T_4 and TSH.

● Patients with increased serum hCG or oestradiol require a testicular ultrasound. If this is normal, further imaging is required (chest radiograph and abdominal CT).

Chapter 21

Female reproductive physiology, amenorrhoea and premature ovarian failure

The menstrual cycle

The menstrual cycle is divided into two phases:
- The *follicular phase* starts with the onset of menses and ends on the day of the luteinizing hormone (LH) surge.
- The *luteal phase* begins on the day of the LH surge and ends at the onset of the next menses.

The average adult menstrual cycle lasts about 28 days, with about 14 days in the follicular phase and about 14 days in the luteal phase. The first day of the cycle is the first day of menses. There is significantly more cycle variability for the first 5–7 years after menarche and for the last 10 years before menopause. The longer menstrual cycles are usually associated with anovulation. There is relatively less cycle variability between the ages of 20 and 40 years. With each normal menstrual cycle, a single mature oocyte is released from a pool of hundreds of thousands of primordial oocytes.

During the early follicular phase, the serum oestradiol and progesterone levels are low (Fig. 21.1). The reduced negative feedback effects of oestradiol, progesterone and probably inhibin A (produced by the corpus luteum of the previous cycle) result in increased *gonadotrophin-releasing hormone* (GnRH) pulse frequency, which in turn increases

serum *follicle-stimulating hormone* (FSH) levels and *LH* pulse frequency.

The increase in FSH stimulates the recruitment and growth of a cohort of *ovarian follicles*. The ovarian follicles consist of oocytes surrounded by granulosa cells and theca cells (Fig. 21.2a). FSH stimulates the enzyme aromatase (in the granulosa cells of the dominant follicle), which converts androgens (synthesized in the theca cells) to oestrogens (Fig. 21.2b).

The increase in oestradiol production initially suppresses serum FSH and LH levels (negative feedback effect on hypothalamic GnRH and pituitary gonadotrophins). Serum inhibin B secreted by the follicles also plays a role in suppressing FSH.

By the late follicular phase, a single dominant follicle is selected, and the rest of the growing follicles undergo atresia. The negative feedback effect of ovarian steroids (particularly oestradiol) switches to a positive feedback effect, resulting in an *'LH surge'* and a smaller rise in serum FSH concentration. The positive feedback is associated with an increased frequency of GnRH secretion and enhanced pituitary sensitivity to GnRH. Just before ovulation, oestradiol secretion reaches a peak and then falls.

The LH surge stimulates the release of the dominant oocyte from the follicle at the surface of the ovary within 36 hours. The granulosa cells begin to produce progesterone and develop into the corpus luteum. During the luteal phase, LH secretion

Lecture Notes: Endocrinology and Diabetes. By A. Sam and K. Meeran. Published 2009 by Blackwell Publishing. ISBN 978-1-4051-5345-4.

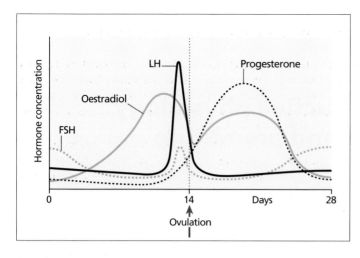

Figure 21.1 Changes in serum luteinizing hormone (LH), follicle-stimulating hormone (FSH), oestradiol and progesterone concentration during the menstrual cycle.

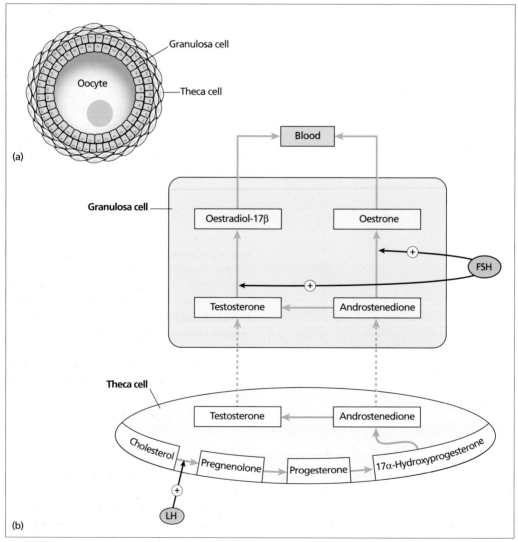

Figure 21.2 (a) Simplified diagram of an ovarian follicle consisting of an oocyte surrounded by granulosa cells and theca cells. (b) Androgens (testosterone and androstenedione) synthesized in the theca cells are converted to oestrogens (oestradiol-17β and oestrone) in granulosa cells by the enzyme aromatase, which is stimulated by follicle-stimulating hormone (FSH). Luteinizing hormone (LH) stimulates the conversion of cholesterol to pregnenolone.

decreases. This in turn results in a gradual fall in progesterone and oestradiol production by the corpus luteum. As progesterone and oestrogen levels fall near the end of the luteal phase, FSH starts to rise to stimulate the development of the next follicle, usually in the contralateral ovary. Inhibin A levels are low in the follicular phase and are increased in the luteal phase.

If, however, the oocyte becomes fertilized and is implanted in the endometrium, the early embryo begins to make chorionic gonadotrophin, which maintains the corpus luteum and progesterone production.

Endometrial changes

The endometrium undergoes marked alterations in response to the changing plasma levels of ovarian hormones. The rising serum oestradiol concentrations during the follicular phase of the menstrual cycle result in proliferation of the uterine endometrium and glandular growth. Hence the follicular phase is also known as the 'proliferative' phase.

After ovulation, increasing serum progesterone secreted by the corpus luteum plays an important role in converting the proliferative endometrium into a secretory lining. Hence the luteal phase is also known as the 'secretory phase'.

As the corpus luteum function declines and the plasma oestrogen and progesterone levels decrease, the arterioles supplying the endometrium undergo vasospasm (caused by locally synthesized prostaglandins), causing ischaemic necrosis, endometrial desquamation and bleeding (the onset of menses at the beginning of the next cycle).

Oestrogens

The principal and most potent oestrogen secreted by the ovary is *oestradiol*. Oestrogens promote the development of secondary sexual characteristics (e.g. breast development), cause uterine growth and play an important role in the regulation of the menstrual cycle (see above).

Oestrogens act by binding to a nuclear receptor (either oestrogen receptor alpha or beta), which binds to specific DNA sequences and regulates the transcription of various genes. There is growing evidence that oestrogen receptors may also alter signal transduction by other mechanisms independent of binding to DNA.

The other oestrogen produced by the ovaries is oestrone, but this is synthesized mainly by the conversion of androstenedione in the peripheral tissues.

Progesterone

Progesterone is the principal hormone secreted by the corpus luteum and is responsible for 'progestational' effects, including induction of secretory activity in the endometrium in preparation for the implantation of a fertilized egg, inhibition of uterine contractions, increased viscosity of cervical mucus and glandular development of the breasts. Changes in progesterone levels also mediate the changes in basal body temperature during the ovulatory cycle. The basal body temperature increases by $0.3–0.5\,°C$ after ovulation, persists during the luteal phase and returns to normal after the onset of menses.

Other ovarian hormones

Inhibin is a glycoprotein consisting of two disulphide-linked subunits, alpha and beta. The beta-subunit can exist in two forms, and therefore there are two forms of inhibin—inhibin A and inhibin B. Inhibin B is secreted by the follicle and inhibits the release of FSH from the pituitary gland. Inhibin A levels are low in follicular phase and are increased in the luteal phase.

Activin is secreted by the follicles. It may enhance FSH secretion and may have local effects on ovarian steroid synthesis. Follistatin binds to and attenuates the action of activin.

Amenorrhoea

Amenorrhoea is the absence of menstrual periods in a woman during her reproductive years.

Amenorrhoea may be primary or secondary:

• *Primary amenorrhoea* is defined as the absence of menstrual periods by age 14 in a girl without breast development or by age 16 in a girl with breast development.

- *Secondary amenorrhoea* is defined as the absence of menstrual periods for more than 3 months in a woman who has previously had an established menstrual cycle.

Epidemiology

The incidence of primary amenorrhoea is about 0.5–1.2%. The incidence of secondary amenorrhoea is about 5%.

Turner's syndrome (see below) occurs in up to 1.5% of conceptions, 10% of spontaneous abortions and 1 in 2000–2500 live births.

Aetiology

Considerable overlap exists between causes of primary and secondary amenorrhoea. All causes of secondary amenorrhoea can also present as primary amenorrhoea.

Amenorrhoea may be due to defects at any level of the reproductive system: hypothalamus, pituitary, ovaries, uterus or vaginal outflow tract. Other causes of menstrual abnormalities include thyroid dysfunction and hyperandrogenism (Box 21.1).

Constitutional delay of puberty is an uncommon cause of delayed puberty and primary amenorrhoea in girls (see Chapter 29). It is difficult to distinguish clinically from congenital GnRH deficiency except that these girls eventually go on to have completely normal pubertal development at a later age.

Hypothalamic and pituitary disorders

Functional hypothalamic amenorrhoea (Box 21.1) is characterized by abnormal hypothalamic GnRH secretion, resulting in decreased gonadotrophin pulsations.

Pituitary/hypothalamic tumours and other infiltrative disorders (Box 21.1) may cause hypogonadotrophic hypogonadism and amenorrhoea (see Chapter 12).

Hyperprolactinaemia may be due to a prolactin-secreting pituitary adenoma or other tumours

---

Box 21.1 Causes of amenorrhoea

Functional hypothalamic amenorrhoea
Stress, weight loss, excessive exercise, eating disorders (anorexia nervosa, bulimia)

Pituitary and hypothalamic tumours and infiltrative lesions
Pituitary adenomas, craniopharyngiomas, haemochromatosis

Hyperprolactinaemia
Prolactinomas or tumours causing pituitary stalk compression

Congenital gonadotrophin-releasing hormone deficiency
Kallmann's syndrome, idiopathic

Premature ovarian failure
Chromosomal abnormalities (e.g. Turner's syndrome), autoimmune, iatrogenic (surgery, chemotherapy, radiation), *FMR1* gene premutation carriers (CGG repeats of between 55–200), galactosaemia

Uterine and vaginal outflow tract disorders
Congenital anatomical abnormalities or acquired (Asherman's syndrome)

Thyroid dysfunction
Hypothyroidism or thyrotoxicosis

Hyperandrogenism
Congenital adrenal hyperplasia, polycystic ovary syndrome

---

causing pituitary stalk compression. This interrupts the transport of dopamine to the anterior pituitary, which normally exerts an inhibitory effect on prolactin secretion. Hyperprolactinaemia can result in hypogonadotrophic hypogonadism by a direct inhibition of gonadotrophin release.

Congenital GnRH deficiency is a rare cause of primary amenorrhoea. Patients with congenital GnRH deficiency have apulsatile and prepubertal low serum gonadotrophin levels. Congenital GnRH deficiency associated with anosmia is called Kallmann's syndrome. Kallmann's syndrome may be due to sporadic or familial mutations of several genes (e.g. *KAL1*, FGFR1 [*KAL2*], *PROK2*) required for the migration of GnRH-secreting neurones into the hypothalamus. Other rare causes include Prader–Willi and Laurence–Moon–Biedel syndromes (see Chapter 29).

Congenital GnRH deficiency can be inherited as an autosomal dominant, autosomal recessive or X-linked condition. However, more than two-thirds of cases are sporadic.

Premature ovarian failure

Amenorrhoea may be due to premature ovarian failure. Premature ovarian failure is defined as primary hypogonadism (lack of folliculogenesis and ovarian oestrogen production) before the age of 40 years. Most cases of premature ovarian failure are idiopathic.

The largest number of patients with primary amenorrhoea and ovarian failure have *Turner's syndrome* (45X0) followed by 46XX gonadal dysgenesis and, rarely, 46XY gonadal dysgenesis.

Turner's syndrome results from the lack or deletion of part of an X chromosome. The ovaries in Turner's syndrome consist of small amounts of connective tissue and no follicles or a few atretic follicles (streak gonads).

The presentation of Turner's syndrome is variable and ranges from no pubertal development and primary amenorrhoea (in most patients) to normal pubertal development and secondary amenorrhoea. Some patients may have no morphologic defects. In general, deletions of the long arm of the X chromosome tend to be associated with ovarian failure, and deletions of the short arm of the X chromosome tend to be associated with short stature and somatic anomalies (see 'Clinical presentations' below).

Although X0 is the most frequent abnormality, other X chromosome abnormalities and mosaicism may be present. In subjects with a mosaic karyotype (45X0/46XX), spontaneous menstruation and pregnancy may occur. The presence of a Y chromosome increases the risk of gonadoblastomas, and gonadectomy should be performed.

Acquired ovarian failure may be *iatrogenic* (due to chemotherapy or radiation) or *autoimmune*. Autoimmune ovarian failure is strongly associated with other autoimmune conditions such as adrenal insufficiency and thyroid disease. Around 3% of cases of spontaneous premature ovarian failure develop autoimmune adrenal insufficiency (a 300-fold increase compared with the general population).

Vaginal outflow tract and uterine disorders

Primary amenorrhoea may be due to *Müllerian agenesis* characterized by congenital absence of the vagina with variable uterine development. Patients have normal growth and development of secondary sexual characteristics. This disorder is usually sporadic. However, various genetic aetiologies have been proposed.

The differential diagnosis of Müllerian agenesis includes *androgen insensitivity*, which is caused by mutations in the androgen receptor. The karyotype is XY, but patients are phenotypically female with normal breast tissue.

Primary amenorrhoea may also be due to an imperforate hymen or a transverse vaginal septum between the cervix and hymenal ring, preventing the egress of menses. These patients have normal growth and development of secondary sexual characteristics, and present with abdominal pain due to retained menses. Treatment is surgical.

Secondary amenorrhoea may be caused by a history of pelvic infection, dilatation and curettage or uterine instrumentation resulting in intrauterine scarring and adhesions (Asherman's syndrome).

Thyroid dysfunction

Both hypothyroidism and thyrotoxicosis are associated with menstrual abnormalities.

Hyperandrogenism

Excessive androgen production is associated with both primary and secondary amenorrhoea, and may be due to either ovarian or adrenal sources.

The most common cause of primary amenorrhoea with excess androgen production is congenital adrenal hyperplasia (CAH), most commonly 21-hydroxylase deficiency (see Chapter 9).

Polycystic ovary syndrome (PCOS) classically presents with a peripubertal onset of menstrual disturbances and variable hyperandrogenism. Some patients may present with primary amenorrhoea, but most present with oligomenorrhoea or secondary amenorrhoea (see Chapter 22). PCOS is strongly associated with insulin resistance.

Androgen-secreting ovarian or adrenal tumours should be considered with serum testosterone levels higher than 5.2 nmol/L and a rapid onset of clinical signs of virilization (see below).

> **Box 21.2 Features of Turner's syndrome**
>
> Lack of secondary sexual characteristics
> Short stature
> Widely spaced nipples
> Low posterior hairline
> Musculoskeletal: high arched palate, wide carrying angle, short fourth and fifth metacarpals
> Cardiovascular: congenital lymphoedema, aortic dissection, bicuspid aortic valve, coarctation of aorta, hypertension
> Gastrointestinal: angiodysplasia, coeliac disease, abnormal liver function tests
> Renal anomalies: horseshoe kidneys, abnormal vascular supply
> Endocrine: increased risk of hypothyroidism and diabetes mellitus

Clinical presentations

After excluding pregnancy, patients should be questioned about the major causes:
- Has there been any recent stress, change in weight, excessive dieting or exercise, or illness that might cause hypothalamic amenorrhoea?
- Is the patient taking any drugs that might be associated with amenorrhoea (e.g. oral contraceptive pills)?
- Are there symptoms of hypothalamic–pituitary disease such as headaches, visual field defects, fatigue or polyuria and polydipsia?
- Is there galactorrhoea (suggestive of hyperprolactinaemia)?
- Are there any symptoms of oestrogen deficiency, for example hot flushes, vaginal dryness, poor sleep or reduced libido?
- Are there any symptoms of thyrotoxicosis or hypothyroidism?
- Is there a history of hirsutism, acne or deepening of the voice (suggestive of hyperandrogenism)?
- Is there a history of lower abdominal pain at the time of expected menses in girls with primary amenorrhoea (suggestive of anatomical vaginal outflow tract abnormalities)?
- Is there a history of dilatation and curettage, or endometritis that might have caused scarring of the endometrial lining (Asherman's syndrome)?

Physical examination should include the following:

- Assessment of pubertal development (Tanner staging).
- Measurements of height and weight, and calculation of body mass index. (Women with a body mass index <18.5 kg/m^2 may have functional hypothalamic amenorrhoea.)
- Signs associated with possible underlying causes:
  — *Hypothalamic/pituitary disease*: visual field defects and anosmia (Kallmann's syndrome).
  — *Ovarian failure*: somatic signs of Turner's syndrome (Box 21.2) and signs of other autoimmune diseases, for example hyperpigmentation in Addison's disease or vitiligo.
  — *Vaginal outflow tract disorders*: evidence of imperforate hymen or haematocolpos in primary amenorrhoea.
  — *Thyroid dysfunction*: signs of hypothyroidism or thyrotoxicosis.
  — *Hyperandrogenism*: patients with classic CAH may present with ambiguous genitalia at birth. Signs of hyperandrogenism in patients with non-classic late-onset CAH and PCOS include acne, hirsutism and alopecia. Patients with androgen-secreting tumours (ovarian or adrenal) may present with progressive virilization (clitoral enlargement, increased muscle mass, deepening of the voice). Patients with PCOS may have acanthosis nigricans (sign of insulin resistance).

Investigations

Initial tests

A *pregnancy test* (serum or urine human chorionic gonadotrophin tests) should be performed in all women with amenorrhoea.

In patients with primary amenorrhoea, *pelvic imaging* (ultrasound and/or magnetic resonance imaging [MRI]) should be done to demonstrate the presence or absence of the uterus and vagina, and vaginal or cervical outlet obstruction.

Serum FSH levels are elevated in premature ovarian failure (due to reduced inhibition by ovarian oestradiol and inhibin). However, it must be remembered that intermittent follicle development and transient normalization of serum FSH may occur in ovarian failure. A low or normal serum FSH suggests functional hypothalamic amenorrhoea, congenital GnRH deficiency or other disorders of the hypothalamic–pituitary axis.

Serum prolactin levels should be measured to exclude hyperprolactinaemia as a cause of secondary hypogonadism. Prolactin levels may be transiently increased by stress or eating. Thus prolactin should be measured at least twice before MRI of the hypothalamic–pituitary area is performed.

Serum thyroid-stimulating hormone (TSH) and *free thyroxine* (T_4) should be checked as patients with hypothyroidism and thyrotoxicosis can present with menstrual abnormalities.

Serum androgens (dehydroepiandrosterone-sulphate [DHEA-S] and testosterone) should be measured if there are signs of hyperandrogenism.

Follow-up of the initial test

Patients with high FSH levels suggestive of primary ovarian failure should have a *karyotype* to look for chromosomal abnormalities (complete or partial deletion of the X chromosome [Turner's syndrome] or the presence of a Y chromosome).

Patients with androgen insensitivity syndrome are phenotypically female but have an XY karyotype and a male-range serum testosterone.

Hypothalamic–pituitary MRI is indicated in women with hypogonadotrophic hypogonadism (low-to-normal FSH) and no clear explanation, and those with visual field defects, headaches or any other signs of hypothalamic–pituitary dysfunction.

In patients with hyperandrogenism, the differential diagnosis includes PCOS, CAH and androgen-secreting tumours. CAH is diagnosed with elevated 17-hydroxyprogestrone levels (basal or after adrenocorticotrophic hormone stimulation: see Chapter 9). The diagnostic criteria for PCOS are discussed in Chapter 22. An androgen-secreting tumour of the ovary or adrenal gland should be suspected and further imaging should be done if serum testosterone is >5.2 nmol/L or DHEA-S is >13.6 μmol/L.

Patients with normal serum prolactin and FSH and a history of uterine instrumentation should be evaluated for Asherman's syndrome. Cyclic oestrogen–progestin therapy can be given to determine whether a functional endometrium is present. If bleeding does not occur, hysteroscopy or hysterosalpingography should be performed to confirm the diagnosis.

Other investigations

Since pituitary iron deposition can cause secondary hypogonadism, serum transferrin saturation should be measured when hereditary haemochromatosis is suspected. This would apply to patients with an appropriate family history or other suggestive features such as bronzed skin, diabetes mellitus or unexplained heart or liver disease.

Further investigations should be targeted toward known complications of the disease established as the cause of the ovarian failure.

Around 30% of patients with *Turner's syndrome* have congenital heart disease (Box 21.2), and the risk of death from aortic aneurysm is high. Initial evaluation with periodic *echocardiography* and cardiology follow-up are needed. Thirty per cent have renal anomalies and a *renal ultrasound scan* should be done at diagnosis. *Thyroid function tests* should be checked every 1–2 years as up to 30% of patients develop thyroid disease.

Patients with likely autoimmune oophoritis (for which there is no diagnostic measurable autoantibody) should be evaluated for autoimmune adrenal insufficiency (by measuring 21-hydroxylase antibodies and, if positive, an adrenocorticotrophic hormone stimulation test) and for autoimmune thyroid disease (by measuring TSH and free T$_4$).

In women with unexplained premature ovarian failure, screening for premutation in the *FMR1* gene may be done only after appropriate genetic counselling and informed consent. This is because women with the *FMR1* premutation are at risk of having a child with mental retardation as premutations are unstable when transmitted by females and can expand to a full mutation, causing fragile X syndrome.

Treatment

All women with primary amenorrhoea should be counselled regarding the aetiology and management of amenorrhoea, and their reproductive potential. Treatment of amenorrhoea depends on the underlying cause.

Hypothalamic/pituitary disorders

Functional hypothalamic amenorrhoea can be reversed in most cases by weight gain, reduction in exercise intensity or resolution of illness or stress. Patients may benefit from cognitive-behavioural therapy and nutritional or psychological counselling.

Pituitary tumours may require surgery (see Chapter 12). The majority of women with prolactinomas are successfully treated with dopamine agonists (see Chapter 14).

Patients with irreversible gonadotrophin deficiency should receive *oestrogen replacement therapy* and *progesterone* if they have a uterus (see the treatment of ovarian failure below). Hormone replacement therapy is also often started in the setting of hypothalamic dysfunction to optimize bone development.

Women who want to become pregnant may receive either exogenous gonadotrophins or pulsatile GnRH. Pulsatile GnRH is more likely than gonadotrophins to result in the development and ovulation of a single follicle, thereby reducing the risk of ovarian hyperstimulation and multiple gestations.

Ovarian failure

In girls with primary amenorrhoea and delayed puberty, oral ethinylestradiol is started at a low dose (2 μg daily) to promote breast development and adult body habitus. The dose is gradually increased. Cyclical oral progesterone is added with the onset of breakthrough bleeding. Progesterone should not be added until breast growth has plateaued. Premature initiation of progesterone therapy can compromise ultimate breast growth.

Oestrogen–progestin replacement therapy is required for the prevention of osteoporosis and symptomatic control (vasomotor symptoms and vaginal dryness) and possibly the prevention of coronary heart disease.

Adult women with premature ovarian failure may be treated with 100 μg of transdermal estradiol or 2 mg of oral estradiol daily. (A dose of 50 μg of transdermal estradiol is considered equivalent to 1 mg of oral estradiol, 5–10 μg of ethinylestradiol and 0.625 mg of conjugated oestrogens per day.)

In all women with a uterus, cyclic progesterone must be added to prevent endometrial hyperplasia due to unopposed oestrogen action (e.g. 5–10 mg of medroxyprogesterone for about 10–14 days). About 90% of women receiving cyclic regimens have monthly withdrawal bleeding. In the majority of women, the bleeding starts after the last dose of progestin, but some have it while still taking the progestin. Hormone therapy is continued until approximately age 50 years (the average age of normal menopause). At that point, a discussion of potential risks and benefits of postmenopausal hormone therapy should take place (see Chapter 23).

Women who desire fertility can carry a fetus in their uterus following in vitro fertilization of their partner's sperm and donor oocytes.

In patients with Y chromosome material, gonadectomy must be performed to prevent the development of gonadal tumours. In androgen insensitivity syndrome, removal of the gonads may be deferred until immediately after pubertal maturation.

For the treatment of short stature in Turner's syndrome, see Chapter 30.

Uterine and vaginal outflow tract disorders

Surgery may be required in patients with congenital anatomical lesions. Surgical correction of a vaginal outlet disorder (e.g. hymenectomy) is essential as soon as the diagnosis is made, to allow passage of menstrual blood. For patients with Müllerian failure, the creation of a neovagina is usually delayed until the woman is emotionally mature. Asherman's syndrome is treated with hysteroscopic lysis of adhesions followed by long-term oestrogen administration to stimulate the regrowth of endometrial tissue.

Women with an absent uterus can have the embryo resulting from in vitro fertilization of their own oocyte transferred to a gestational carrier.

Thyroid dysfunction and hyperandrogenism

For the management of hypothyroidism, thyrotoxicosis, PCOS and CAH, see the appropriate chapters.

Key points:

- Amenorrhoea may be due to defects at any level of the reproductive system: hypothalamus, pituitary, ovaries, uterus or vaginal outflow tract. Other causes of menstrual abnormalities include thyroid dysfunction and hyperandrogenism.
- The most common cause of primary amenorrhoea is gonadal dysgenesis caused by chromosomal abnormalities, particularly Turner's syndrome (due to the lack or deletion of part of an X chromosome).
- Initial investigations in amenorrhoea include a pregnancy test, serum FSH, prolactin, TSH, free T_4 and androgens (DHEA-S and testosterone).
- The underlying cause of amenorrhoea must be identified and treated, for example by weight gain and a reduction in exercise intensity in functional hypothalamic amenorrhoea, and dopamine agonists for prolactinomas.
- Patients with irreversible gonadotrophin deficiency should receive oestrogen replacement therapy (and progesterone if they have a uterus).
- In patients with Y chromosome material, gonadectomy must be performed to prevent the development of gonadal tumours.

Chapter 22

Polycystic ovary syndrome

The Rotterdam criteria for the diagnosis of polycystic ovary syndrome (PCOS) include two out of the following three:

- *Oligomenorrhoea/amenorrhoea*
- *Hyperandrogenism*: clinical (acne, hirsutism, male-pattern hair loss) and/or biochemical (elevated serum androgen levels)
- *Polycystic ovaries on ultrasound* (see 'Investigations' below).

In addition, other causes of menstrual irregularity (e.g. hyperprolactinaemia, thyroid dysfunction) and hyperandrogenism (e.g. congenital adrenal hyperplasia, Cushing's syndrome, androgen-secreting tumours) must be excluded.

PCOS is frequently associated with obesity, *insulin resistance* (impaired glucose intolerance, diabetes) and dyslipidaemia.

Epidemiology

PCOS is the most common cause of infertility in women. It affects 6–8% of women. The prevalence of PCOS is increased in patients with obesity, insulin resistance, diabetes mellitus and a positive family history for PCOS among first-degree relatives. PCOS may first become apparent at the onset of puberty.

Lecture Notes: Endocrinology and Diabetes. By A. Sam and K. Meeran. Published 2009 by Blackwell Publishing. ISBN 978-1-4051-5345-4.

Aetiology

Both environmental factors (e.g. related to diet and the development of obesity) and a number of different genetic variants (possibly in genes regulating gonadotrophin, insulin and androgen synthesis, secretion and action, weight and energy regulation) may influence the development of PCOS.

Clinical presentations

Clinical presentations of PCOS include:

- *menstrual abnormalities*: infrequent or absent menses (oligomenorrhoea or amenorrhoea), infertility and occasionally dysfunctional uterine bleeding resulting from chronic anovulation
- *hyperandrogenism*: acne, hirsutism and male-pattern hair loss.

Hirsutism (Fig. 22.1) is defined as excess hair growing in a male distribution (e.g. on the upper lip and chin, in the midsternum, periareolarly, along the linea alba of the lower abdomen). Obesity, signs of insulin resistance, for example acanthosis nigricans (hyperpigmented skin, usually in the neck [Fig. 22.2], axilla or groin), impaired glucose intolerance/diabetes mellitus and dyslipidaemia are frequently seen in patients with PCOS. Other clinical manifestations include obstructive sleep apnoea and non-alcoholic steatohepatitis.

Androgen-secreting ovarian or adrenal tumours and ovarian hyperthecosis (see below) should be

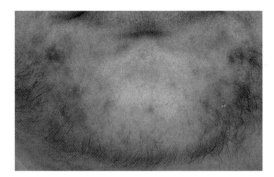

Figure 22.1 Hirsutism and acne in a patient with polycystic ovary syndrome.

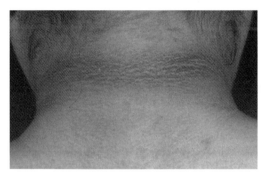

Figure 22.2 Acanthosis nigricans in a patient with polycystic ovary syndrome.

suspected in patients with progressive hirsutism, amenorrhoea and signs of virilization such as clitoral enlargement, increased muscle mass and deepening of the voice.

Investigations

• A *pregnancy test* should be done in all women who have missed an expected menstrual period.

• *Luteinizing hormone* (LH): high serum LH levels (due to an increased frequency and amplitude of the LH pulse) and a high (>3) ratio of LH to follicle-stimulating hormone (FSH) are seen in many women with PCOS. However, these are not part of the diagnostic criteria for PCOS. Serum LH levels are affected by the timing of the blood sample relative to the last menstrual period.

• *FSH*: serum FSH levels should be measured to rule out 'premature ovarian failure' (see Chapter 21).

• *Androgens*: testosterone, androstenedione and dehydroepiandrosterone sulphate (DHEA-S) are usually raised in PCOS. The excess androgens can be derived from the ovary, the adrenal cortex or both. It is important to check androgen levels to screen for androgen-secreting ovarian and adrenal tumours (see below).

• *Sex hormone-binding globulin* (SHBG): elevated insulin levels and androgen levels both inhibit the hepatic production of SHBG. Lower SHBG levels (seen in about 50% of patients) result in an increase in circulating free androgens.

Exclude *other causes* of menstrual irregularity or hyperandrogenism by performing the following tests:

• *Hyperprolactinaemia*: serum prolactin.

• *Hypo/hyperthyroidism*: free thyroxine and thyroid-stimulating hormone.

• *Congenital adrenal hyperplasia*: 17-hydroxyprogesterone (9 a.m., follicular phase).

• Cushing's syndrome (only if there is a high clinical suspicion of Cushing's syndrome): two or three 24-hour urine collections for free cortisol measurement or an overnight dexamethasone suppression test.

• *Androgen-secreting ovarian or adrenal tumours*: serum testosterone levels are nearly always higher than 5.2 nmol/L. Those with adrenal tumours usually have serum DHEA-S levels above 21 μmol/L. Their serum LH levels are low.

About 8% of hyperandrogenic patients have no identified cause despite thorough investigation and are said to have idiopathic hyperandrogenaemia.

Look for *impaired glucose tolerance/diabetes mellitus*. About 45% of patients with PCOS have impaired glucose tolerance or type 2 diabetes mellitus. Ideally, an oral glucose tolerance test (OGTT) should be performed in all patients. If this is not practical, a fasting glucose and glycated haemoglobin level should be done. If either one is abnormal, an OGTT should be performed to distinguish between impaired glucose tolerance and diabetes mellitus. A fasting lipid profile should also be requested in all women with PCOS.

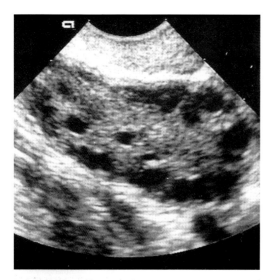

Figure 22.3 Ovarian ultrasound in a patient with polycystic ovary syndrome.

Ultrasound

The presence of 12 or more follicles in each ovary measuring 2–9 mm, and/or an increased ovarian volume of more than 10 mL (calculated by the formula: $0.5 \times$ length $\times$ width $\times$ thickness), is part of the Rotterdam criteria for the diagnosis of PCOS (Fig. 22.3). Ovarian ultrasound may show increased ovarian stroma. The transvaginal approach should be used. However, these ultrasonographic criteria may be difficult to document if an experienced ultrasonographer is not available.

Treatment

The management of PCOS depends on the patient's symptoms (hirsutism, oligomenorrhoea, obesity, glucose intolerance) and goals (e.g. desire to become pregnant).

Hirsutism

Oral contraceptive pills are the treatment of choice for hirsutism or other androgenic symptoms. The oestrogen component increases serum SHBG, which binds to and decreases serum free androgen. In addition, inhibition of gonadotrophin secretion

by oral contraceptive therapy results in a decrease in ovarian androgen secretion. Adrenal androgen secretion is also reduced, although the exact mechanism of this is not fully understood.

Many endocrinologists start with a preparation containing 30–35 µg of ethinylestradiol plus a progestin with minimal androgenic effect (e.g. norethindrone, norgestimate, desogestrel) or anti-androgenic effect (e.g. cyproterone acetate, drospirenone). Norgestrel- and levonorgestrel-containing preparations should be avoided due to their androgenic activity. In breast-feeding women, progestin-only contraceptives should be used (no earlier than 6 weeks postpartum) as combined oestrogen–progestin contraceptives suppress milk production.

In adolescents, oral contraceptives should be continued for 5 years after menarche or until a substantial amount of excess weight has been lost. At this time, a trial off treatment may be tried to document the persistence of the syndrome.

If the patient is not satisfied with the clinical response after 4–6 months, *spironolactone* may be added. Antiandrogens should not be prescribed without reliable contraception (ideally an oral contraceptive pill or intrauterine progestogen-only system) to women of reproductive age due to potential teratogenic effects.

Given the comparable efficacy of all the antiandrogens in the treatment of hirsutism, spironolactone is the first-line treatment chosen by many endocrinologists because of its safety. It inhibits testosterone binding to its receptors and also decreases ovarian androgen production. The usual dose is 50–100 mg twice a day. The effects may be noticeable within 2 months, and reach a peak at 6 months. The side-effects of spironolactone include hyperkalaemia (rarely a problem in those with normal renal function) and gastrointestinal discomfort.

Other antiandrogens used in treatment of hirsutism include the following:
- *Flutamide* also inhibits testosterone binding to its receptors and may be more potent than spironolactone. However, its use may result in hepatotoxicity.
- *Finasteride* inhibits 5α-reductase, which catalyzes the conversion of testosterone to dihydrotes-

tosterone. Finasteride is as effective as or less effective than spironolactone.

• *Cyproterone acetate* is a progestin with antiandrogenic activity, and may be given alone or with ethinylestradiol in the contraceptive pill Dianette. There is a perceived increase in risk of hepatotoxicity.

Medical management is combined with *cosmetic treatment* for removal of hair by means such as shaving, waxing, depilatories, electrolysis or laser treatment.

Eflornithine hydrochloride (Vaniqa) cream is a relatively new topical treatment used to inhibit hair growth. Eflornithine inhibits the enzyme ornithine decarboxylase, which regulates cell division by catalyzing the first step in polyamine biosynthesis.

Oral contraceptives and antiandrogen therapy may also reduce acne, but an occasional woman needs antibiotic or other therapy as advised by a dermatologist.

Oligomenorrhoea

Chronic anovulation is associated with endometrial hyperplasia and possibly increased risk of endometrial cancer. The progestin component of the *oral contraceptive pill* inhibits endometrial proliferation, preventing hyperplasia and the associated risk of carcinoma. The oestrogen component reduces excess androgen, which improves menstrual irregularity and dysfunctional uterine bleeding.

For those who choose not to or cannot take oral contraceptives, intermittent progestin therapy may be given for endometrial protection (10 mg of medroxyprogesterone acetate for 7–10 days every 1–2 months). Progestin therapy alone will not reduce the symptoms of acne or hirsutism, and will not provide contraception.

Infertility

Patients with PCOS who desire pregnancy should be advised to lose weight. In patients who are unable to lose weight, or in whom modest weight loss does not restore ovulatory cycles, ovulation induction may be initiated with *clomiphene citrate*. Clomiphene is superior to metformin in achieving live birth. However, multiple birth is a complication. It binds to oestrogen receptors in the hypothalamus. This is sensed as a state of hypo-oestrogenaemia, resulting in an increased release of gonadotrophin-releasing hormone (GnRH). If this is unsuccessful, other ovulation induction strategies should be considered (see Chapter 21).

Obesity

Lifestyle changes (diet and exercise) and modest weight loss may result in a restoration of ovulatory cycles and an improvement in hyperandrogenism and insulin resistance. *Metformin* is a reasonable adjunct to diet and exercise for patients with PCOS who are obese. It is associated with a reduction in blood pressure, low-density lipoprotein cholesterol and fasting insulin levels. It also improves ovulation in 50%, and modestly reduces androgen levels.

Diabetes mellitus

Diabetes mellitus and impaired glucose tolerance should be treated as for patients with these disorders who do not also have PCOS.

Other causes of hirsutism

The causes of hirsutism are summarized in Box 22.1.

Box 22.1 Causes of hirsutism

Idiopathic hirsutism
Polycystic ovary syndrome
Congenital adrenal hyperplasia (most often 21-hydroxylase deficiency)
Cushing's syndrome
Ovarian tumours (Sertoli–Leydig cell tumours, granulosa–theca cell tumours, hilus cell tumours)
Adrenal tumours
Ovarian hyperthecosis
Drugs (e.g. danazol, oral contraceptives containing androgenic progestins)
Severe insulin resistance syndromes

Congenital adrenal hyperplasia and Cushing's syndrome are discussed in separate chapters.

Ovarian hyperthecosis

Ovarian hyperthecosis is characterized by the presence of islets of luteinized theca cells in the ovarian stroma, resulting in an increased production of androgens. Women with hyperthecosis have more severe hirsutism and are much more likely to have clitoral enlargement, temporal balding and deepening of the voice. Ovarian hyperthecosis can occur in postmenopausal women (unlike PCOS, which occurs only during the reproductive years). Increased ovarian secretion of androgen also results in increased peripheral oestrogen production and an increased risk of endometrial hyperplasia.

Patients have high serum testosterone levels (≥ 7 nmol/L), similar to those seen with androgen-secreting adrenal or ovarian tumours. Pelvic ultrasonography must be performed to exclude virilizing ovarian tumours and to measure endometrial thickness. In practice, the diagnosis of ovarian hyperthecosis is made by histological examination of the ovaries following a wedge biopsy performed to rule out virilizing ovarian tumours.

The treatment of hyperthecosis includes weight reduction, oral contraceptives and spironolactone. GnRH agonists may reduce intraovarian androgen levels and restore sensitivity to exogenous gonadotrophins, with subsequent ovulation.

Key points:

- PCOS is characterized by oligomenorrhoea/amenorrhoea and hyperandrogenism.
- PCOS is frequently associated with obesity and insulin resistance.
- Hirsutism is treated with oral contraceptive pills, antiandrogens (e.g. spironolactone), eflornithine cream and cosmetic treatment.
- Antiandrogens should not be prescribed without reliable contraception due to potential teratogenic effects.
- Menstrual irregularity and dysfunctional uterine bleeding are treated with oral contraceptive pills.
- Metformin is a reasonable adjunct to diet and exercise in women with PCOS who are obese.
- Clomiphene is superior to metformin in achieving live birth.

Chapter 23

Menopause

Menopause is the time of ovarian failure and cessation of menstrual periods that occurs in normal women at a mean age of 51 years.

Menopause occurs between the ages of 45 and 55 years in 90%, between ages 40 and 45 years in 5% and after age 55 in 5% of women.

Endocrinology of menopause

In the early menopausal transition, levels of inhibin B released from the ovaries start to decrease due to a fall in follicular number. This results in an increase in serum follicle-stimulating hormone (FSH) levels due to a loss of the negative feedback effect of inhibin B on FSH secretion. Oestradiol levels are initially relatively preserved, possibly due to increased aromatase activity stimulated by the elevated FSH levels (FSH stimulates the aromatization of androgens to produce oestrogen). It is important to note that, during menopausal transition, there are significant fluctuations in serum FSH and oestradiol levels.

After menopause, when the ovarian follicles are depleted, the ovaries no longer secrete oestradiol but continue to secrete androgens under the continued stimulation of luteinizing hormone.

Lecture Notes: Endocrinology and Diabetes. By A. Sam and K. Meeran. Published 2009 by Blackwell Publishing. ISBN 978-1-4051-5345-4.

Clinical presentations

The menopausal transition starts with variation in the length of the menstrual cycle (>7 days different from normal cycle length). The menopausal transition ends with the final menstrual period. Menopause is diagnosed clinically as amenorrhoea for 12 months in a woman over age 45 in the absence of other causes.

Menopausal symptoms include:
- *hot flushes*
- *urogenital symptoms*: vaginal dryness, dysuria, frequency, stress incontinence and recurrent urinary tract infections
- *mood changes* and *sleep disturbances*.

Diagnosis and differential diagnoses

The best approach to diagnosing the menopausal transition is to evaluate the menstrual cycle history and menopausal symptoms. Serum FSH levels increase across the menopausal transition. FSH levels increase more than those of luteinizing hormone, presumably because of the loss of inhibin as well as the oestrogen negative feedback. However, since serum FSH and oestradiol levels fluctuate during the menopausal transition, a single elevated serum FSH value and even undetectable oestradiol and inhibin levels do not mean that menopause has occurred. Menopause is diagnosed clinically in a woman over age 45 who has had amenorrhoea for 12 months in the absence of other causes.

Other causes of menstrual cycle changes such as pregnancy, hyperprolactinaemia and thyroid dysfunction should be ruled out.

Atypical hot flushes and night sweats may also be associated with certain medications, phaeochromocytoma, thyrotoxicosis, carcinoid syndrome, underlying infection or malignancy.

Management

Hormone replacement therapy (HRT) with *oestrogen* is the most effective treatment for the relief of menopausal symptoms. However, unopposed oestrogen can result in endometrial hyperplasia and carcinoma, and therefore a *progestin* must be added to the oestrogen in women who have not had a hysterectomy. HRT is not recommended in those with a previous history of breast cancer, coronary heart disease, stroke or venous thromboembolism, or risk factors for these conditions.

Hormone replacement therapy

Sequential cyclical regimen

In this regimen, oestrogen (e.g. 0.625 mg of conjugated oestrogens) is given continuously, and a progestin (e.g. 5–10 mg of medroxyprogesterone) is added for the first 12–14 days of each month.

Around 90% of women have a monthly withdrawal bleed. Newly postmenopausal or younger women may prefer this regimen to avoid the irregular bleeding caused by the continuous combined regimen (see below). Uterine bleeding usually starts after the ninth day of progestin therapy.

Women with three or more cycles of uterine bleeding before the ninth day of progestin therapy or those with a change in the duration or intensity of uterine bleeding should have a transvaginal ultrasound performed by an experienced sonographer to look at *endometrial thickness*. An endometrial thickness of less than 5 mm excludes disease in 96–99% of cases. If the endometrial thickness is

more than 5 mm, an endometrial biopsy is required to exclude carcinoma.

Continuous combined regimen

In this regimen, oestrogen (e.g. 0.625 mg conjugated oestrogens) and lower doses of a progestin (e.g. 2.5–5 mg medroxyprogesterone) are given on a daily basis. Uterine bleeding is light, but the timing is unpredictable. Uterine bleeding stops within 12 months in 90% of women as daily progestin results in an atrophic endometrium. This regimen is preferred by older women who do not want monthly withdrawal bleeds.

If bleeding is heavy within the first 12 months, if it continues after 12 months or if it starts after a period of amenorrhoea, a transvaginal ultrasound should be performed to assess endometrial thickness (see above).

In any woman with previous long-term exposure to unopposed oestrogen or a previous history of irregular bleeding, a pre-treatment biopsy should be performed to rule out atypical endometrial hyperplasia or carcinoma.

Women's Health Initiative trials

HRT is not recommended in women with history of breast cancer, coronary heart disease, stroke or venous thromboembolism or risk factors for these conditions. *Women's Health Initiative (WHI) trials* reported that continuous combined oestrogen–progestin therapy increased the risk of breast cancer, coronary heart disease events, stroke and venous thromboembolism. The risks of fracture and colorectal cancer were, however, reduced.

In the unopposed oestrogen trial (in women with a previous hysterectomy), the risk of only stroke and venous thromboembolism was increased. It is possible that progestin may have played a role in the increased breast cancer risk and coronary heart disease in the studies with combined oestrogen–progestin.

A limitation of the WHI trials was the 'timing of exposure'. The WHI population had a mean age of 63 years, and HRT may have been started in an older population with more atherosclerotic lesions susceptible to the prothrombotic and proinflammatory effects of oestrogen. It must also be remembered that the absolute risk of an adverse event was extremely low (19 additional events per year per 10 000 women).

Hot flushes

Women with mild hot flushes do not usually require any pharmacological treatment. HRT may be given to women with moderate-to-severe symptoms and no history of breast cancer, cardiovascular or thromboembolic disease. HRT may be continued for 1–3 years, but generally not for more than 5 years.

For treatment of hot flushes, oestrogen should be given continuously. The effective daily dose equivalents are:
- 0.625 mg oral conjugated equine oestrogens
- 1 mg oral estradiol
- 50 µg transdermal estradiol.

Transdermal patches avoid first-pass hepatic metabolism, and are therefore ideal in women with liver disease or hypertriglyceridaemia. However, 10% of women develop skin reactions.

These doses given daily are sufficient to abolish hot flushes in 80% of women, and to reduce the frequency and severity of hot flushes in the rest. In women who have not had a hysterectomy, oestrogen should always be given in combination with a progestin to prevent the occurrence of endometrial hyperplasia.

HRT does not provide contraception during the menopausal transition. For perimenopausal women between the ages of 40 and 50 years who are troubled by menopausal symptoms and also desire contraception, a low-oestrogen (20 µg of ethinylestradiol) combined oral contraceptive pill is an appropriate treatment if there are no risk factors for venous and arterial disease. When these women reach age 51 years, the oral contraceptive pill is either stopped or changed to HRT if necessary for symptom control.

Stopping HRT

Many women are able to stop their oestrogen abruptly. If the patient is troubled by recurrent symptoms, HRT may be restarted and a 6-week taper may be tried by reducing by one pill per week. Women who are unable to tolerate this tapering regimen may require resumption of their HRT and a much slower taper, for example over 1 year by reducing one pill every 2 months. Various preparations of transdermal estradiol can also be used to decrease the dose gradually.

Women with a history of severe hot flushes before starting HRT often require a gradual taper over 6–12 months.

Other treatments

Women in whom oestrogen is contraindicated or not tolerated, and those who experience recurrent symptoms after stopping oestrogen and do not want to be restarted on HRT, may benefit from serotonin–noradrenaline reuptake inhibitors, selective serotonin reuptake inhibitors or gabapentin (given at bedtime in women with predominantly night-time symptoms). Hot flushes gradually subside in most postmenopausal women, and any drug can be gradually tapered after 1–2 years.

Urogenital symptoms

Women with mild symptoms are treated with regular vaginal moisturizing agents and lubricants during intercourse. Patients with moderate-to-severe symptoms and no history of breast cancer are treated with low-dose vaginal oestrogen. The choice of the vaginal delivery system, i.e. tablet, ring or cream, depends on the patient's preference.

Osteoporosis

Oestrogen is not the first-line treatment for osteoporosis in postmenopausal women. Bisphosphonates (alendronate, risedronate) are first-line treatments for postmenopausal osteoporosis (see Chapter 27). In postmenopausal women with osteoporosis who cannot tolerate bisphosphonates, raloxifene may be given if there are no fragility fractures. Parathyroid hormone therapy may be considered for those with at least one fragility fracture.

Postmenopausal women with osteoporosis should receive adequate calcium and vitamin D (1000 mg of elemental calcium and 800 IU of vitamin D daily). Patients should be informed of the importance of the relevant lifestyle measures including exercise and smoking cessation, and should receive counselling on fall prevention.

Key points:

- Menopause is the time of ovarian failure and cessation of menstrual periods that occurs in normal women at a mean age of 51 years.
- During menopausal transition, there are significant fluctuations in serum FSH and oestradiol levels.
- Menopausal symptoms include hot flushes, urogenital symptoms, mood changes and sleep disturbances.
- WHI trials reported that continuous combined oestrogen–progestin therapy increased the risk of breast cancer, coronary heart disease events, stroke and venous thromboembolism.
- HRT may be given to women with moderate-to-severe symptoms and no history of breast cancer, cardiovascular or thromboembolic disease.
- Oestrogen is not the first-line treatment for osteoporosis in postmenopausal women.

Chapter 24

Hypocalcaemia

Hypocalcaemia may be caused by either decreased calcium entry into the circulation or increased loss of free calcium from the circulation (due to deposition in the tissues or increased binding of calcium in the serum).

Aetiology

Causes of decreased calcium entry into the circulation include:

- *vitamin D deficiency* (decreased vitamin D synthesis, intake or action): the role of vitamin D in calcium homeostasis is discussed in Chapter 25. Causes of vitamin D deficiency are summarized in Box 24.1
- *hypoparathyroidism* (decreased secretion or action of parathyroid hormone [PTH]): the role of PTH in calcium homeostasis is discussed in Chapter 25. Causes of hypoparathyroidism are summarized in Box 24.1. Magnesium depletion may cause reduced PTH secretion and bone resistance to PTH.
- *pseudohypoparathyroidism*: characterized by target organ (kidney and bone) resistance to PTH.

Causes of extravascular calcium deposition include:

- *rhabdomyolysis* and *tumour lysis syndrome*: excess tissue breakdown results in acute hyperphosphataemia and consequently calcium deposition, mostly in bone but also in extraskeletal tissue
- *acute pancreatitis*: calcium soaps (calcium bound to free fatty acids) are precipitated in the abdominal cavity
- *widespread osteoblastic metastases* (e.g. breast or prostate cancer): calcium is deposited in the metastases
- *hungry bone syndrome*: calcium is deposited in bone after parathyroidectomy in patients with primary hyperparathyroidism.

Causes of increased intravascular calcium binding include:

- *acute respiratory alkalosis*: elevated extracellular pH results in increased binding of calcium to albumin and lower plasma free calcium levels
- *massive blood transfusion*: the citrate used to inhibit coagulation in banked blood chelates calcium in the serum
- *foscarnet* (used to treat cytomegalovirus): chelates calcium in the serum.

Hypocalcaemia may be caused by a number of drugs (see Box 24.1). *Sepsis* can be associated with hypocalcaemia due to impaired secretion of both PTH and calcitriol, and due to end-organ resistance to the action of PTH (probably due to hypomagnesaemia). These may be mediated by actions of inflammatory cytokines on the parathyroid glands, kidneys and bone. In addition, increased lactate levels in sepsis chelate calcium in the serum.

Lecture Notes: Endocrinology and Diabetes. By A. Sam and K. Meeran. Published 2009 by Blackwell Publishing. ISBN 978-1-4051-5345-4.

Box 24.1 Causes of hypocalcaemia

Vitamin D deficiency
Lack of sun exposure
Poor intake or malabsorption (e.g. coeliac disease)
Liver failure (decreased 25-hydroxylation of vitamin D), medications increasing vitamin D metabolism, e.g. phenytoin
Chronic kidney disease
Impaired activation of vitamin D due to mutations in the 1α-hydroxylase gene (vitamin D-dependent rickets type 1)
Target organ resistance due to mutations in the vitamin D receptor gene (vitamin D-dependent rickets type 2)

Hypoparathyroidism
Post thyroid or parathyroid surgery (hypoparathyroidism may be transient or permanent)
Autoimmune, e.g. part of autoimmune polyglandular syndrome type 1 (see Chapter 6)
Infiltrative diseases of the parathyroid glands: haemochromatosis, Wilson's disease, granulomas, metastatic cancer
Congenital: DiGeorge syndrome (defective development of the pharyngeal pouch system, resulting in cardiac defects, cleft palate and abnormal facies, hypoplastic thymus and hypoparathyroidism)
Hypomagnesaemia: due to malabsorption, chronic alcoholism, prolonged parenteral fluid administration, diuretics, aminoglycosides and cisplatin
HIV infection

Pseudohypoparathyroidism (end-organ parathyroid hormone resistance): type 1a, type 1b, type 2

Extravascular calcium deposition
Hungry bone syndrome
Pancreatitis
Rhabdomyolysis
Tumour lysis syndrome
Widespread osteoblastic metastases

Increased intravascular calcium binding
Respiratory alkalosis
Massive blood transfusions

Sepsis

Drugs
Combination chemotherapy with 5-fluorouracil and leucovorin (decreases calcitriol production), fluoride poisoning (inhibits bone resorption), bisphosphonates (suppress the formation and function of osteoclasts)

Calcium-sensing receptor gene mutations (autosomal dominant) or **autoantibodies** directed against the calcium-sensing receptor

---

Rarer causes of hypocalcaemia include calcium-sensing receptor gene mutations (autosomal dominant) or autoantibodies directed against the calcium-sensing receptor, resulting in hypocalcaemia and hypercalciuria.

Pseudohypocalcaemia may be seen in patients who have had some of the gadolinium-based contrast agents for magnetic resonance angiography, due to interference with the colorimetric assays for calcium.

Clinical presentations

Box 24.2 summarizes the clinical manifestations of hypocalcaemia.

Box 24.2 Clinical presentations of hypocalcaemia

Musculoskeletal

Tetany, muscle spasms/cramps, paraesthesia (perioral/peripheral), myopathy

Chvostek's sign: tapping the facial nerve in front of the ear causes contraction of the facial muscles ipsilaterally

Trousseau's sign: inflating the blood pressure cuff to above systolic blood pressure causes carpal spasm

Neuropsychiatric/eyes

Seizures, fatigue, depression, anxiety, in children mental retardation

Movement disorders: dystonia, hemiballismus, basal ganglia calcifications

Eyes: cataracts, papilloedema with severe hypocalcaemia, keratoconjunctivitis

Cardiovascular

Cardiac failure, hypotension, prolonged QT interval, decreased digoxin effect

Gastrointestinal

Reduced gastric acid secretion, steatorrhoea

Skin

Dry and coarse skin and hair, brittle nails

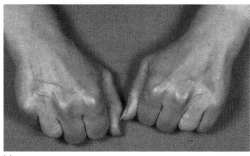

(a)

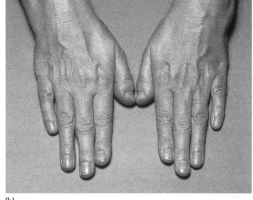

(b)

Figure 24.1 Shortening of the fourth (a) and fifth (b) fingers due to short metacarpals.

Pseudohypoparathyroidism

Pseudohypoparathyroidism is characterized by PTH resistance usually caused by mutations in the *GNAS* gene (encoding the alpha subunit of the G protein, coupled to the PTH receptor), resulting in an inability of PTH to activate adenylate cyclase.

- In *type 1a disease*, patients with maternally inherited mutations have hypocalcaemia (due to PTH resistance in the kidney) as well as phenotypic abnormalities (short stature, obesity, round face, short fourth/fifth metacarpals (Fig. 24.1), subcutaneous calcification, occasionally mental retardation), known as Albright's hereditary osteodystrophy (AHO).

Patients with paternally inherited mutations have the phenotypic abnormalities of AHO (due to impaired PTH action in bone) but have normal serum calcium levels. This is an example of tissue-specific genetic imprinting.

- *Type 1b* is characterized by hypocalcaemia but not the phenotypic abnormalities of AHO (as PTH resistance is confined to the kidney).

- *Type 2*: the molecular defect in the rare type 2 pseudohypoparathyroidism has not been identified (see 'Investigations' below).

Investigations

Total serum calcium is the sum of free (ionized) calcium and calcium bound to albumin. Changes in serum albumin result in a change in the amount of bound calcium and total calcium, but not free (ionized) calcium. Therefore the 'total serum calcium' measurement should always be adjusted for albumin levels.

Approximately 40% of circulating calcium is bound to albumin in a ratio of 0.02 mmol/L of calcium per 1.0 g/L of albumin. Therefore to calculate 'adjusted' (corrected) total calcium: add 0.02 mmol/L to total calcium levels for every g/L of albumin below 40 and subtract 0.02 mmol/L from total calcium for every g/L of albumin over 40.

Useful tests in determining the cause of hypocalcaemia include serum *phosphate, magnesium, alkaline phosphatase, creatinine, alanine transaminase*, a *coeliac screen, 25-hydroxyvitamin D, 1,25-dihydoxyvitamin D* and intact *PTH*. In hypoparathyroidism, phosphate levels may be normal or high, and PTH is low or inappropriately normal despite low serum calcium. In vitamin D deficiency, serum phosphate levels are low or normal, urinary calcium excretion may be low, bone-specific alkaline phosphatase is elevated and PTH is raised (secondary hyperparathyroidism).

In patients with type 1 pseudohypoparathyroidism, the infusion of PTH fails to induce an increase in urinary cyclic AMP and phosphate excretion (the Ellsworth–Howard test). Patients must be vitamin D replete before the test. In rare type 2 pseudohypoparathyroidism, there is a normal cyclic AMP response without a concomitant increase in phosphate excretion.

Treatment

Patients with an adjusted total calcium of more than 1.9 mmol/L are usually asymptomatic and can be treated by increasing dietary calcium intake by 1 g per day (except in those with hyperphosphataemia).

Many patients become symptomatic when serum total calcium concentration is less than 1.9 mmol/L. Intravenous calcium is required particularly in patients with tetany, seizures, ECG changes and reduced cardiac function.

Calcium gluconate is preferred over calcium chloride as it causes less local tissue necrosis. If the patient is symptomatic, treatment is started with 10 mL 10% w/v calcium gluconate (diluted in 100 mL 0.9% saline or 5% dextrose) infused over 10–20 minutes (with cardiac monitoring). This will increase the serum calcium levels for 2–3 hours, and should be followed by a slow infusion of calcium. A dose of 100 mL 10% calcium gluconate is added to 1 L of 0.9% saline (or 5% dextrose). The infusion may be started at 50 mL per hour and titrated to maintain serum calcium in the low-normal range.

A solution of 10% calcium gluconate contains 10 g of calcium gluconate in 100 mL, and 10 g of calcium gluconate contains about 900 mg of elemental calcium. Therefore adding 100 mL of 10% calcium to 1 L of fluid gives a preparation close to 1 mg/mL of elemental calcium. Calcium infusion is usually given at 0.5–1.5 mg/kg per hour of elemental calcium.

Concomitant hypomagnesaemia should be corrected with intravenous magnesium sulphate. Magnesium sulphate 2 g (8 mmol) is given over 10–20 minutes, followed by another 4 g in the next 4 hours if necessary.

Intravenous calcium should be continued until the patient is receiving an effective regimen of oral calcium and vitamin D. Calcitriol (1,25-dihydroxycholecalciferol) is the preferred preparation of vitamin D for patients with severe acute hypocalcaemia because of its rapid onset of action. Calcitriol should be started immediately at a dose of 0.5–1 μg per day. The doses of calcitriol and oral calcium are adjusted to maintain serum calcium in the low-normal range (2.0–2.1 mmol/L). This is because patients with hypoparathyroidism have decreased calcium reabsorption in the distal tubules. Raising plasma calcium above 2.1 mmol/L may result in marked hypercalciuria and calcium stone formation.

Even in stable patients, serum and urinary calcium should be checked every 6 months to check for hypercalcaemia and hypercalciuria.

In patients with the rare mutations in the calcium-sensing receptor, vitamin D results in further hypercalciuria, nephrocalcinosis and renal impairment. Therefore asymptomatic patients are generally left untreated.

Key points:

- The 'total serum calcium' measurement should always be adjusted for albumin levels.
- Clinical presentations of hypocalcaemia include tetany, paraesthesia, cardiac dysfunction and seizures.
- Hypocalcaemia may be caused by either decreased calcium entry into the circulation (e.g. due to hypoparathyroidism or vitamin D deficiency) or increased loss of free calcium from the circulation (due to deposition in tissues or increased binding of calcium in serum).
- Investigation of hypocalcaemia should include serum phosphate, magnesium, alkaline phosphatase, creatinine, 25-hydroxyvitamin D and PTH levels.
- Symptomatic patients or those with calcium of below 1.9 mmol/L should receive intravenous calcium gluconate. Chronic hypocalcaemia, for example due to hypoparathyroidism, is treated with calcitriol and calcium supplements.
- The goal of treatment in chronic hypocalcaemia is to maintain serum calcium in the low-normal range without causing hypercalciuria.

Chapter 25

Hypercalcaemia and primary hyperparathyroidism

Calcium homeostasis

Most of the body's calcium exists as hydroxyapatite, which is the main mineral component of bone. In the plasma, 40% of calcium is bound to albumin, 15% is complexed with citrate, sulphate or phosphate, and 45% exists as the physiologically important free (ionized) calcium.

The plasma concentration of free calcium is regulated by *parathyroid hormone* (PTH) and *vitamin D*. The physiological roles of calcitonin in the regulation of calcium and phosphate balance are incompletely understood.

Parathyroid glands and PTH

PTH is a polypeptide secreted from the parathyroid glands. There are four parathyroid glands (one superior and one inferior gland on each side). They are about 6 mm long in their greatest diameter, and are embedded in the back of the thyroid gland. The superior glands develop from the fourth branchial pouch. The inferior glands develop from the third pouch. The thymus also develops from the third pouch, and may occasionally drag the inferior glands with it to the mediastinum.

PTH release is stimulated by a decrease in plasma free calcium levels. Changes in plasma free calcium

Lecture Notes: Endocrinology and Diabetes. By A. Sam and K. Meeran. Published 2009 by Blackwell Publishing. ISBN 978-1-4051-5345-4.

are sensed by a specific calcium-sensing receptor on the plasma membrane of the parathyroid cells. PTH increases plasma calcium by stimulating:
- *bone resorption*, resulting in the release of calcium and phosphate
- *intestinal absorption* of calcium by stimulating 1α-hydroxylation of 25-hydroxyvitamin D in the kidney and the formation of calcitriol (see below)
- *renal reabsorption* of calcium (in the distal tubule and connecting segment).

PTH reduces proximal tubular phosphate reabsorption by decreasing the activity of the type II sodium–phosphate co-transporter.

Vitamin D_3

Vitamin D_3 (cholecalciferol) is a fat-soluble steroid. Sources of vitamin D_3 include diet and synthesis in the skin from 7-dehydrocholesterol in the presence of ultraviolet light.

Vitamin D_3 is activated by 25-hydroxylation in the liver followed by 1α-hydroxylation in the kidney. 1,25-dihydroxyvitamin D (calcitriol) is the most active form of vitamin D. 1α-Hydroxylation is stimulated by PTH. Calcitriol stimulates bone resorption, intestinal absorption and renal reabsorption.

Hypercalcaemia

Hypercalcaemia is a relatively common clinical problem. Common causes of hypercalcaemia include the following.

Malignancy is the most common cause of hyper-calcaemia among hospitalized patients (about 65% of cases). Hypercalcaemia may be due to a local resorption of bone caused by metastases (mediated by the release of cytokines, tumour necrosis factor, interleukin-1) or the production of PTH-related protein (which activates osteoclasts).

Hyperparathyroidism is the most common cause of hypercalcaemia in ambulatory patients (>90% of cases). The effect of PTH on calcium levels is dis-cussed above. Hyperparathyroidism is discussed in more detail below.

In *hypervitaminosis D*, the source of excess vitamin D may be exogenous (excess intake of supplements) or endogenous (i.e. increased pro-duction of calcitriol in chronic granulomatous disorders such as tuberculosis, sarcoidosis and lym-phoma). Occasionally, the condition may be idio-pathic. The effect of vitamin D on plasma calcium levels is discussed above.

Familial hypocalciuric hypercalcaemia is an auto-somal dominant disorder caused by inactivating mutations in the gene encoding the calcium-sensing receptor on the parathyroid cells and in the kidneys. This results in mild resistance of the parathyroid cells to calcium, and reduced capacity of the kidneys to increase calcium excretion. Patients have mild hypercalcaemia with inappro-priately normal-to-slightly-increased serum PTH concentrations. Although this condition is rare, it must be excluded as a differential diagnosis of hyperparathyroidism as patients with this condi-tion have few if any symptoms of hypercalcaemia and require no treatment.

Less common causes of hypercalcaemia include:
- *drugs:* lithium (causes increased secretion of PTH), thiazide diuretics (lower urinary calcium excretion and usually unmask underlying hyper-parathyroidism), theophylline toxicity
- *immobility:* due to increased bone resorption
- *milk-alkali syndrome:* a high intake of milk or calcium carbonate (used to treat dyspepsia) may lead to hypercalcaemia mediated by the high calcium intake plus metabolic alkalosis, which augments calcium reabsorption in the distal tubule
- *other endocrine causes:* adrenal insufficiency, acromegaly, phaeochromocytoma (due to concur-rent hyperparathyroidism if part of multiple endocrine neoplasia [MEN] type 2 or due to the production of PTH-related protein), thyrotoxicosis or hypervitaminosis A (due to increased bone resorption).

Primary hyperparathyroidism

Most patients have only small elevations in serum calcium concentrations (<2.75 mmol/L), and many have mostly high-normal values with intermittent hypercalcaemia.

Aetiology

Primary hyperparathyroidism is due to either a solitary adenoma (80–85%), multiple adenomas or four-gland hyperplasia. Parathyroid carcinoma is a very rare cause of primary hyperparathyroidism (<0.5%).

Primary hyperparathyroidism is usually sporadic but may be associated with the following inherited syndromes:
- *MEN type 1*, characterized by hyperparathyroid-ism (in 90–95% of patients by the age of 50), pan-creatic endocrine tumours (30–80%) and pituitary adenomas (15–50%).
- *MEN type 2a*: up to 25% of patients have parathy-roid hyperplasia associated with medullary thyroid carcinoma (100%) and phaeochromocytoma (50%).

Other rare forms of inherited primary hyper-parathyroidism usually present at a younger age and include familial isolated hyperparathyroidism and hyperparathyroidism–jaw tumour syndrome (fibro-osseous tumours of the jaw associated with renal cysts or Wilms' tumour). Sporadic parathy-roid carcinomas frequently have *HRPT2* mutations that are likely to be of pathogenetic importance.

Epidemiology

The incidence of primary hyperparathyroidism has increased since the introduction of multi-channel autoanalyzers. More individuals have been diagnosed with primary hyperparathyroid-ism whose disease would not previously have been recognized simply because serum calcium was not routinely measured.

Clinical presentations

Most patients currently diagnosed with primary hyperparathyroidism have serum calcium levels less than 0.25 mmol/L above the reference range and are usually asymptomatic at diagnosis.

Symptomatic patients generally have serum calcium levels of 3.0 mmol/L or more. Patients may present with nausea, constipation, polydipsia and polyuria, depression and generalized aches and pains ('bones, stones, abdominal moans and groans'). However, many of these symptoms are common in the general population, and it is not clear whether they are causally related to primary hyperparathyroidism. The abnormalities most directly associated with hyperparathyroidism are nephrolithiasis (seen in 15–20% of newly diagnosed patients) and bone disease (see below).

Osteoporosis is a common feature of primary hyperparathyroidism and affects cortical bone, for example the distal radius, more than trabecular bone such as the vertebral bodies.

Osteitis fibrosa cystica is now rarely seen (<2% of patients), probably because routine serum calcium checks identify patients with primary hyperparathyroidism before this skeletal complication develops. Osteitis fibrosa cystica is characterized by generalized skeletal demineralization, subperiosteal bone resorption (e.g. on the radial aspect of the middle phalanges) and brown tumours (osteoclastomas) manifested as lytic lesions.

Patients with parathyroid carcinomas are more likely to have a marked hypercalcaemia, neck mass and symptoms of bone and kidney disease.

Investigations

In all patients with hypercalcaemia serum phosphate, vitamin D and PTH levels should be measured. Patients with primary hyperparathyroidism may have low or low-normal phosphate levels. Vitamin D deficiency should be excluded as the cause of raised PTH levels.

- In patients with *suppressed PTH*: myeloma, malignancy and granulomatous conditions causing excess production of 1,25-dihydroxyvitamin D (i.e. tuberculosis, sarcoidosis, lymphoma) should be excluded. Measure serum protein electrophoresis and urinary Bence Jones protein (to look for multiple myeloma) and serum angiotensin-converting enzyme (raised in sarcoidosis), and request further imaging (to look for malignancy).
- In patients with *high or inappropriately normal PTH levels*: the calcium-to-creatinine clearance ratio should be measured to differentiate between primary hyperparathyroidism (ratio >0.01) and familial hypocalciuric hypercalcaemia (ratio <0.01). This is calculated from simultaneous measurements of urine and serum calcium and creatinine concentrations, using the following formula:

$$\frac{\text{Urine calcium}(\text{mmol/L}) \times [\text{Plasma creatinine}(\mu\text{mol/L})/1000]}{\text{Plasma calcium}(\text{mmol}) \times \text{Urine creatinine}(\text{mmol/L})}$$

Patients with parathyroid carcinomas are more likely to have a marked hypercalcaemia with very high serum PTH levels.

A 24-hour urine collection should be sent for creatinine clearance and calcium measurement.

Imaging

Patients with confirmed primary hyperparathyroidism should also have a renal ultrasound at baseline to look for renal calculi.

Ultrasound of the neck and ^{99m}technetium sestamibi scan (Fig. 25.1) should be performed as part of preoperative localization when surgical intervention is indicated (see below).

More extensive preoperative imaging including magnetic resonance imaging, computed tomography, angiography and selective venous sampling may be required in patients with recurrent disease or ectopic parathyroid adenoma (e.g. mediastinal, intrathyroid, lateral neck, retro-oesophageal).

Treatment

The only curative treatment for primary hyperparathyroidism is surgery. However, surgery is not

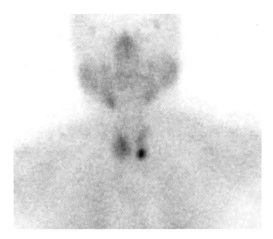

Figure 25.1 A left inferior parathyroid adenoma on a sestamibi scan.

appropriate in all patients. The potential benefits must be weighed against the risks in each case.

Indications for surgery

Guidelines for surgical intervention have been developed based on risk of disease progression and end-organ effects. Parathyroidectomy improves bone density and may have modest effects on some quality of life symptoms. The US National Institutes of Health guidelines (2002) for surgical intervention include:
- symptomatic patients
- asymptomatic patients with:
  — Age below 50 years (in a study of patients treated conservatively over 10 years, the disease progressed in 27% of asymptomatic patients, most of whom were younger than 50 years and age was the only predictive index)
  — Bone mineral density: T-score less than –2.5 (hip, spine, forearm)
  — Calculi (renal stones)
  — Creatinine clearance reduced by 30%
  — Difficult to do follow-up periodically
  — Elevated serum calcium more than 0.25 mmol/L above the upper limit of normal or 24-hour urinary calcium above 10 mmol. This is a relative indication for surgery. It is recognized that urinary calcium excretion correlates poorly with the development of renal stones.

It is important to note that the National Institutes of Health guidelines do not apply to familial primary hyperparathyroidism syndromes.

Bilateral neck exploration

Parathyroidectomy should be performed only by surgeons who are highly experienced and skilled in this operation. The standard surgical approach for most patients is bilateral neck exploration with identification of all four glands, usually under general anaesthesia. The amount of parathyroid tissue removed varies with the cause of hyperparathyroidism:
- The gland containing a *parathyroid adenoma* is removed. The other glands may be biopsied.
- For *four-gland hyperplasia*, three and one-half glands are removed, leaving one-half of the most normal-appearing gland marked with a clip.
- In patients with *MEN type 1*, total parathyroidectomy may be performed (with surgical implantation of parathyroid tissue in the forearm in some centres) because of the high recurrence rate.

Minimally invasive parathyroidectomy

Minimally invasive parathyroidectomy may be the procedure of choice in patients with unilateral pathology (detected by imaging), with no family history of MEN and in the high-risk elderly.

Minimally invasive parathyroidectomy may be performed if ^{99m}technetium sestamibi and ultrasound scans both show an adenoma in the same location ('concordant' imaging). The location is marked on the skin, and surgery is performed through a 2–4 cm incision under local anaesthetic.

Minimally invasive parathyroidectomy requires an intraoperative test to confirm that the adenoma removed is the only source of abnormal glandular activity. The short plasma half-life of PTH (3–4 minutes) and a rapid assay for PTH make it a useful test for this purpose. A reduction of over 50% in serum PTH measured shortly after the resection compared with preincision levels is considered successful, and the operation is terminated. Alternatively, technetium-labelled sestamibi may be administered intravenously 1–2 hours preoperatively. After the suspected adenoma has been removed, a gamma probe is used to measure the radioactivity of the excised tissue, which is compared with the radioactivity of the surgical bed.

Minimally invasive surgery is not an option for patients with non-concordant imaging, multi-gland disease or a history of previous surgery. The cure rates of bilateral neck exploration and minimally invasive parathyroidectomy are similar (95–98%), and complication rates with both are low with an experienced surgeon.

For parathyroid carcinomas, surgery is the initial therapy. Treatment becomes limited to the control of hypercalcaemia with hydration or a bisphosphonate when the tumour is no longer amenable to surgical intervention. Cinacalcet (a calcimimetic agent) has recently been approved for the treatment of hypercalcaemia in patients with parathyroid cancer. Some patients have germline *HRPT2* mutations, and genetic evaluation can play an important role in management of such patients and their family members.

Postoperative hypocalcaemia

Serum corrected calcium and magnesium should initially be checked at least daily. Following parathyroidectomy, calcium starts to fall 4–12 hours after the surgery. The nadir is reached by 24 hours. If the patient becomes hypocalcaemic, it may be due to the following:
• *Functional hypoparathyroidism* (due to the suppression of other parathyroid glands, parathyroid gland ischaemia, hypomagnesaemia): PTH levels checked after day 3 (postoperatively) are detectable. This transient hypoparathyroidism may develop in up to 70% of patients and usually resolves within 1–3 weeks. Patients may require oral calcium supplements and a 1α-hydroxylated vitamin D metabolite.
• *Hungry bone syndrome* causes severe hypocalcaemia, hypophosphataemia and hypomagnesaemia due to extensive skeletal remineralization.
• *Permanent hypoparathyroidism*: PTH levels checked after day 3 (postoperatively) will be undetectable (<1 pg/mL). Patients with permanent hypoparathyroidism (<2%) require lifelong treatment with a 1α-hydroxylated vitamin D metabolite.

In severe hypocalcaemia (calcium <1.6 mmol/L), intravenous calcium gluconate should initially be given with cardiac monitoring (see Chapter 24). Hypomagnesaemia should be treated with intravenous magnesium sulphate. Oral calcium (e.g. calcium carbonate) is started at a dose of 2.0–2.4 g daily, and calcitriol (or alfacalcidol) is given at a dose of 1 μg per day.

The goal is to relieve symptoms and to achieve a serum calcium concentration in the low-normal range (2.0–2.1 mmol/L). This is because these patients lack the normal stimulatory effect of PTH on renal tubular calcium reabsorption, and therefore excrete more calcium than normal subjects at the same serum calcium concentration. Therefore completely correcting hypocalcaemia may result in hypercalciuria, nephrolithiasis, nephrocalcinosis and chronic renal insufficiency. The diet also should be limited in phosphate to minimize hyperphosphataemia.

The dose of calcium and vitamin D should be adjusted according to the patient's serum calcium values. Urinary calcium excretion should be measured periodically, and the dose of calcium reduced if it is elevated. Patients are usually weaned off calcium supplementation and calcitriol (or alfacalcidol) is continued.

Medical management

Patients who do not meet surgical criteria or who prefer to avoid surgery are managed conservatively with periodic follow-up (see below). Patients should be advised to:
• avoid factors that can exacerbate hypercalcaemia, including thiazide diuretic and lithium therapy, dehydration, prolonged bed rest and inactivity
• maintain adequate hydration (at least 6–8 glasses of water per day)
• maintain a moderate calcium intake (1000 mg per day). A low-calcium diet may lead to increased PTH secretion and aggravate bone disease. A high-calcium diet may exacerbate hypercalcaemia
• maintain moderate vitamin D intake (400–600 IU daily). Vitamin D deficiency stimulates PTH secretion and bone resorption.

About 25% of patients with primary hyperparathyroidism managed conservatively for 10 years develop an indication for surgery (worsening hypercalcaemia, hypercalciuria, renal calculi, osteoporosis) and will benefit from surgical intervention.

In patients with osteopenia or osteoporosis who are not candidates for surgery, bisphosphonates should be given to preserve bone mass.

Cinacalcet is a calcimimetic agent that increases the sensitivity of the calcium-sensing receptors to extracellular calcium, resulting in reduced PTH secretion. Cinacalcet may become the preferred medical therapy for patients who are not candidates for surgery if longer-term studies demonstrate persistent improvements in biochemical abnormalities and neurocognitive function, stabilization of bone mineral density and a good safety profile.

Follow-up and monitoring

Patients with primary hyperparathyroidism who are managed conservatively should have:
- a baseline 24-hour urine collection for calcium and creatinine clearance measurement
- a baseline renal ultrasound to look for renal calculi
- serum calcium measured every 6 months
- serum creatinine measured once a year
- a dual-energy X-ray absorptiometry scan every 2 years.

Management of severe hypercalcaemia

Patients with severe symptomatic hypercalcaemia require rehydration with 3–6 L 0.9% saline in the first 24 hours. Once rehydrated, 0.9% saline infusion is continued, and furosemide (20–40 mg every 2–4 hours) may be given to encourage calciuresis. Potassium must be added to fluids to avoid hypokalaemia if furosemide is used.

If rehydration fails to correct symptoms or the calcium level remains above 2.8 mmol/L, or if there is a known underlying malignancy at the outset, intravenous pamidronate (a bisphosphonate) may be given. The dose of pamidronate depends on the level of hypercalcaemia (30 mg over 2 hours with calcium <3 mmol/L or significant renal impairment, 60 mg over 4 hours with calcium 3.0–3.4 mmol/L, and 90 mg over 6 hours with calcium >3.4 mmol/L). The pamidronate infusion should be made up in a concentration no greater than 60 mg in 250 mL of 0.9% saline.

The use of intravenous pamidronate results in a decrease in plasma calcium over 3–5 days. Doses should not be repeated sooner than a minimum of 7 days.

Patients with humoral hypercalcaemia of malignancy due to production of PTH-related protein by the tumour may have a better response to zoledronic acid or gallium nitrate.

Bisphosphonates are not necessary in patients with hypercalcaemia secondary to primary hyperparathyroidism as they often respond to rehydration. Bisphosphonates should particularly be avoided if parathyroid surgery is imminent as their use can cause profound hypocalcaemia postoperatively.

Glucocorticoids (prednisolone 40–60 mg per day orally) should be considered if hypercalcaemia is secondary to sarcoidosis, hypervitaminosis D or myeloma.

> **Key points:**
>
> - The plasma concentration of free calcium is regulated by PTH and vitamin D.
> - Malignancy is the most common cause of hypercalcaemia among hospitalized patients.
> - Hyperparathyroidism is the most common cause of hypercalcaemia in ambulatory patients.
> - Primary hyperparathyroidism may be due to a solitary adenoma (85%), multiple adenomas or four-gland hyperplasia.
> - Hyperparathyroidism may be part of MEN type 1 or 2a.
> - The only curative treatment for primary hyperparathyroidism is surgery.
> - The accepted criteria for parathyroid surgery include symptoms, age below 50 years, osteoporosis, reduced creatinine clearance and renal calculi.
> - Parathyroid surgery may be complicated by hypocalcaemia.
> - Patients who do not meet surgical criteria or who prefer to avoid surgery are managed conservatively with periodic follow-up and adequate oral fluid intake.

Chapter 26

Osteomalacia

Osteomalacia is a disorder of *mineralization* of bone matrix ('osteoid'). Rickets is a disorder of defective mineralization of cartilage in the epiphyseal growth plates of children.

Aetiology

Osteoclasts begin the bone remodelling cycle by excavating a cavity on the bone surface. Osteoblasts lay down the organic matrix ('osteoid').

The process of bone mineralization begins in the 'matrix vesicles'. Matrix vesicles are extracellular organelles derived from the plasma membrane of chondrocytes. Calcium is transported from the extracellular space into the matrix vesicles. Phosphatases (e.g. alkaline phosphatase) increase the inorganic phosphate levels inside the matrix vesicles. The increase in intravesicular calcium and phosphate results in a deposition of calcium phosphate, which undergoes conversion to hydroxyapatite. The hydroxyapatite crystals are subsequently released from the matrix vesicles.

Defective bone mineralization in osteomalacia is mostly due to reduced calcium and phosphate levels in the extracellular fluid. This may be due to *vitamin D deficiency* or *phosphate deficiency* secondary to primary renal phosphate wasting.

Lecture Notes: Endocrinology and Diabetes. By A. Sam and K. Meeran. Published 2009 by Blackwell Publishing. ISBN 978-1-4051-5345-4.

Vitamin D deficiency

Vitamin D_3 (cholecalciferol) may either be taken in the diet (e.g. fish, eggs) or synthesized in the skin from 7-dehydrocholesterol by the ultraviolet light in sunshine (Fig. 26.1). Vitamin D is activated by hydroxylation in the liver (25-hydroxylation) and the kidneys (1α-hydroxylation), resulting in 1,25-dihydoxyvitamin D.

Causes of vitamin D deficiency are summarized in Box 26.1.

The exact concentrations of 25-hydroxyvitamin D associated with osteomalacia are still not entirely clear. Variability of the assays and the lack of standardization are still a problem in this area. 25-Hydroxyvitamin D concentrations less than 8 ng/mL (20 nmol/L) are generally associated with osteomalacia. Vitamin D deficiency is defined as 25-hydroxyvitamin D levels less than 20 ng/mL (<50 nmol/L). Vitamin D levels between 20 and 30 ng/mL (50–75 nmol/L) are termed 'insufficient'.

Vitamin D insufficiency is extremely common and may contribute to the development of osteoporosis, falls and fractures.

Renal phosphate wasting

Primary renal phosphate wasting can occur in:
• *renal tubular acidosis* (type 2) due to defective proximal tubular transport. This may be congenital (Fanconi's syndrome, Wilson's disease, cystino-

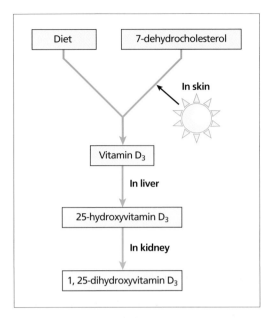

Figure 26.1 Vitamin D₃ may either be taken in the diet or synthesized in the skin from 7-dehydrocholesterol by the effect of ultraviolet light in sunshine. Vitamin D₃ is activated by hydroxylation in the liver and kidneys.

sis) or acquired (e.g. in patients with multiple myeloma)

- *X-linked hypophosphataemic rickets*: mutations in a gene named *PHEX*, which codes for a cleaving enzyme, result in reduced inactivation of hormone-like substances ('phosphatonins') such as fibroblast growth factor-23 (FGF23) that promote phosphate excretion
- *autosomal dominant hypophosphataemic rickets*: mutations in the gene for FGF23 interfere with its cleavage
- *oncogenic (tumour-induced) osteomalacia*: excess FGF23 is produced by the tumour (usually mesenchymal tumours).

Rarer causes

These include inadequate alkaline phosphatase activity (hypophosphatasia), inhibition of mineralization by excess fluoride ingestion and abnormal bone matrix, for example in osteogenesis imperfecta or fibrogenesis imperfecta.

Box 26.1 Causes of osteomalacia

Vitamin D deficiency
Reduced synthesis, intake or absorption
Inadequate sunlight exposure
Malabsorption: small bowel disease (e.g. coeliac disease, inflammatory bowel disease), extensive bowel surgery, gastrectomy, pancreatic insufficiency

Reduced 25-hydroxylation of vitamin D
Liver disease
Anticonvulsants

Reduced 1α-hydroxylation
Chronic kidney disease
Hypoparathyroidism (reduced stimulation of vitamin D 1α-hydroxylation by PTH)
Vitamin D-dependent rickets type 1 (an autosomal recessive disorder caused by mutations in the gene encoding the enzyme 1α-hydroxylase)
Vitamin D-dependent rickets type 2 (an autosomal recessive disorder caused by mutations in the gene encoding the vitamin D receptor, resulting in target organ resistance to vitamin D)

Primary renal phosphate wasting
Type 2 renal tubular acidosis: Fanconi's syndrome, multiple myeloma
Hereditary hypophosphataemic rickets (X-linked and autosomal dominant)
Oncogenic osteomalacia

Rarer causes
Abnormal bone matrix: osteogenesis imperfecta, fibrogenesis imperfecta
Hypophosphatasia (associated with periodontal disease)
Mineralization inhibitors: high doses of fluoride (e.g. in certain teas), aluminium, bisphosphonates

Clinical presentations

Osteomalacia may be asymptomatic and present radiologically as osteopenia. Clinically, patients with osteomalacia may present with diffuse bone pain and tenderness, fractures with little or no trauma (typically in the ribs, vertebrae and long bones) and proximal muscle weakness, which may be associated with a waddling gait.

History and physical examination should look for symptoms and signs of the possible underlying cause.

Children with rickets may present with hypotonia, growth retardation and skeletal deformities.

The laying down of uncalcified osteoid at the metaphases leads to widening of the ends of the long bones. This may be seen as 'rachitic rosary' in the ribs (enlarged ends of the ribs resembling beads at the costochondral junction) and at the level of the ankle and the wrist. Other skeletal deformities include frontal bossing, pectus carinatum and bowing of the long bones.

Investigations

Radiographic findings

A *spine X-ray* may show decreased bone density, with blurring and deformity of the spine that makes the films appear of low quality. Concavity of the vertebral bodies is seen in more advanced disease.

Looser's zones or 'pseudofractures' are the characteristic radiological finding in osteomalacia. These are narrow radiolucent lines (2–5 mm in width) with sclerotic borders that often lie perpendicular to the cortical margins of the bones. They are usually found at the femoral neck, on the medial part of the femoral shaft and on the pubic rami. They may also occur at the ulna, scapula, clavicle, rib and metatarsal bones. It has been proposed that Looser's zones may represent stress fractures that have been repaired by inadequately mineralized osteoid. They have also been suggested to be the result of erosion by arterial pulsations.

More severe disease can lead to shortening and bowing of the tibia, fractures and coxa profunda hip deformity (in which the femoral head comes deeply into the pelvis).

Laboratory findings

Patients with vitamin D deficiency may have:
- low plasma phosphate levels
- low-normal to low plasma calcium levels
- an increased alkaline phosphatase level
- low levels of 25-hydroxyvitamin D
- increased PTH (secondary hyperparathyroidism).

Patients with primary renal phosphate wasting have:
- low plasma phosphate levels
- increased phosphate excretion: if the renal phosphate wasting is not the cause of the hypophosphataemia, the fractional excretion of phosphate should be well below 5%
- a normal anion gap (hyperchloraemic) metabolic acidosis if the patients have renal tubular acidosis.

Patients with hypophosphatasia have low alkaline phosphatase levels but normal plasma calcium and phosphate concentrations.

In patients with tumour-induced osteomalacia, a thorough search for the tumour must be undertaken with magnetic resonance imaging or technetium scans.

Osteomalacia can be accurately diagnosed by bone biopsy using double tetracycline labelling. Tetracycline is deposited at the mineralization front as a band. After two courses of tetracycline (separated by a period of days), the distance between the bands of deposited tetracycline is reduced in osteomalacia. However, despite its accuracy, bone biopsy is not usually performed as osteomalacia can be diagnosed from the history, examination, laboratory and radiological studies.

Treatment

Treatment should include reversal of the underlying disorder (e.g. a gluten-free diet in coeliac disease) and supplementation with vitamin D and calcium (at least 1000 mg per day). Vitamin D replacement reduces fracture rate and improves bone tenderness and muscle weakness.

Vitamin D replacement

Patients with nutritional vitamin D deficiency may initially be treated with 50 000 IU of oral vitamin D_2 (ergocalciferol) or D_3 (cholecalciferol) once a week for 6–12 weeks, followed by maintenance doses of 800–1000 IU of vitamin D_3 daily. Vitamin D_2 is made by ultraviolet irradiation of ergosterol obtained from yeast. A dose of 300 000 IU of intramuscular ergocalciferol in one or two doses per year is an alternative option when poor compliance is suspected.

25-Hydroxyvitamin D concentrations should be measured approximately 3 months after initiating therapy. The dose of vitamin D may require adjustment depending upon individual absorption.

In patients with a gastrectomy or malabsorption, high doses of vitamin D (10000–50000 IU daily) may be necessary. The adequacy of the calcium and vitamin D supplementation should be confirmed by measurements of serum calcium, phosphate, 25-hydroxyvitamin D and parathyroid hormone (PTH).

Vitamin D-deficient and -insufficient pregnant women are treated more slowly, by giving 800–1000 IU of vitamin D_3 daily. Urinary calcium excretion increases in pregnancy, and it should be monitored when treating vitamin D deficiency, particularly in women with a history of renal stones.

Patients with defective vitamin D_3 hydroxylation (e.g. due to chronic renal failure or liver disease) are treated with alfacalcidol or calcitriol (0.25–1.0 μg per day), which have a rapid onset of action and a shorter half-life (around 6 hours).

Patients with hereditary hypophosphataemic rickets are treated with a combination of oral phosphate supplementation and calcitriol.

Patients with vitamin D insufficiency may be treated with 800–1000 IU of vitamin D_3 daily. Vitamin D replacement in patients with coexisting vitamin D insufficiency and primary hyperparathyroidism is controversial. A recent small study of vitamin D replacement in patients with coexisting vitamin D insufficiency and primary hyperparathyroidism (with mild hypercalcaemia) showed a decrease in PTH level and no increase in mean calcium concentrations.

Follow-up and monitoring

In hypocalcaemic patients, serum calcium is monitored every 2 weeks until normocalcaemic (to permit early detection of hypercalcaemia from excessive dosing). The 24-hour urinary calcium should be monitored initially after 3 months and less frequently as plasma calcium stabilizes. Maintenance of normal urinary calcium levels often indicates that treatment is effective.

Serum calcium, phosphate, alkaline phosphatase, PTH levels and vitamin D (25-hydroxyvitamin D or 1,25-dihydroxyvitamin D depending on the aetiology of the osteomalacia) should be rechecked after 3 months of therapy and at regular intervals thereafter. The dose of vitamin D should be adjusted accordingly.

Key points:

- Osteomalacia is a disorder of decreased mineralization of bone matrix.
- Defective mineralization in osteomalacia is mostly due to reduced calcium and phosphate levels in the extracellular fluid, which may be caused by vitamin D deficiency or primary renal phosphate wasting.
- Osteomalacia may present with diffuse bone pain and tenderness, fractures and proximal muscle weakness.
- Looser's zones or 'pseudofractures' are the characteristic radiological finding in osteomalacia.
- Patients with osteomalacia may have low plasma phosphate, low plasma calcium, increased alkaline phosphatase and low levels of 25-hydroxyvitamin D or increased phosphate excretion.
- Treatment should include reversal of the underlying disorder and supplementation with vitamin D and calcium.
- Patients with hereditary hypophosphataemic rickets may be treated with a combination of oral phosphate supplementation and calcitriol.

Chapter 27

Osteoporosis

Bone remodelling

Bone is continuously formed and resorbed. This 'remodelling' process is important in the prevention of fatigue damage and the maintenance of calcium homeostasis. Around 10% of the skeleton is 'remodelled' each year in adults.

The bone remodelling cycle consists of three phases (Fig. 27.1):
- *Resorption:* osteoclasts remove matrix and mineral on the trabecular surface or within the cortical bone.
- *Reversal:* mononuclear cells, possibly of monocyte/macrophage lineage, appear on the bone surface and may provide signals for osteoblast differentiation and migration. A layer of glycoprotein-rich material is laid down on the resorbed surface, to which the new osteoblasts can adhere. Osteopontin may be a key protein in this process.
- *Formation:* osteoblasts lay down bone to replace resorbed bone.

Cellular signals regulating bone remodelling

Cells of the osteoblast lineage express a factor called RANKL (receptor activator of nuclear factor kappa B ligand), which interacts with a receptor on osteoclast precursors called RANK and results in the activation and differentiation of osteoclasts. RANKL can also bind to a protein produced by osteoblasts and other marrow cells called osteoprotegerin or osteoclastogenesis inhibitory factor. The role of osteoprotegerin in the pathogenesis of osteoporosis is uncertain

Osteoporosis

Osteoporosis is a skeletal disease characterized by reduced bone mass and microarchitectural deterioration, resulting in increased bone fragility and fracture risk.

Epidemiology

According to the International Osteoporosis Foundation, osteoporosis affects approximately 1 in 3 women and 1 in 8 men worldwide. After the age of 50 years, the risk of osteoporotic fractures is 40% in women and 15% in men. This risk is termed the 'lifetime fracture risk'. In both men and women, the incidence of hip fractures increases exponentially with age, although the increase begins approximately 5–10 years later in men.

Aetiology

Osteoporosis is characterized by increased bone turnover. However, an imbalance between rates of bone formation and resorption results in bone loss

Lecture Notes: Endocrinology and Diabetes. By A. Sam and K. Meeran. Published 2009 by Blackwell Publishing. ISBN 978-1-4051-5345-4.

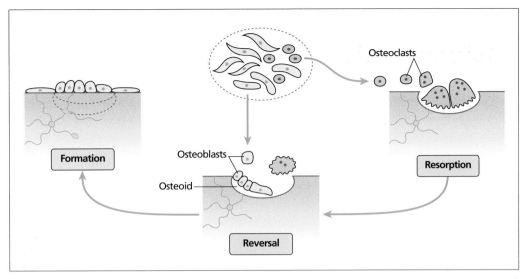

Figure 27.1 The process of bone remodelling. Osteoclast precursors are attracted to the site to be resorbed. They differentiate and fuse to form multinucleated osteoclasts, which resorb bone by secreting acid and proteolytic enzymes. Osteoblast precursors are attracted to the site that has undergone resorption. They differentiate and lay down uncalcified bone matrix (osteoid), which then calcifies to form mature bone.

and consequent trabecular thinning and perforation, with loss of bone strength.

Bone mineral density (BMD) changes with age (Fig. 27.2). The maximum BMD ('peak bone mass') is achieved by the age of 30–40 years. Thereafter, bone is lost in both men and women at a rate of about 1% per year. Women experience a phase of accelerated bone loss for 3 years after the menopause. A decrease in spine BMD of 1 standard deviation (or 12%) doubles the risk of fracture. Box 27.1 summarizes the factors that increase the rate of bone loss.

Clinical presentations

Osteoporosis does not cause pain or deformity per se but increases the risk of fractures that can then result in pain, deformity, increased dependence and mortality. Osteoporosis-related fractures associated with minor trauma tend to occur at sites comprising more than 50% trabecular bone (i.e. less than 50% cortical bone). These sites include the:

• *vertebral bodies*: these fractures result in backache that usually subsides after 3 months. Chronic pain

> **Box 27.1 Factors associated with increased bone loss**
>
> Family history
> Lifestyle: reduced exercise, excess alcohol, smoking
> Drugs: corticosteroids, cyclosporine, cytotoxic agents, heparin
> Endocrine causes: hypogonadism, hyperparathyroidism, Cushing's syndrome, osteomalacia, thyrotoxicosis
> Malabsorption: coeliac disease
> Myeloma
> Liver disease
> Renal disease
> Anorexia nervosa
> Rheumatoid arthritis and other inflammatory conditions

may occur due to secondary osteoarthritis. Vertebral fractures also result in kyphosis, loss of height and abdominal protrusion. Vertebral fractures may appear as wedge deformity (loss of anterior height), end-plate deformity (loss of middle height) or compression deformity (loss of anterior, posterior and middle height)

• *proximal femur*: mortality is increased by 20% in the first year following a hip fracture

• *distal radius* (Colles' fracture).

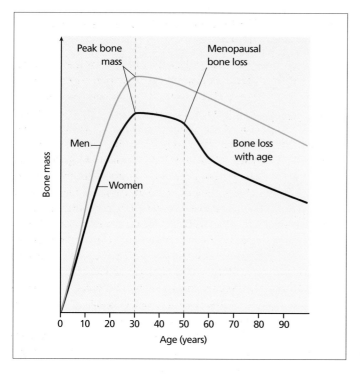

Figure 27.2 Changes in bone mass with age in men and women.

Investigations

Diagnosis

In patients presenting with osteoporosis-related fractures, BMD is measured using *dual-energy X-ray absorptiometry* (DEXA). It is worthwhile measuring BMD in patients with low-trauma fractures and those with strong risk factors, for example taking long-term corticosteroids.

Low doses of X-rays of two different energy levels are directed toward areas of interest (lumbar spine, proximal femur, distal radius) and are absorbed to different extents by bone and soft tissue. This principle is used to calculate bone density in g/cm².

The *T-score* compares the patient's BMD with that of a young reference population. The World Health Organization (WHO) has selected a T-score of −2.5 or less to define osteoporosis in healthy postmenopausal women and men aged 50 years and older. The diagnosis of osteoporosis is made by DEXA using the lowest T-score of the lumbar spine (L1–L4), proximal femur or distal radius. A T-score of between −2.5 and −1.0 is referred to as osteopenia.

The *Z-score* compares the patient's BMD to that of an age-matched reference population. In premenopausal women and younger men, the relationship between BMD and risk of fracture is not well established. For premenopausal women and men under age 50 years, Z-scores rather than T-scores should be used. In these patients, a clinical diagnosis of osteoporosis may be made in the presence of a fragility fracture, or when there is low BMD and risk factors for fracture, such as long-term steroid therapy or hyperparathyroidism.

Secondary causes

Patients with osteoporosis-related fractures resulting from minor trauma should be investigated to look for secondary causes (Box 27.2).

Other investigations

Markers of bone turnover are not useful in the diagnosis of osteoporosis as there is substantial

Box 27.2 Investigations for secondary causes of osteoporosis

Endocrine causes

Hypogonadism: luteinizing hormone, follicle-stimulating hormone, oestradiol (premenopausal women) or testosterone (men)

Primary hyperparathyroidism: calcium, phosphate, parathyroid hormone

Osteomalacia: calcium, phosphate, alkaline phosphatase, 25-hydroxyvitamin D, 1,25-dihydroxyvitamin D (if indicated)

Thyrotoxicosis: thyroid-stimulating hormone, free thyroxine

Cushing's syndrome: 24-hour urine free cortisol or overnight dexamethasone suppression test (if clinically indicated)

Myeloma

Erythrocyte sedimentation rate, serum protein electrophoresis, urinary Bence Jones protein

Malabsorption

Full blood count, coeliac screen

overlap in normal subjects and patients with osteoporosis. Bone biopsy is rarely used but can be in unusual forms of osteoporosis in young adults. It may provide information about the presence of rare secondary forms of osteoporosis (e.g. systemic mastocytosis).

Treatment

The aims of treatment are:

• alleviation of symptoms (with adequate analgesics)

• reduction of the risk of further fractures (currently available drugs for osteoporosis reduce the incidence of fractures by up to 50%)

• treatment of the underlying cause: this often leads to a partial recovery of bone mass.

All patients with low BMD should receive adequate calcium (1200 mg per day), vitamin D (800 U per day), advice regarding lifestyle modifications, i.e. weight-bearing exercise, smoking cessation and avoidance of excessive alcohol use, and fall prevention counselling.

WHO Fracture Risk Assessment Tool (FRAX)

The *FRAX* calculator (http://www.sheffield.ac.uk/FRAX/index.htm) may be used to calculate the 10-year probability of hip fracture and major osteoporotic (clinical spine, forearm, hip, shoulder) fracture. The FRAX calculator requires information regarding age, sex, weight, height, previous fractures, parental fractured hip, current smoking, alcohol (≥3 units per day), glucocorticoids (>3 months at a dose of prednisolone ≥5 mg per day), rheumatoid arthritis, secondary osteoporosis (due to untreated longstanding hyperthyroidism, hypogonadism, chronic malnutrition/malabsorption, chronic liver disease, type 1 diabetes, osteogenesis imperfecta in adults) and BMD at the femoral neck (if available).

If the fracture risk is calculated in the absence of BMD, the patient may be classified to be at low, intermediate or high risk (Fig. 27.3):

• *For patients at low risk:* reassure, give lifestyle advice and re-evaluate in 5 years or less depending on the clinical context.

• *For patients at intermediate risk:* measure BMD and recalculate the fracture risk to determine whether an individual's risk lies above or below the intervention threshold (see below).

• *For patients at high risk:* consider pharmacological treatment.

When the BMD of the femoral neck is available, it can be included in the calculation of the fracture risk to determine whether the individual lies above or below the intervention threshold. Treatment should be strongly considered in individuals with probabilities of a hip fracture and/or major osteoporotic fracture above the intervention threshold (Fig. 27.4). Where both probabilities fall below the treatment threshold, a further assessment is recommended in 5 years or less depending on the clinical context.

The differences in the magnitude of fracture reduction caused by different treatments are not clear. Therefore the choice of agent is determined by the spectrum of anti-fracture effects across skeletal sites, side-effects and cost. Bisphosphonates are often used as first-line therapy. In patients who are intolerant of alendronate or in whom it is

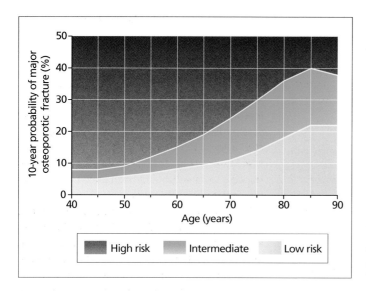

Figure 27.3 Classification of patients into low-, intermediate- and high-risk groups according to their 10-year probability of major osteoporotic fracture.

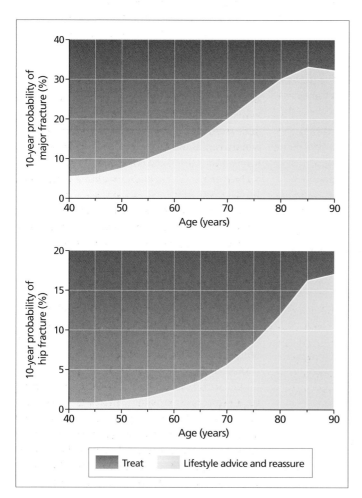

Figure 27.4 Intervention threshold depending on the 10-year probability of hip or major osteoporotic fracture calculated by FRAX.

contraindicated, strontium ranelate or raloxifene (in postmenopausal women) may be appropriate alternatives. The high cost of parathyroid hormone (PTH) peptides restricts their use to those at very high risk (see below).

Bisphosphonates

Alendronate (70 mg weekly) or *risedronate* (35 mg once weekly) are often used as first-line therapy. If the patient's diet does not contain sufficient amount of calcium, a calcium supplement (500 mg per day) should be given in the evening. Bisphosphonates must be taken with a full glass of water half an hour before breakfast to help absorption. Patients must be advised not to lie down after taking the tablet in order to avoid oesophagitis. These strict dosing instructions may reduce compliance in the elderly. These bisphosphonates prevent fracture of the hip, spine and forearm.

Intravenous zolendronic acid may occasionally be used in patients who cannot tolerate oral bisphosphonates, or cannot comply with administration instructions (e.g. an inability to sit upright for 30–60 minutes). Long-term safety data beyond 3 years in patients with osteoporosis are lacking.

Strontium ranelate

In patients who do not tolerate bisphosphonates, *strontium ranelate* may be given in a dose of 2 g per day in water at bedtime. It reduces the risk of vertebral and, to a lesser extent, non-vertebral fractures.

Raloxifene

Another alternative in postmenopausal women with osteoporosis is raloxifene (a selective oestrogen receptor modulator), which may be given in a dose of 60 mg per day. It reduces the risk of spine (but not other) fractures. Raloxifene may reduce the risk of breast cancer. It may increase the risk of deep vein thrombosis.

Hormone replacement therapy

Hormone replacement therapy is no longer a first-line treatment for osteoporosis (see Chapter 23).

Anabolic treatment

Teriparatide is a recombinant fragment of PTH that is administered subcutaneously (20 μg per day). It increases BMD and reduces fracture risk. It is recommended in patients with severe osteoporosis (T-score <−2.5 and at least one fragility fracture) who do not tolerate bisphosphonates or do not respond to them (i.e. who continue to have fractures after 1 year of therapy).

Previous or current bisphosphonate use blunts the response to PTH. Thus PTH should be started about 3 months after bisphosphonates have been discontinued. PTH treatment should not be continued beyond 24 months at present because of concerns about the development of osteosarcomas. For patients at high risk of subsequent fracture after discontinuing PTH, a bisphosphonate may be started after the PTH has been discontinued.

Premenopausal women

In premenopausal women, isolated low bone mass may or may not be associated with a decrease in bone strength or quality. However, those with secondary causes of low bone mass are more likely to have an increased risk of fracture. Therefore a secondary cause of low BMD should be determined and treated. The DEXA scan should be repeated in 1 year. Those with no accelerated bone loss, fragility fractures and no known secondary cause may not require any pharmacological treatment.

Men

Secondary causes of osteoporosis are commonly found among men. Therefore men should be thoroughly investigated, and a secondary cause of low BMD should be determined and treated.

Men with osteoporosis and hypogonadism should receive testosterone replacement therapy. Bisphosphonates remain a reasonable alternative in these men. PTH therapy may be considered for men with severe osteoporosis (T-score <−2.5 and at least one fragility fracture) who are unable to tolerate bisphosphonates or who continue to have fractures after 1 year of bisphosphonate therapy.

Preventing osteoporosis

Prevention of osteoporosis should aim to maximize peak bone mass and reduce the rate of bone loss. Preventative measures include using adequate calcium (at least 1000 mg per day) and vitamin D intake (400–800 IU per day), regular (although not excessive) weight-bearing exercise, and avoidance of smoking and alcohol. Hip fractures can be prevented in elderly patients by the use of hip protectors.

The need for bisphosphonates (alendronate and risedronate 35 mg once weekly) depends on the fracture risk, determined by a combination of low BMD and risk factors (advanced age, prior fragility fracture, a parental history of hip fracture, corticosteroid use, excess alcohol intake, rheumatoid arthritis, current cigarette smoking).

Markers of bone turnover may be useful in predicting the rate of future bone loss and risk of fractures in patients with osteopenia. Patients with osteopenia (a T-score between −2.5 and −1) may be treated if their bone turnover markers are above the upper limits of normal for premenopausal women. Bone density measurement should be repeated after 2 years in patients with osteopenia.

Follow-up and monitoring

There is no consensus on the optimal monitoring for osteoporosis. However, most guidelines recommend follow-up DEXA scan (of the hip and spine) 1 year after starting treatment. The same DEXA instrument should be used for serial BMD testing whenever possible, as it is not possible to make quantitative comparisons of BMD measured on different instruments unless a cross-calibration study has been done. If BMD is stable or improved, the frequency of monitoring may be reduced thereafter.

Fasting urinary cross-linked N-terminal telopeptides of type 1 collagen (NTX) or serum cross-linked C-terminal telopeptides of type 1 collagen (CTX) may be used to monitor the response to antiresorptive treatment, particularly if a repeat DEXA scan cannot be performed at 1 year. A 50% decrease in fasting urinary NTX or serum CTX 6 months after treatment indicates compliance with antiresorptive treatment. Treatment is continued, and follow-up DEXA scans are repeated after 2–3 years. A decrease of less than 50% may be due to non-compliance or poor absorption (e.g. due to an insufficient time interval between drug intake and food ingestion).

Monitoring patients on PTH treatment should include measurement of serum calcium, renal function and uric acid prior to the initiation of therapy and at least once during the course of treatment.

Key points:

- Osteoporosis is characterized by reduced bone mass and microarchitectural deterioration resulting in increased bone fragility and fracture risk (particularly of the hip, vertebrae and distal radius).
- The WHO definition of osteoporosis is based on a T-score of −2.5 or less (measured using DEXA) in healthy postmenopausal women and men age 50 years and older.
- Secondary causes of osteoporosis include hypogonadism, hyperparathyroidism, osteomalacia, thyrotoxicosis and Cushing's syndrome.
- The WHO FRAX tool may be used to calculate the 10-year probability of hip and major osteoporotic fractures and helps in treatment decision plans.
- Alendronate or risedronate is often used as the first-line therapy for osteoporosis. Other therapies include strontium ranelate and raloxifene.
- Teriparatide should be considered in patients with a T-score less than −2.5 and at least one fragility fracture who do not tolerate bisphosphonates or continue to have fractures after 1 year of bisphosphonate therapy.

Chapter 28

Paget's disease of bone

Paget's disease of bone is a skeletal disorder characterized by increased bone turnover.

Epidemiology

It is difficult to estimate the incidence of Paget's disease of bone because most patients are asymptomatic. Studies of autopsies and plain radiographs of unselected patients admitted to hospitals have shown Paget's disease in 3–4% of patients over the age of 40 years. The incidence appears to increase with age. Men and women are equally affected.

Paget's disease is more common in areas of the world with large concentrations of people of Anglo-Saxon origin, and it is rare in Asia, Africa and Scandinavia.

Aetiology

The aetiology of Paget's disease is unknown. Genetic factors and viral infection may play a role, as suggested by familial and pathologic studies.

Excessive bone resorption by abnormally large osteoclasts is followed by increased bone formation by osteoblasts in a disorganized fashion. This results in an abnormal ('mosaic') pattern of lamellar bone. The marrow spaces are filled by an excess

Lecture Notes: Endocrinology and Diabetes. By A. Sam and K. Meeran. Published 2009 by Blackwell Publishing. ISBN 978-1-4051-5345-4.

of fibrous tissue with a marked increase in blood vessels.

Clinical presentations

Around 90% of patients with Paget's disease are asymptomatic. The diagnosis is usually suspected from a plain radiograph obtained for some other reason, or from routine biochemistry screen showing an elevated serum alkaline phosphatase. Any part of the skeleton may be involved. However, the most commonly affected areas are the pelvis, spine, skull and long bones (proximal and distal areas).

The changes of Paget's disease spread through individual bones (at an annual rate of about 1 cm). However, it is rare for the disease to move between bones. Therefore when patients present with Paget's disease, the distribution within their skeleton is likely to remain fixed.

Pain

Pain may be due to periosteal stretching caused by bone enlargement, microfractures or secondary degenerative arthritis. Bone pain often worsens upon weight-bearing and at night. Patients may complain of headache due to skull involvement. Pain may also arise from complications including nerve impingement or osteosarcoma. Increased blood flow in the affected areas may also cause a warm sensation.

Deformities

The bone changes result in enlarged and abnormally contoured bones, for example anterior bowing of the tibia and anterolateral bowing of the femur. Involvement of the skull may be seen as enlargement of the frontal and occipital areas.

Fractures

The abnormal bone is weak and prone to fractures. Fractures may be associated with substantial acute blood loss.

Osteosarcoma

Osteosarcomas occur in up to 1% of cases. These may present with increased pain with or without an enlarging mass. Such patients have a poor prognosis, with a 5-year survival rate of 10–15%.

Neurological complications

Nerve compression may be caused by enlarging bones. Compression of the VIIIth, VIIth and IInd nerves can result in hearing loss, facial palsy and visual disturbance respectively. Involvement of the base of the skull can lead to invagination of the skull by cervical vertebrae (platybasia), and possibly to hydrocephalus due to blockage of the aqueduct of Sylvius.

Involvement of the spine can result in nerve impingement. Increased blood flow to highly vascularized and hypermetabolic Pagetic bone may cause ischemic myelitis (vascular 'steal syndrome').

Cardiac complications

High-output cardiac failure can occur in Paget's disease with involvement of more than 20% of the skeleton. Signs of calcific aortic stenosis and conduction abnormalities are more common in patients with severe Paget's disease (with ≥75% involvement of three or more major bones).

Investigations

Laboratory findings

Patients with Paget's disease have an elevated concentration of serum alkaline phosphatase (a marker of increased bone formation). Serum calcium, phosphate and 25-hydroxyvitamin D concentrations are normal. Hypercalcaemia can occur with immobilization or fracture due to an unopposed increase in bone resorption.

Patients with polyostotic Paget's disease have an increased urinary excretion of hydroxyproline (a reflection of accelerated bone resorption), but this test is not readily available.

Radiographs

The diagnosis of Paget's disease is primarily based on plain radiographs. In the early stages, bone resorption at localized areas may be seen as lytic areas. Later, chaotic new bone formation results in a lack of distinction between the cortex and medullary bone. The affected bones are expanded. This feature is helpful in differentiating Paget's disease from sclerotic metastases, in which the bone is of normal size.

Plain radiographs also show the adjacent joints, fractures and the extent of deformity. Involvement of the skull begins with radiolucent areas (osteoporosis circumscripta) followed, many years later, by a 'cotton wool' appearance due to a disruption of normal bone architecture.

Radioisotope bone scan

Radioisotope bone scanning is useful for determining the extent of skeletal involvement, but is not specific for diagnosis. Pagetic bone lesions are seen as focal areas of markedly increased uptake ('hot spots').

Differentiating Paget's disease from metastatic bone disease is sometimes difficult. Previous laboratory tests and radiographs can be helpful. If, for example, laboratory and radiographic studies from the previous year were normal, the diagnosis of Paget's disease is unlikely. In rare cases, usually affecting a single vertebra, distinguishing between Paget's disease and metastasis may require computed tomography-guided biopsy.

Treatment

The primary indication for treatment in Paget's disease is the presence of symptoms.

Long-term studies are needed to determine whether treatment prevents complications. However, many endocrinologists also treat patients with involvement of sites where there is an increased risk of complications, i.e. the skull (deafness), long bones (deformity, fracture, arthritis) and spine (cord compression, vascular steal syndrome).

If there is doubt regarding the origin of pain when both Paget's disease and osteoarthritis are present, the arthritis may be treated first with paracetamol or non-steroidal anti-inflammatory drugs.

All drugs used to treat Paget's disease suppress osteoclastic activity. Many endocrinologists use bisphosphonates as first-line therapy because of their superior efficacy compared with calcitonin and their minimal side-effects.

Bisphosphonates

Three courses of intravenous pamidronate may be given fortnightly (60 mg in 1 L of saline over 4 hours). Treatment usually suppresses disease activity for 12–18 months. Recurrent disease (clinical symptoms or increasing alkaline phosphatase) usually responds to re-treatment.

The side-effects of pamidronate include low-grade fever and flu-like symptoms in the first 1–2 days in 20% of patients. Hypocalcaemia may occasionally occur, and can be ameliorated by the administration of 1000 mg calcium per day for 1–2 weeks. Rarer side-effects include ocular complications (conjunctivitis, uveitis, scleritis) and osteonecrosis of the jaw.

Oral risedronate (30 mg per day for 2 months) is an effective alternative to intravenous pamidronate, but may cause oesophagitis. It should be taken with a full glass of water (250 mL) half an hour before breakfast. Patients should remain in the upright position for at least half an hour after taking their tablet in order to minimize the risk of oesophagitis.

Calcitonin

Salmon calcitonin may be given initially at a dose of 100 U per day subcutaneously at bedtime. Biochemical improvement (a 50% reduction in serum alkaline phosphatase) occurs in 3–6 months. The dose is then reduced to 50–100 U every other day. The optimum duration of treatment has not been established. Intermittent therapy may be tried. Patients with severe disease may require indefinite treatment.

Around 20% of patients become resistant to salmon calcitonin due to the development of antibodies. Human calcitonin has been developed to avoid this problem, but is somewhat less potent than salmon calcitonin. Both salmon and human calcitonin are expensive, and 20% of patients have side-effects such as nausea, facial flushing and a metallic taste. Rare side-effects include diarrhoea, abdominal pain and allergic reactions.

Surgery

Elective surgery for joint replacement, tibial osteotomy and internal fixation of pathological fractures may benefit patients with refractory pain. Patients with spinal cord compression, spinal stenosis or basilar invagination complicated by neural compromise may require decompression procedures. Pre-treatment with calcitonin or bisphosphonates (for a minimum of 2–3 months) may prevent excessive bleeding and postoperative hypercalcaemia.

Follow-up and monitoring

Patients should be clinically monitored for an improvement in symptoms such as pain and symptoms of nerve compression. Effective therapy results in a reduction in serum alkaline phosphatase and urinary hydroxyproline levels. Serum alkaline phosphatase should be measured initially every other month, and once stabilized once or twice a year as long as there is a good clinical response.

Repeat bone scans and radiographs are not necessary unless the patient has new or progressive symptoms. Neurological complications may improve with early treatment. Bowed extremities will not change.

Key points:

- Paget's disease of bone is a skeletal disorder characterized by increased bone turnover.
- 90% of patients with Paget's disease are asymptomatic. The diagnosis is usually suspected from a plain radiograph obtained for some other reason, or from a routine biochemistry screen showing an elevated serum alkaline phosphatase.
- Complications of Paget's disease include pain, deformities, fractures, osteosarcoma, nerve compression (e.g. VIIIth cranial nerve) and high-output cardiac failure.
- The diagnosis of Paget's disease is primarily based on plain radiographs, which may show lytic areas (in the early stages), a lack of distinction between cortex and medullary bone and expanded bones.
- The primary indication for treatment in Paget's disease is the presence of symptoms.
- Many endocrinologists use bisphosphonates as first-line therapy.

Chapter 29

Disorders of puberty

Puberty

Puberty is the process of acquisition of secondary sexual characteristics and attainment of reproductive function. Puberty is associated with a growth spurt (accelerated linear growth). Secondary sexual characteristics include the development of genitalia, pubic and axillary hair in boys and girls, the development of breasts in girls and an increase in testicular volume in boys.

Normal puberty occurs between the ages of 8 and 13 years in girls and 9 and 14 years in boys, and usually lasts for 3–4 years.

Endocrinology of puberty

The first step in initiation of puberty is activation of the hypothalamic *gonadotrophin-releasing hormone (GnRH) pulse generator* and the pulsatile secretion of GnRH. This results in an increase in plasma concentrations of luteinizing hormone (LH), follicle-stimulating hormone (FSH) and sex steroids, i.e. testosterone in boys and oestradiol in girls.

The initial change in gonadotrophin secretion during the early stages of puberty is a nocturnal increase in serum LH levels during sleep. In the

later stages of puberty, daytime LH levels also increase, gradually changing to the adult pattern of one pulse every 90 minutes throughout the day and night.

The activation of the GnRH pulse generator and onset of puberty is likely to be influenced by multiple neuronal and hormonal signals that are not completely understood.

It has been proposed that a critical body weight or composition is necessary for the development of puberty. *Leptin* is a hormone produced largely in adipocytes and may act as a signal of the availability of the metabolic reserve necessary for pubertal development.

Kisspeptin is a hypothalamic neuropeptide that binds to the GPR54 receptor. Kisspeptin/GPR54 signalling has also been shown to be crucial for the development of puberty. Mutations in GPR54 cause autosomal recessive hypogonadotrophic hypogonadism in humans.

Tanner staging

Normal puberty occurs between the ages of 8 and 13 years in girls, and 9 and 14 years in boys. Although girls enter puberty at an earlier chronological age than boys, their onset of fertility is usually later.

The sequence of pubertal changes in secondary sexual characteristics may be categorized into five *Tanner stages*. Box 29.1 describes the five Tanner

Lecture Notes: Endocrinology and Diabetes. By A. Sam and K. Meeran. Published 2009 by Blackwell Publishing. ISBN 978-1-4051-5345-4.

Box 29.1 Tanner staging of pubertal changes

Boys

Genital changes

Stage 1: Prepubertal

Stage 2: Scrotum and testes enlarge, and scrotum skin reddens and changes in texture

Stage 3: Penis enlarges (length at first) and the testes grow further

Stage 4: Size of the penis increases with a growth in breadth and development of the glans; the testes and scrotum become larger, and the scrotum skin becomes darker

Stage 5: Adult genitalia

Pubic hair

Stage 1: Prepubertal (velus hair similar to the abdominal wall)

Stage 2: Sparse growth of long, slightly pigmented hair, straight or curled, at the base of the penis

Stage 3: Darker, coarser and more curled hair, spreading sparsely over the junction of the pubes

Stage 4: Hair adult in type but covering a smaller area than in the adult, and no spread to the medial surface of the thighs

Stage 5: Adult in type and quantity

Girls

Breast development

Stage 1: Prepubertal

Stage 2: Breast bud stage with elevation of breast and papilla; enlargement of the areola

Stage 3: Further enlargement of the breast and areola; no separation of their contour

Stage 4: Areola and papilla form a secondary mound above the level of the breast

Stage 5: Mature stage with projection of papilla only, related to recession of the areola

Pubic hair

Stage 1: Prepubertal (velus hair similar to the abdominal wall)

Stage 2: Sparse growth of long, slightly pigmented hair, straight or curled, along the labia

Stage 3: Darker, coarser and more curled hair, spreading sparsely over the junction of the pubes

Stage 4: Hair adult in type but covering a smaller area than in adult; no spread to the medial surface of the thighs

Stage 5: Adult in type and quantity

stages for the development of pubic hair (both males and females), breasts (in girls) and genital changes (in boys).

- In *girls*, the first sign of puberty is the onset of *breast development* (thelarche). Breast enlargement is followed by the development of pubic hair (pubarche). Menarche occurs 2–3 years after the onset of puberty. The first 1–2 years following menarche involve anovulatory cycles associated with irregular and usually painful periods. Peak growth velocity (the growth spurt) occurs within the first year after the onset of puberty.
- In *boys*, the first sign of puberty is an increase in *testicular volume* ($\geq 4\,mL$). Testicular enlargement is followed by penile and pubic hair development. Spermatogenesis begins at Tanner stage 3 (see below). Peak growth velocity occurs 2 years after the onset of puberty (Tanner stage 3–4, at a testicular volume of about $12\,mL$). Boys experience a greater peak height velocity than girls.

In both sexes, puberty progresses through distinct stages in an orderly and consistent manner.

Delayed puberty

Delayed puberty is defined as the absence or incomplete development of secondary sexual characteristics by an age at which 95% of children of that sex and culture have initiated sexual maturation.

- In boys, delayed puberty may be diagnosed when there is no testicular enlargement by age 14.
- In girls, delayed puberty may be diagnosed when there is no breast development by age 13.

Aetiology

Causes of delayed puberty are summarized in Box 29.2.

Constitutional delay of growth and puberty

Constitutional delay of growth and puberty (CDGP) is one of the most common conditions presenting to paediatric endocrinologists. It is a normal variant of growth and puberty, and is char-

Constitutional delay of growth and puberty

Hypogonadotrophic hypogonadism
*Pituitary/hypothalamic tumours and other sellar/
parasellar disorders*
Adenomas, cysts, craniopharyngiomas, germinomas,
   meningiomas, gliomas, astrocytomas
Infiltrative diseases (haemochromatosis, granulomatous
   diseases, histiocytosis)
Trauma
Pituitary apoplexy

Functional gonadotrophin deficiency
Anorexia nervosa, excessive exercise
Systemic illness, malnutrition
Hyperprolactinaemia
Hypothyroidism

*Congenital gonadotrophin-releasing hormone
deficiency*
Idiopathic without anosmia
May be associated with anosmia (Kallmann's syndrome),
   congenital adrenal hypoplasia or mental retardation/
   obesity (Laurence–Moon–Biedl and Prader–Willi
   syndrome)

Hypergonadotrophic hypogonadism
Congenital
Chromosomal abnormalities: 45X0 in girls (Turner's syn-
   drome), 47XXY in boys (Klinefelter's syndrome)

Acquired
Gonadal damage: infection, trauma, iatrogenic (chemotherapy, radiotherapy), autoimmune

acterized by a delayed onset of puberty, pubertal growth spurt and skeletal maturation (i.e. delayed bone age).

In the years preceding the expected time of puberty, the growth pattern of these children is normal (usually along the lower growth percentiles). The height of the child begins to drift from the growth curve because the onset of the pubertal growth spurt is delayed. However, the child's height is appropriate for the bone age. Physical examination and biochemical investigations are normal and prepubertal.

Patients often have a family history of a late onset of puberty in one or both parents. The pre-dicted height for the child is in the appropriate range for the parental heights. It may be difficult to distinguish between CDGP and congenital GnRH deficiency as gonadotrophin levels are low in both conditions, and the diagnosis may only be made with time and serial observations. Persistent hypogonadism beyond age 18 is highly suggestive of congenital GnRH deficiency.

Hypogonadotrophic hypogonadism

Hypogonadotrophic (or secondary) hypogonadism is due to an impaired secretion of hypothalamic GnRH and/or impaired FSH and LH levels. Hypogonadotrophic hypogonadism may be acquired or congenital (see Box 29.2).

Congenital hypogonadotrophic hypogonadism may be associated with the following:
• *Anosmia:* in *Kallmann's syndrome*, which is usually X-linked (although autosomal dominant transmission can also occur). Kallmann's syndrome may be due to the sporadic or familial mutations of several genes (e.g. *KAL1*, FGFR1 [*KAL2*], *PROK2*) encoding cell surface adhesion molecules or their receptors required for the migration of GnRH-secreting neurones into the brain and hypothalamus. Kallmann's syndrome may be associated with midline facial abnormalities (e.g. cleft palate), red–green colour blindness, hearing loss, urogenital tract abnormalities and synkinesis (mirror movements of the hands).
• *Mental retardation and obesity:* in Prader–Willi syndrome (caused by deletion of part of paternally derived chromosome 15q) and Laurence–Moon–Biedl syndrome (also associated with polydactyly and retinitis pigmentosa).
• *Congenital adrenal hypoplasia:* due to a mutation of the *NROB1* (DAX-1) gene.

Hypergonadotrophic hypogonadism

Hypergonadotrophic (or primary) hypogonadism may be associated with high FSH and LH levels due to a lack of negative feedback of the sex steroids. Hypergonadotrophic hypogonadism may be congenital or acquired (Box 29.2).

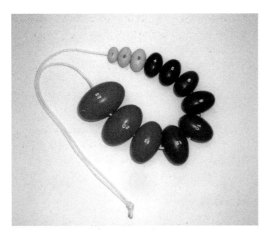

Figure 29.1 Prader orchidometer.

Clinical evaluation

History should enquire about the features associated with the possible underlying causes of delayed puberty (Box 29.2).

Physical examination should include the following:

• Assessment of secondary sex characteristics and staging according to the Tanner criteria (see Box 29.1). Testicular volume is measured using a Prader orchidometer, which comprises a series of plastic ellipsoids with a volume from 1 to 25 mL (Fig. 29.1). The symmetry of the testes must be carefully examined as gonadal tumours may present at puberty with asymmetrical gonadal development and defects in sexual maturation.

• Measurement and plotting of height on a growth chart that includes normal growth patterns with centiles. Height velocity must be documented for at least 6 months.

• Measurement of weight and calculation of body mass index.

• General examination to look for any features of an underlying cause, for example visual field defects due to a pituitary tumour, systemic illness or Kallmann's, Turner's or Klinefelter's syndromes (Box 29.2).

If the first signs of puberty (i.e. breast buds in girls and a testicular volume of more than 4 mL in boys) are present, normal spontaneous puberty usually occurs in more than 95% of patients.

However, follow-up is essential since some children with genetic causes of idiopathic hypogonadotrophic hypogonadism can exhibit cessation after some initial signs of pubertal development.

Investigations

The investigation of patients with delayed puberty should include:

• full blood count, urea and electrolytes, liver function tests and erythrocyte sedimentation rate

• serum LH and FSH, oestradiol (girls) or testosterone (boys)

• prolactin

• free thyroxine and thyroid-stimulating hormone

• karyotype (to evaluate the possibility of Klinefelter's syndrome in boys and Turner's syndrome in girls).

Bone age is determined by the comparison of a radiograph of the patient's bones in the left hand and wrist with the bones in a standard atlas, usually 'Greulich and Pyle'. Bone age allows an assessment of skeletal maturation and the potential for future skeletal growth.

Brain magnetic resonance imaging (MRI) should be performed if there are associated neurological symptoms or signs, or if the blood tests suggest a pituitary/hypothalamic disease.

Pelvic or testicular ultrasonography should be performed when an ovarian or testicular mass is detected on the physical examination. Pelvic ultrasound determines the presence or absence of a uterus (the uterus is absent in patients with androgen insensitivity and disorders of the Müllerian duct system).

Treatment

Treat the underlying disorder if identified, for example levothyroxine for hypothyroidism, a dopamine agonist for prolactinomas and the excision of craniopharyngiomas. Patients with features of chronic illness or anorexia nervosa should be referred to the appropriate specialist teams.

CDGP and congenital GnRH deficiency

It is difficult to distinguish between CDGP and congenital GnRH deficiency. The initial therapeutic approach may be similar for both disorders. The diagnosis can only be made with serial observations.

In patients with significant psychosocial concerns, a short-term (6-month) course of low-dose sex steroid therapy may be given to promote secondary sexual characteristics and growth without inducing premature closure of the epiphyses. Boys may be treated with 50 mg testosterone enanthate or cypionate intramuscularly monthly. Girls may be treated with 2 μg ethinylestradiol orally daily.

Patients should be assessed after cessation of therapy. Spontaneous pubertal development (an enlargement of testicular volume in boys and spontaneous menstruation in girls) indicates CDGP. In contrast, patients with hypogonadotrophic hypogonadism show little pubertal development. These patients need replacement therapy with sex steroids (i.e. testosterone in boys, and oestrogen and progesterone in girls). It is important to remember the normal timescale of pubertal development.

Treatment should be started with low doses of sex steroid replacement (as above), the dose being increased gradually at appropriate intervals. In boys, the dose of testosterone is gradually increased to the adult dose (250 mg intramuscularly monthly). The side-effects of testosterone therapy include acne and rarely priapism.

In girls, the dose of oestrogen is gradually increased. Cyclical oral progesterone is added with the onset of breakthrough bleeding. Progesterone should not be added until breast growth has plateaued. Premature initiation of progesterone therapy can compromise ultimate breast growth.

Primary (hypergonadotrophic) hypogonadism

Primary (hypergonadotrophic) hypogonadism must also be treated with a gradually increasing dose of sex steroids over 2–3 years to complete puberty.

Precocious puberty

Precocious puberty is defined as the onset of secondary sexual characteristics before the age of 8 years in girls or 9 years in boys.

Children with untreated precocious puberty have increased growth velocity, advanced bone age and smaller predicted final adult heights due to epiphyseal fusion at an early age.

Epidemiology

The incidence of precocious puberty is 20 per 10 000 girls and fewer than 5 per 10 000 boys (using the above diagnostic age limit).

Aetiology

Precocious puberty may be GnRH dependent or GnRH independent (Box 29.3).

Box 29.3 Causes of precocious puberty

Gonadotrophin-releasing hormone (GnRH)-dependent (central precocious) puberty
Central nervous system disorders
Hydrocephalus
Hamartomas (containing GnRH neurones)
Tumours (astrocytomas, ependymomas, pineal tumours, gliomas)
Trauma
Radiotherapy
Inflammatory disease
Congenital midline defects (e.g. septo-optic dysplasia)

Idiopathic (80–90%)

GnRH-independent precocious puberty
Increased sex steroids secreted from the ovaries
Ovarian cysts and tumours (granulosa cell tumours and gonadoblastomas)

Increased testosterone secreted from the testes
Leydig cell tumours (benign testosterone-secreting tumours)
Human chorionic gonadotrophin-secreting germ cell tumours (gonadal, pineal, hepatic, retroperitoneal, mediastinal)
Testotoxicosis

Increased sex steroids secreted from the adrenal glands
Congenital adrenal hyperplasia
Adrenal (androgen- and oestrogen-secreting) tumours

McCune–Albright syndrome

Exogenous sex steroids

GnRH-dependent ('central') precocious puberty

GnRH-dependent ('central') precocious puberty is caused by earlier activation of the hypothalamic–pituitary–gonadal axis. Pubertal development is 'consonant' with normal puberty, i.e. patients have a normal sequence and pace of pubertal milestones. The secondary sexual characteristics are appropriate for the child's gender ('iso-sexual'). Children with GnRH-dependent precocious puberty may have a central nervous system disorder, but 80% have no identifiable cause. Boys are more likely to have occult intracranial pathology.

GnRH-independent precocious puberty

GnRH-independent precocious puberty is caused by the autonomous endogenous secretion of sex steroids from the gonads or adrenal glands or excess exogenous sex steroids. Human chorionic gonadotrophin-secreting germ cell tumours can also increase testosterone production via activation of the LH receptors on the Leydig cells.

In these children, pubertal development may not be consonant with normal puberty (i.e. there may be deviations from the normal sequence and pace of puberty) because of the unregulated pattern of sex steroid secretion. The sexual characteristics may be appropriate for the child's gender ('iso-sexual precocity') or inappropriate, with the virilization of girls and feminization of boys ('contrasexual precocity').

Testotoxicosis is an autosomal dominant disorder caused by an activating mutation of the LH receptor gene, resulting in premature Leydig cell maturation and increased testosterone secretion in boys.

McCune–Albright syndrome is a rare disorder characterized by precocious puberty, café-au-lait skin pigmentation and fibrous dysplasia of bone. It is due to an activating mutation of the gene (*GNAS*) encoding the alpha subunit of the stimulating G protein that couples transmembrane receptors to adenylate cyclase. The mutation may result in continued stimulation of LH/FSH receptors (causing precocious puberty). It may be associated with acti-

vation of a number of pituitary hormone receptors, resulting in other endocrinopathies such as gigantism, Cushing's syndrome and thyrotoxicosis.

Incomplete precocity

Premature thelarche (breast development with no other signs of puberty) and premature adrenarche (the appearance of pubic and/or axillary hair with no other signs of puberty) are variants of normal puberty. Growth velocity and bone age are normal. Close monitoring is essential as a significant number of these children will develop central precocious puberty.

Isolated breast development may be a presentation of primary hypothyroidism. Increased thyrotrophin-releasing hormone may stimulate FSH, causing ovarian cyst development and increased oestradiol secretion.

Clinical evaluation

The evaluation of patients includes a thorough medical history, a physical examination and a range of investigations to determine the aetiology of precocious puberty.

Medical history

Medical history should enquire about:
- details of pubertal development: when the initial pubertal changes were first noted (for the patient, as well as for his/her parents and siblings). Deviation from the normal sequence and pace suggests a GnRH-independent cause.
- a previous history of central nervous system disease, radiotherapy, trauma or presence of any neurological symptoms, such as headaches or seizures
- a history of exposure to exogenous androgens or oestrogens
- the presence of abdominal pain (ovarian disease).

Physical examination

Physical examination should include the following:

- Measurements of height and height velocity (cm per year) to look for accelerated linear growth.
- Pubertal (Tanner) staging: staging breast development in girls, testicular volume (and symmetry) and penile size in boys, and pubic hair development in both sexes. Physical examination also determines whether the secondary sexual characteristics are iso-sexual (appropriate for the patient's gender) or contrasexual—virilization in females (hirsutism, cliteromegaly, deepening of the voice) or feminization in males. Boys who have an adrenal cause will not have testicular enlargement (i.e. testicular volume will be <4 mL).
- Neurological examination including fundoscopy (to look for papilloedema, a sign of increased intracranial pressure) and visual field assessment.
- Dermatological examination to look for café-au-lait spots (associated with McCune–Albright syndrome).

Investigations

Investigation of a patient with precocious puberty should include the following:
- *Bone age* (determined from a radiograph of the left hand/wrist): to look for advanced skeletal maturation, i.e. bone age higher than chronological age. Children with incomplete precocity (see above) have a normal bone age.
- *Sex steroid* (oestrogen and testosterone) levels are often uninformative, and low levels do not exclude precocious puberty.
- *LH and FSH levels*: in a GnRH-dependent (central) precocious puberty, basal levels of LH and FSH are at pubertal levels and will increase with GnRH stimulation (increment >3–4 IU/L for LH and >2–3 IU/L for FSH). In GnRH-independent precocious puberty, baseline LH and FSH levels are low and will not increase with GnRH stimulation.
- *Thyroid function tests* should be performed in all girls presenting with early breast development to exclude primary hypothyroidism.
- *GnRH dependent (central) precocious puberty*: a brain MRI scan is indicated to determine whether there is an identifiable central nervous system cause. Pelvic ultrasonography may show multicystic ovaries and an enlarging uterus in girls.

- *GnRH-independent precocious puberty*: measure testosterone, oestradiol, dehydroepiandrosterone sulphate (elevated in adrenal tumours) and 17-hydroxyprogesterone (elevated in the common form of congenital adrenal hyperplasia).
- Pelvic ultrasound may identify the presence of an ovarian cyst or tumour in girls.

Treatment

Central precocious puberty

If a cause has been found, it should be treated appropriately. If there is no identifiable cause, the decision to treat depends on the predicted final adult height (based upon a measurement of height velocity) and the psychosocial effects of the precocity.

GnRH analogue therapy (monthly leuprorelin acetate or goserelin given intramuscularly) is effective and safe. It induces the downregulation of pituitary GnRH receptors and results in the suppression of pulsatile gonadotrophin secretion. It slows accelerated puberty and improves final height. Bone density should be monitored during therapy.

GnRH-independent precocious puberty

The underlying pathology should be treated, i.e. surgical removal of tumours of the testis, adrenal gland or ovary. Children with human chorionic gonadotrophin-secreting tumours may require some combination of surgery, radiotherapy and chemotherapy depending on the site and histology.

Children with congenital adrenal hyperplasia should be treated with glucocorticoids (see Chapter 9).

Patients with McCune–Albright syndrome are treated with drugs that inhibit gonadal steroid synthesis or action rather than surgery, in order to preserve fertility. Girls may be treated with testolactone (which inhibits the aromatization of androgen to oestrogen). Successful treatment has also been achieved with tamoxifen (an anti-oestrogen). Boys may be treated with ketoconazole (which inhibits androgen synthesis) or a combination of spirono-lactone (which inhibits androgen action) and testolactone. Bone pain and increased fractures caused by the fibrous dysplasia of bone may improve with the intravenous pamidronate.

Incomplete precocity

Patients with premature thelarche or premature adrenarche do not require any treatment but should be followed up regularly to detect possible progression to central precocious puberty.

Key points:

- Normal puberty occurs between the ages of 8 and 13 years in girls and 9 and 14 years in boys, and usually lasts for 3–4 years.
- The first step in the initiation of puberty is activation of the hypothalamic GnRH pulse generator and the pulsatile secretion of GnRH.
- Leptin is a hormone produced largely in adipocytes that may act as a signal of the availability of the metabolic reserve necessary for pubertal development.
- Kisspeptin/GPR54 signalling has also been shown to be crucial for the development of puberty.
- The sequence of pubertal changes in secondary sexual characteristics may be categorized into five Tanner stages.
- Delayed puberty may be diagnosed when there is no testicular enlargement by age 14 in boys or no breast development by age 13 in girls.
- Delayed puberty may be due to constitutional delay of growth and puberty, hypogonadotrophic hypogonadism or hypergonadotrophic hypogonadism.
- Precocious puberty may be GnRH dependent or GnRH independent (due to increased sex steroids secreted from the gonads or adrenal glands, McCune–Albright syndrome or exogenous sex steroids).

Chapter 30

Growth and stature

Normal growth

There are three phases of postnatal growth:
- The *infantile phase* is characterized by rapid but decelerating growth during the first 2 years of life. Infants often cross percentile lines in the first 2 years and settle onto their childhood centile position at age 2–3 years. Overall growth during this period is about 30–35 cm. Nutrition is an important factor for growth in this phase.
- The *childhood phase* is characterized by growth at a relatively constant velocity of 5–7 cm per year. There is often a slight slowing later in childhood. Normal children do not cross percentile lines. Growth hormone (GH) is the most significant endocrine factor for growth in this phase.
- The *pubertal phase* is characterized by a growth spurt of 8–14 cm per year due to the synergistic effects of increasing gonadal steroid and GH secretion. Bone maturation occurs during puberty, and growth stops as the epiphyses fuse. Limb growth ceases before spinal growth.

Prediction of height potential

Mid-parental height

The mid-parental height can be used to estimate a child's adult height:

Lecture Notes: Endocrinology and Diabetes. By A. Sam and K. Meeran. Published 2009 by Blackwell Publishing. ISBN 978-1-4051-5345-4.

- For *boys*, 13 cm is added to the mother's height and averaged with the father's height.
- For *girls*, 13 cm is subtracted from the father's height and averaged with the mother's height.

The 13 cm represents the average difference in height of men and women. For both girls and boys, 8.5 cm on either side of this calculated value represents the 3rd to 97th percentiles for anticipated adult height.

Mid-parental height is useful in assessing genetic influences on height. However, it is important to remember that illnesses or other factors in parents may have prevented them from reaching their genetic potential. The mid-parental height is less accurate than the *bone age* method (see below), because it does not reflect environmental contributions to growth or disease processes.

Bone age

Bone age is a measure of skeletal maturity. It is obtained by assessing the appearance and shape of the bones of the hand and wrist from a radiograph. The methods used most commonly for determining bone age are the 'Greulich and Pyle' atlas and the Tanner–Whitehouse method.

At any given bone age, an individual is at a certain percentage of adult height. Thus multiplying the present height by the reciprocal of this percentage (of adult height) predicts the adult height.

Short stature

Short stature is defined as a height 2 standard deviations or more below the mean height for children of that gender and chronological age. This translates into being below the 3rd percentile for height.

Concerns about short stature are a common reason for referral to a paediatrician. However, most children referred are found to be normal.

Aetiology

Causes of short stature are summarized in Box 30.1.

Low birth weight and illnesses in infancy

Children with low birth weight or loss of growth potential in infancy due to various illnesses have short stature but normal growth velocity.

Box 30.1 Causes of short stature

Low birth weight and illnesses in infancy

Familial

Constitutional delay of growth and puberty

Endocrine abnormalities
Thyroid disease
Growth hormone or insulin-like growth factor-1 deficiency or insensitivity
Cushing's syndrome
Vitamin D deficiency or resistance

Dysmorphic syndromes associated with abnormal skeletal growth
Turner's syndrome
Noonan's syndrome
Down's syndrome
Achondroplasia

Chronic illness, malnutrition

Psychosocial problems

Idiopathic

Familial short stature

Children with *familial (genetic) short stature* have short parent(s) with a history of normal puberty. These children have normal growth velocity, timing of puberty and bone age.

Constitutional delay of growth and puberty

Constitutional delay of growth and puberty (CDGP) is the one of the most common conditions presenting to paediatric endocrinologists. It is a normal variant of growth and puberty, and is characterized by a delayed onset of puberty, the pubertal growth spurt and skeletal maturation (i.e. delayed bone age).

The growth chart and growth velocity of a boy with CDGP is shown in Fig. 30.1. In the years preceding the expected time of puberty, the growth pattern of these children is normal (usually along the lower growth percentiles). The height of the child begins to drift from the growth curve because the onset of pubertal growth spurt is delayed. However, the child's height is appropriate for his bone age. Physical examination and biochemical investigations are normal and prepubertal. Patients often have a family history of late onset of puberty in one or both parents. The predicted height for the child is in the appropriate range for the parental heights.

Endocrine abnormalities

Children with abnormalities in the *endocrine* control of growth have reduced growth velocity and are usually overweight for height.

GH deficiency

GH deficiency is the most common endocrine cause of short stature. GH deficiency may be isolated or associated with other pituitary hormone deficiencies (see Chapters 12 and 13).

GH secretion is stimulated by hypothalamic GH-releasing hormone (GHRH). GH stimulates epiphyseal prechondrocyte differentiation and linear bone growth in children. GH also stimulates skel-

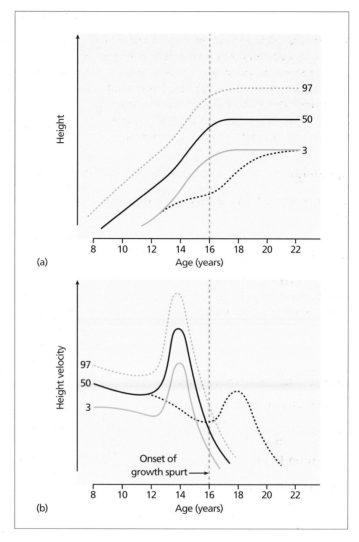

(a)

(b)

Figure 30.1 (a) Serial height measurements of a boy with constitutional delay of growth and puberty (CDGP; dotted black line) are plotted on a growth chart with 3rd, 50th and 97th percentile lines. Note that the height of the child falls below the 3rd percentile line during the early teenage years because of the delay in onset of the pubertal growth spurt. (b) Growth velocity of a boy with CDGP (dotted black line) is plotted on a growth velocity chart with 3rd, 50th and 97th percentile lines. Note the delayed onset of the growth spurt (arrow) and reduced peak height velocity.

etal growth through a stimulation of the hepatic synthesis and secretion of *insulin-like growth factor-1* (IGF-1), which is a potent growth and differentiation factor. GH deficiency usually results from a deficiency of GHRH, but can be secondary to sellar and parasellar tumours such as germinoma.

Rare causes of short stature include an inactivating mutation of the GHRH receptor inherited in an autosomal recessive manner, homozygous GH gene deletion, abnormalities of the GH receptor (Laron's syndrome) and abnormal IGF-1 secretion or action.

Hypothyroidism

Hypothyroidism is a well-recognized cause of short stature. The skeletal age is usually as delayed as the height age, and as a result many children with hypothyroidism have a reasonably normal growth potential.

Cushing's syndrome

Cushing's syndrome in children is usually iatrogenic, due to glucocorticoid therapy for asthma, inflammatory bowel disease or immunological renal disease. Endogenous Cushing's syndrome is rare but should be considered if the child has both weight gain and growth retardation. Bone age is normal at diagnosis in most patients.

Dysmorphic syndromes associated with abnormal skeletal growth

Abnormalities in skeletal growth are features of certain syndromes such as Turner's syndrome (see Chapter 21), Down's syndrome (trisomy 21) and achondroplasia (caused by an autosomal dominant mutation in the gene encoding fibroblast growth factor receptor-3, resulting in abnormal cartilage formation).

Malnutrition or chronic illness

Malnutrition or chronic illnesses such as congenital heart disease, asthma, cystic fibrosis, coeliac disease, inflammatory bowel disease, chronic kidney disease, vitamin D deficiency or HIV infection can result in short stature. These children are usually underweight for height.

Psychosocial problems

Psychosocial problems in childhood can contribute to short stature. These children have reduced growth velocity.

Idiopathic

Idiopathic short stature is the term applied to children with short stature in whom no endocrine, metabolic or other diagnosis can be made. These children have normal (often at the lower limit) growth velocity. Mutations in the short stature homeobox (*SHOX*) gene are responsible for up to 15% of cases of apparent 'idiopathic' short stature.

Clinical evaluation

A full medical history should be taken to determine:
- birth weight and history of any illnesses during infancy/childhood
- the parents' height (heights reported by adults

may be inaccurate and should be measured)
- the stage of puberty
- a family history of delayed puberty
- nutrition and any features of systemic illness
- psychosocial problems.

A thorough clinical examination should be performed to look for the following:
- *Reduced growth velocity*: accurate serial measurement of height and plotting of the measurements on a growth chart is essential to determine the growth velocity (Fig. 30.2).
- *Underweight/overweight*: children with systemic illness or malnutrition are usually underweight for height, whereas children with endocrine abnormalities are overweight for height.
- *Pubertal development* (see Chapter 29).
- *Dysmorphic features*: particularly features of Down's syndrome and Turner's syndrome (see Chapter 21). Patients with achondroplasia have short stature with disproportionately short arms and legs, a large head and characteristic facial features with frontal bossing and mid-face hypoplasia.
- *Features of chronic illness*.
- *Features of endocrine abnormalities* (GH deficiency, hypothyroidism, Cushing's syndrome).

Investigations

Children with reduced growth velocity should be thoroughly investigated for the following conditions:
- *Systemic illness:* initial blood tests should include full blood count, urea and electrolytes, liver function tests, bone profile, glucose, coeliac serology and erythrocyte sedimentation rate.
- *Turner's syndrome:* a *karyotype* analysis should be performed in girls.
- *GH deficiency or resistance:* serum IGF-1 and *IGF-binding protein-3* (IGFBP-3) should be measured. If IGF-1 and IGFB-3 levels are low, provocative GH testing (using insulin-induced hypoglycaemia or arginine) may be performed. However, provocative GH testing has a number of limitations, including the arbitrary cut-off level of 'normal' (GH concentration of 10 µg/L), variable accuracy of the GH assays, the risk of insulin-induced hypoglycaemia

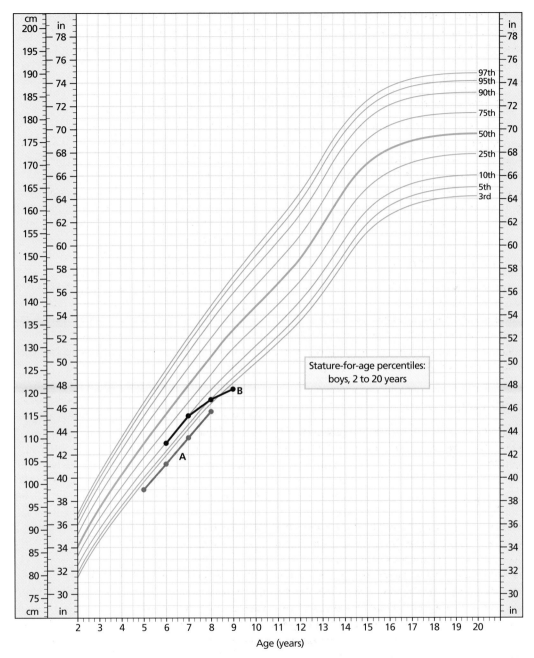

Figure 30.2 The serial height measurements of two boys with short stature are plotted on the growth chart for boys. Child A has normal growth velocity. Child B has reduced growth velocity.

and inadequate documentation of test reproducibility. Children with GH insensitivity (Laron's syndrome) have high serum GH concentrations but low serum IGF-1 and IGFBP-3 concentrations. When sellar/parasellar disorders are suspected, a *magnetic resonance imaging* (MRI) scan of the hypothalamic–pituitary area should be performed.

• *Hypothyroidism:* serum *thyroid-stimulating hormone* and free *thyroxine* should be measured. It is important to remember that if the child is hypothyroid, provocative GH testing should be postponed until thyroxine has been adequately replaced.

• *Cushing's syndrome:* investigations (see Chapter 16) should only be performed if there is a high clinical suspicion.

The bone age can be determined from a radiograph of the left hand and wrist (using a scoring system of epiphyseal maturation). This is useful in estimating adult height (see above) and differentiating children with familial short stature (normal bone age) and constitutional delay of growth and puberty (delayed bone age).

Treatment

Affected children may miss important psychosocial milestones if they continue to differ from their peers with respect to stature and degree of adolescent development.

Growth rate can be improved by treating the underlying condition. For example, thyroxine replacement in hypothyroidism and a gluten-free diet in coeliac disease result in normal growth if the child is compliant with the treatment.

GH is administered as a daily subcutaneous injection and is usually continued until the growth rate slows at the end of puberty. Only a small proportion may benefit from GH replacement therapy as adults. Thus it is mandatory to retest GH-deficient children after completion of growth. Children with multiple pituitary hormone deficiencies rarely recover the ability to secrete GH as an adult.

Few adverse events have been reported during treatment. Benign intracranial hypertension (around 1 in 1000) and carpal tunnel syndrome may occur, possibly due to sodium and water retention. Other adverse effects include pancreatitis, and an increase in the growth and pigmentation of naevi. The development of glucose intolerance and type 2 diabetes mellitus may occur in children receiving GH therapy, but the absolute risk appears to be low.

There are several indications for GH replacement therapy, described below.

GH deficiency

GH therapy (40 μg/kg per day) is monitored using the growth response and IGF-1 levels. The goal is to achieve IGF-1 levels of about 1 standard deviation above the mean for age and/or Tanner stage of pubertal development. With adequate replacement, adult height should be within the parental target range.

Turner's syndrome

Children with Turner's syndrome are treated with slightly higher doses of GH (45 –50 μg/kg per day) because they have a degree of GH resistance. GH therapy should be started as soon as the height of a girl with Turner's syndrome falls below the 5th percentile for age (usually between 2 and 5 years of age). In girls 9–12 years of age, combination therapy with GH and oxandrolone (an anabolic steroid) at a dose of 0.0625 mg/kg per day is recommended. GH therapy is continued until growth slows to less than 2 cm per year and the bone age exceeds 15 years.

Growth failure associated with chronic kidney disease

Treatment with GH has been shown to stimulate growth in prepubertal children with renal failure. GH should be started when the patient falls below the 3rd percentile for height and no spontaneous catch-up growth is seen with stabilization of other factors contributing to uraemic growth failure.

Children with chronic kidney disease are treated with slightly higher doses of GH (45–50 μg/kg per day), because they have a degree of GH resistance. The response to GH is better in children with preterminal chronic kidney disease than those on renal replacement therapy. Therefore GH therapy should be commenced well before the need for dialysis. GH therapy is continued until final height is reached or a well-functioning renal transplant has been achieved. The minimal therapeutic aim is a height greater than the 3rd percentile of the general population.

Children born small for gestational age

It is critical to discuss realistic expectations with the patient and family. GH therapy is likely to result in only modest gains in height compared with no treatment (an increase in adult height of approximately 6 cm, provided the treatment is started early and continued for at least 7 years). Adult height will usually be below average despite therapy. GH is started at doses of approximately 40 µg/kg per day based on ideal body weight. The dose is adjusted to maintain IGF-1 levels at approximately 1 standard deviation above the mean.

Prader–Willi syndrome

GH treatment (35 µg/kg per day) should be offered to all children and adolescents with clinical evidence of growth failure, unless there are contraindications (severe obesity, respiratory compromise, severe sleep apnoea). Sudden deaths have been reported in severely obese children with Prader–Willi syndrome shortly after starting GH.

GH therapy improves linear growth, body composition and bone density. The treatment may be continued until the epiphyses have closed. The optimal age to begin treatment has not been established. Patients should be closely monitored for the development of respiratory obstruction, particularly during the first few months of treatment.

Idiopathic short stature

GH is licensed in the USA for use in children with idiopathic short stature. Although the adult height is increased, the reported gains are small.

> **Box 30.2 Causes of tall stature**
>
> **Normal growth velocity**
> Constitutional tall stature
> Obesity
> Klinefelter's syndrome
> Marfan's syndrome
> Homocystinuria
>
> **Increased growth velocity**
> Precocious puberty (central or peripheral)
> Growth hormone-secreting pituitary adenoma
> Thyrotoxicosis

Tall stature

Most tall children are normal children of tall parents. Causes of tall stature are summarized in Box 30.2.

Obesity may be accompanied by an early onset of puberty and modest overgrowth. Obese children often have diminished overall GH production but high normal serum IGF-1 and GH-binding proteins, resulting in tall stature for age prior to puberty.

Klinefelter's syndrome is characterized by the presence of one or more extra X chromosomes (most commonly 47XXY). Prepubertal boys have relatively long legs and are often tall for their age. Other features of Klinefelter's syndrome include gynaecomastia, small testes and learning disabilities (mainly expressive language).

Marfan's syndrome is an autosomal dominant condition caused by mutations in the gene encoding fibrillin-1. Features of Marfan's syndrome include upward lens dislocation, arm span exceeding height, arachnodactyly (long thin fingers), skeletal abnormalities and aortic dilatation/regurgitation.

Homocystinuria is an autosomal recessive condition caused by a deficiency of the enzyme cystathionine synthetase. Features of homocystinuria include downward lens dislocation, mental retardation, thromboembolic phenomena and osteoporosis.

Causes of tall stature associated with increased growth velocity include *precocious puberty* (central or peripheral), *GH-secreting pituitary adenoma* and *thyrotoxicosis*.

Children with precocious puberty have accelerated childhood growth and epiphyseal maturation (i.e. accelerated bone age). These children have precocious sexual development and high serum sex steroid hormone levels (for their age). If their growth is not halted, these tall children will be short adults as early epiphyseal closure stops linear growth.

A GH-secreting pituitary adenoma is suspected when increased growth velocity is seen without manifestations of premature puberty. An arm span larger than standing height suggests an onset of disease before fusion of the epiphyses.

Investigations

A *karyotype* analysis should be performed in boys to look for Klinefelter's syndrome (47XXY). *Genetic tests* for the inherited conditions associated with tall stature (e.g. Marfan's syndrome) may be carried out if clinically suspected. *IGF-1* and *IGFBP-3* levels are elevated in children with GH-secreting adenomas. An oral glucose tolerance test will show a failure of GH suppression in these children. If a GH-secreting pituitary adenoma is suspected, a pituitary *MRI* should be performed. Serum *free thyroxine* and *thyroid-stimulating hormone* should be measured to exclude thyrotoxicosis.

Treatment of tall stature

The underlying disorder should be corrected if possible. The treatment of tall children and adolescents is controversial, and treatment is discouraged except in extreme cases. Psychosocial problems influence the final decision about treatment.

Sex steroids promote premature epiphyseal fusion by a direct effect at the epiphysis and an indirect action mediated by the GH–IGF-1 axis.

In *girls*, oestrogen (in the form of estradiol or ethinylestradiol) may be started before a bone age of 14–15 years (usually when the bone age is 10–12 years) at a dose of 15–30 μg per day, and increased to 50 μg per day if well tolerated and clinically indicated. Cyclic progestin therapy is indicated if breakthrough bleeding occurs. Treatment should be continued until the epiphyses fuse.

The risk–benefit ratio of oestrogen therapy must be discussed with the child and parents. Adverse effects include nausea, weight gain, oedema and hypertension. Oestrogen treatment may also have a negative impact on later fertility.

In *boys*, androgens also accelerate epiphyseal fusion, presumably via aromatization to oestrogens. Testosterone therapy as a treatment of constitutional tall stature in boys is extremely uncommon.

> ### Key points:
>
> - Short stature is defined as a height 2 standard deviations or more below the mean height for children of that gender and chronological age. This translates into being below the 3rd percentile for height.
> - Causes of short stature include familial, constitutional delay of growth and puberty, endocrine abnormalities (thyroid disease, GH or IGF-1 deficiency or insensitivity, Cushing's syndrome), dysmorphic syndromes associated with abnormal skeletal growth (e.g. Turner's syndrome, Down's syndrome, achondroplasia), chronic illness, malnutrition and psychosocial problems.
> - Initial investigations in children with reduced growth velocity should include blood tests to look for systemic illness, karyotype analysis (in girls), serum IGF-1 and IGFBP-3, and thyroid function tests.
> - When sellar/parasellar disorders are suspected, an MRI of the hypothalamic–pituitary area should be performed.
> - The bone age is a measure of skeletal maturity and is determined from a radiograph of the left hand and wrist (using a scoring system of epiphyseal maturation).
> - Indications for GH replacement therapy include GH deficiency, Turner's syndrome, growth failure associated with chronic kidney disease, children born small for gestational age and Prader–Willi syndrome.
> - Most tall children are the normal children of tall parents.

Chapter 31

Endocrine disorders of pregnancy

Disorders of thyroid function

Thyroid function during normal pregnancy

Maternal thyroid function

It is important to recognize the physiological changes that occur in the maternal thyroid function during normal pregnancy. These include:
- increased serum 'total' thyroxine (T_4) and triiodothyronine (T_3) levels due to an increase in serum T_4-binding globulin production caused by elevated oestrogen levels
- a slight increase in serum free T_4 and T_3 levels (usually within the normal range), and appropriate reductions in serum thyroid-stimulating hormone (TSH) levels in the first trimester. This is caused by human chorionic gonadotrophin (hCG, produced by the placenta), which is a weak stimulator of the TSH receptor. A first-trimester TSH reference range of 0.01–2.5 mU/L appears appropriate. A transient subclinical hyperthyroidism (normal free T_4 and suppressed TSH) may be seen in 10–20% of normal women during the period of highest serum hCG levels (10–12 weeks' gestation).

Thyroid hormone requirements increase during pregnancy. This may be due to:

Lecture Notes: Endocrinology and Diabetes. By A. Sam and K. Meeran. Published 2009 by Blackwell Publishing. ISBN 978-1-4051-5345-4.

- increased weight
- placental deiodinase activity
- transfer of T_4 to the fetus.

Fetal thyroid function

Maternal TSH does not cross the placenta. However, maternal thyroid hormones cross the placenta in small quantities, and are important for fetal growth and cognitive development during early pregnancy. Fetal TSH appears around the 10th week of gestation. However, little thyroid hormone synthesis occurs until the 18–20th week.

Hypothyroidism in pregnancy

Significance

Hypothyroidism in pregnancy is associated with several complications, including early pregnancy loss, placental abruption, pre-eclampsia, preterm delivery, low birth weight, perinatal mortality and neuropsychological impairment (which may occur even in women with subclinical hypothyroidism).

Treatment and follow-up

If hypothyroidism has been diagnosed before pregnancy, the preconception levothyroxine dose should be adjusted to reach a TSH level of less than 2.5 mU/L. As mentioned above, T_4 requirements increase during pregnancy. However, women with hypothyroidism are unable to increase their T_4 and T_3 secretion. Therefore the dose of levothyroxine should be increased by 30–50% by 4–6 weeks' gestation.

Serum TSH should be measured 4–6 weeks after conception, 4–6 weeks after any change in the dose of levothyroxine, and at least once each trimester. Further dose changes are based upon serum TSH concentrations (aim for a serum TSH of less than 2.5 mU/L).

If overt hypothyroidism is diagnosed during pregnancy, levothyroxine should be started and titrated rapidly to reach and thereafter maintain serum TSH concentrations at less than 2.5 mU/L.

Subclinical hypothyroidism (high serum TSH with a normal free T_4) has been shown to be associated with an adverse outcome for both mother and offspring (neuropsychological impairment). Therefore women with subclinical hypothyroidism must be treated with levothyroxine and monitored as above.

After delivery, the dose of levothyroxine can be reduced to pre-pregnancy levels. However, serum TSH should be measured 4–6 weeks later to confirm that the reduction in dose was appropriate.

Screening

Although professional societies have previously recommended checking thyroid function in pregnant women who are symptomatic or have a family history of thyroid disease, this approach may miss up to one third of women with hypothyroidism. Therefore universal screening for thyroid dysfunction is advisable in pregnant women or those hoping to become pregnant.

Hyperthyroidism in pregnancy

Significance

Poorly controlled hyperthyroidism in pregnancy is associated with an increased risk of pregnancy loss, premature labour, low birth weight, pre-eclampsia and maternal cardiac failure.

Diagnosis

The clinical diagnosis of hyperthyroidism during pregnancy may be difficult as many of the symptoms of hyperthyroidism (e.g. heat intolerance, increased sweating) are similar to the non-specific symptoms associated with pregnancy. In addition, high serum hCG levels during early pregnancy and in women with hyperemesis gravidarum (see below) or multiple pregnancies may result in transient subclinical or rarely overt hyperthyroidism. Hyperthyroidism in these cases rarely requires antithyroid drugs.

Although hyperthyroidism from any cause can complicate pregnancy, Graves' disease is the most common cause. Patients with Graves' disease may have ophthalmopathy, a family history of Graves' disease and a history of other autoimmune conditions.

The diagnosis of hyperthyroidism in pregnant women should be based primarily on a *serum TSH less than 0.01 mU/L* and a *high serum free T_4* and/or free T_3. Radioisotope administration is contraindicated in pregnancy.

Measurement of TSH-receptor antibodies (TRAbs) may be helpful in making the diagnosis of Graves' disease during pregnancy. In addition to mothers with current Graves' disease, TRAbs should also be measured before pregnancy or by the end of the second trimester in those with a history of Graves' disease and treatment with radio-iodine or thyroidectomy, or with a previous neonate with Graves' disease (see 'Fetal and neonatal assessment' below).

Treatment and follow-up

Overt hyperthyroidism due to Graves' disease or hyperfunctioning thyroid nodules should be treated with antithyroid drugs. Patients should be reviewed at 4-week intervals with measurements of free T_4 levels. The dose of the antithyroid drug should be adjusted appropriately. A block and replace regime (with high-dose antithyroid drug and levothyroxine) must not be used as it will result in fetal hypothyroidism.

Antithyroid drugs

Propylthiouracil (PTU) is usually used as a first-line drug. Carbimazole is very rarely associated with congenital anomalies (aplasia cutis), but may be given to patients who have had an adverse reaction to PTU. In patients with severe hyperthyroidism, an initial PTU dose of 150 mg twice a day (or carbimazole 30 mg once a day) may be given to normalize thyroid function. The dose is then adjusted according to the free T_4 levels measured every 2–4 weeks. The aim is to maintain the maternal free T_4 levels in the high-normal range. As pregnancy progresses, most patients require lower PTU doses (50 mg twice a day or less). Doses in excess of 200 mg per day should be avoided in the second and third trimesters due to the risk of fetal goitre and hypothyroidism.

Antithyroid drugs may be stopped in women who have been euthyroid for at least 4 weeks on the lowest dose, and thyroid function tests should be monitored every 4 weeks. Antithyroid drugs are usually not stopped during pregnancy in women with ophthalmopathy and a large goitre (i.e. those with a high chance of recurrence).

Graves' disease usually becomes less severe during the later stages of pregnancy, possibly due to a change in the activity of TRAbs from stimulatory to blocking. It is possible to discontinue the antithyroid drug during the third trimester in one third of women. However, Graves' hyperthyroidism can worsen postpartum. A beta-blocker (propranolol 20–40 mg three times a day) may be used for a few weeks in women with moderate-to-severe symptoms.

There is no evidence that the treatment of subclinical hyperthyroidism improves pregnancy outcome, and treatment could potentially adversely affect fetal outcome.

Breast-feeding mothers should be treated with the lowest possible dose of PTU.

Surgery

Subtotal thyroidectomy may be indicated in hyperthyroid women during pregnancy who cannot tolerate antithyroid drugs because of allergy or agranulocytosis. The optimal timing of surgery is in the second trimester. Radio-iodine treatment is absolutely contraindicated in pregnancy.

Fetal and neonatal assessment

TRAbs can cross the placenta. The fetuses of women treated with antithyroid drugs and those with elevated TRAbs should be monitored by sonography for signs of fetal thyrotoxicosis (fetal heart rate >160 beats per minute, goitre, growth restriction). Treatment is by giving antithyroid drugs to the mother and monitoring fetal heart rate (aiming for <140 beats per minute), growth and goitre size.

Around 1–5% of neonates born to women with Graves' disease have hyperthyroidism due to the transplacental transfer of TSH receptor-stimulating antibodies. The incidence is unrelated to maternal thyroid function. All newborns of mothers with Graves' disease should be evaluated for thyroid dysfunction and treated if necessary.

Hyperemesis gravidarum

Hyperemesis gravidarum is characterized by nausea, vomiting and weight loss ($\geq$5%) during early pregnancy. It may be caused by high serum hCG and oestradiol concentrations, or the secretion of hCG with increased biological activity. Many women with hyperemesis gravidarum have either subclinical or mild overt hyperthyroidism. Features that distinguish the transient hyperthyroidism of hyperemesis gravidarum from Graves' disease are the vomiting, absence of goitre and ophthalmopathy, and absence of the symptoms and signs of thyrotoxicosis (diarrhoea, muscle weakness, tremor). In addition, in hyperemesis gravidarum serum free T_4 is minimally elevated and serum T_3 is usually not elevated.

The hyperthyroidism in hyperemesis gravidarum does not require treatment with antithyroid drugs and resolves as hCG production falls. Patients are treated with intravenous fluids, antiemetics and nutritional support. If overt hyperthyroidism persists for more than several weeks or beyond the first trimester, it is probably not hCG-mediated and may be due to coincident Graves' disease, which should be treated with antithyroid drugs.

Trophoblastic disease

hCG-mediated hyperthyroidism also occurs in about 60% of women with a hydatidiform mole or choriocarcinoma. The hyperthyroidism may be severe, and is primarily treated by evacuation of the mole or therapy directed against the choriocarcinoma.

Goitre, thyroid nodules and cancer

Iodine depletion (due to increased maternal renal clearance and fetal uptake of iodide) may lead to mild thyroid enlargement. However, significant thyroid growth during pregnancy should be considered abnormal, requiring further investigation.

A pregnant woman with a thyroid nodule should be evaluated in the same way as if she were not pregnant (i.e. with fine needle aspiration and cytological examination). Thyroid radioisotope uptake scanning is absolutely contraindicated. Women with benign nodules are followed up. Those whose thyroid nodules enlarge should have another fine needle aspiration.

Women with malignant or suspicious cytology require surgery. The safest time for surgery during pregnancy is the second trimester. However, because of the usually indolent nature of most well-differentiated thyroid cancers, some delay surgery until the postpartum period.

Thyroid peroxidase antibodies

An increased rate of fetal loss and premature delivery has been reported in euthyroid women with high serum antithyroid peroxidase antibody levels. However, most pregnant women are unlikely to know their antithyroid antibody status because universal screening is not routinely done.

Prolactinomas in pregnancy

Prolactinomas usually result in infertility due to the inhibitory effect of prolactin on gonadotrophin secretion. However, treatment of hyperprolactinaemia enables most women to become pregnant.

Increased oestrogen levels in pregnancy cause lactotroph hyperplasia. In normal pregnant women, pituitary size increases throughout pregnancy (more than double). In patients with prolactinomas, the increase in the size of the tumour may result in compression of the optic chiasm and visual impairment. The management of women with prolactinoma during pregnancy varies according to the size of the adenoma.

Microprolactinomas (<1 cm)

The risk of a clinically important enlargement of a microprolactinoma during pregnancy is small (1.5–5.5% may develop neurological symptoms). Patients are treated with dopamine agonists prior to pregnancy.

Bromocriptine is preferred by some endocrinologists as there is greater experience with it. Patients can attempt to become pregnant when the serum prolactin concentration is normal and menstrual periods have occurred regularly for a few months. When periods have resumed, patients should be advised to have a pregnancy test as soon as they miss a period. The dopamine agonist is discontinued as soon as pregnancy has been confirmed.

Monitoring and follow-up

Pregnant women with microprolactinomas should be followed up every 3 months to enquire about headaches and changes in vision. Patients who develop these symptoms should be investigated with formal visual field testing and pituitary magnetic resonance imaging (MRI).

Serum prolactin levels are difficult to interpret as they are elevated during normal pregnancy. Serum prolactin should be measured 2 months after the delivery or cessation of breast-feeding, and if it is similar to the pre-treatment value, dopamine agonist therapy can be resumed. If serum prolactin levels are higher than pre-pregnancy levels, the size of microprolactinomas should be assessed by MRI.

Macroprolactinomas (≥1 cm)

Patient should be advised of the higher risk of clinically important tumour enlargement during pregnancy before conception (neurological symptoms may occur in up to 36%).

If the adenoma does not elevate the optic chiasm

The patient should be treated with bromocriptine or cabergoline to shrink the tumour substantially before she can attempt to become pregnant. The dopamine agonist may be stopped when pregnancy has been confirmed.

The patient should be carefully monitored with monthly visual field testing. If she develops symptoms of tumour enlargement (headache, visual impairment), a pituitary MRI should be performed. If the adenoma has enlarged, the woman should be treated with bromocriptine throughout the remainder of her pregnancy. If there is no response to bromocriptine, it may be substituted with cabergoline.

In patients who do not respond to cabergoline therapy, and whose vision is severely compromised, trans-sphenoidal surgery may be considered in the second trimester. Surgery for persistent visual symptoms in the third trimester should be deferred until delivery if possible as it is associated with a significant risk of fetal loss.

MRI should be performed in the postpartum period to look for tumour growth. Administration of bromocriptine during the first month of pregnancy does not harm the fetus. However, there are insufficient data regarding the use of bromocriptine later in pregnancy. Cabergoline use in early pregnancy appears to be safe, although data are limited.

If the adenoma is very large, elevates the chiasm or is unresponsive to dopamine agonists

Pregnancy should be strongly discouraged until the patient has been treated by trans-sphenoidal surgery and perhaps by postoperative radiotherapy and dopamine agonists. This approach reduces the risk of symptomatic expansion during pregnancy to 4–7%.

Breast-feeding

Breast-feeding does not increase the risk of lactotroph adenoma growth. Therefore, breast-feeding is an option for women with micro- and macro-adenomas that remained stable in size during pregnancy.

Breast-feeding is contraindicated in women who have neurological symptoms (suggesting tumour growth) at the time of delivery, because they should be treated with a dopamine agonist.

Adrenal disorders in pregnancy

Addison's disease in pregnancy

The fetus produces and regulates its own adrenal steroids. Therefore pre-existing primary adrenal insufficiency in the mother is not associated with fetal morbidity.

The treatment of Addison's disease in pregnant women is the same as that of non-pregnant patients. Hydrocortisone is the preferred glucocorticoid as it is metabolized by placental 11β-hydroxysteroid dehydrogenase, and thus fetal adrenal suppression is avoided. The glucocorticoid dose does not need to be increased during pregnancy. Patients should continue on their usual oral hydrocortisone and oral fludrocortisone as per their pre-pregnancy doses. Patients with severe hyperemesis gravidarum during the first trimester require temporary parenteral hydrocortisone. Patients should be warned about this to avoid precipitation of a crisis.

At the time of delivery, high-dose intramuscular hydrocortisone should be given to cover the stress of labour. During uncomplicated labour, 100 mg of hydrocortisone is given intramuscularly 6-hourly for 24 hours, and is then reduced to maintenance dose over 72 hours. Patients should be kept well hydrated. Fludrocortisone may be discontinued while the patient is on high doses of hydrocortisone and restarted when the hydrocortisone doses are tapered.

Addison's disease developing in early pregnancy may be missed as vomiting, fatigue, hyperpigmentation and hypotension may be wrongly attributed to pregnancy. However, clinicians should be alerted by persistent symptoms. Addison's disease developing in pregnancy may present with an adrenal crisis, particularly at the time of delivery.

Congenital adrenal hyperplasia in pregnancy

Only the most common form of congenital adrenal hyperplasia (CAH) due to 21-hydroxylase deficiency is discussed here.

Reduced fertility in women with CAH may be due to inadequate vaginal introitus despite reconstructive surgery and/or anovulation caused by hyperandrogenaemia. However, with improvements in surgical, medical and psychological treatments, more women with classic CAH can successfully complete pregnancies. About 80% of women with the simple virilizing form of CAH and 60% of those with the severe salt wasting form are fertile. Women with CAH are more likely to require caesarean section due to cephalopelvic disproportion.

No major complications in pregnancy are known in women with CAH. Management is similar to that of non-pregnant women, and steroids are increased at the time of delivery as for Addison's disease.

Serum androstenedione, testosterone, 17-hydroxyprogesterone and electrolytes should be monitored every 6 weeks. The glucocorticoid dosage should be adjusted, if necessary, to maintain the concentrations of these hormones within the normal ranges for the stage of pregnancy.

The unaffected female offspring of women with classic CAH are not at risk of virilization. This is because the placenta aromatizes maternal androgens to oestrogens. However, the affected female offspring (i.e. those with 21-hydroxylase deficiency) are at risk of virilization in utero due to excess androgen production by the fetal adrenals (see Chapter 9).

The male partner must be screened for CAH using basal and adrenocorticotrophic hormone (ACTH)-stimulated 17-hydroxyprogesterone (see Chapter 9). If 17-hydroxyprogesterone levels are elevated, genotyping must be done. If the male partner is heterozygote, the fetus is at risk of inheriting CAH and developing virilization. Thus prenatal treatment is recommended (see below). Prenatal treatment is also recommended in women who have had a previous child with CAH from the same partner.

The aim of the prenatal treatment is to prevent virilization of an affected female. *Dexamethasone* (20 μg/kg per day divided into three doses) is given to the mother as soon as the pregnancy is recognized. Because virilization occurs within the first 12 weeks of gestation, one cannot wait until the sex and diagnosis of the fetus are known. Dexamethasone crosses the placenta, suppresses fetal ACTH secretion and prevents overproduction of fetal adrenal androgens.

Dexamethasone treatment is discontinued if chorionic villus sampling (done at 8–12 weeks' gestation) or amniocentesis (done at 18–20 weeks' gestation) indicates that the fetus is male, or if genetic analysis indicates that the fetus is unaffected.

With treatment, 50% of affected female fetuses do not require reconstructive surgery. There are no known fetal congenital malformations associated with glucocorticoid treatment.

The prenatal treatment of women with non-classic CAH with dexamethasone is controversial. There have been no reports of women with non-classic CAH giving birth to a virilized female. However, infants should be screened in the neonatal period by measuring 17-hydroxyprogesterone levels.

Phaeochromocytomas in pregnancy

Phaeochromocytomas are rare in pregnancy but are potentially disastrous for both mother and fetus. The highest risk of hypertensive crisis and death is during labour (precipitated by anaesthesia or even normal delivery). Maternal mortality may be as high as 17% and fetal mortality may be up to 30% if not treated promptly.

The main sign of the disease is hypertension, but this is also common in pregnancy. However, phaeochromocytomas should be suspected in patients with hypertension (persistent or intermittent) with no proteinuria or oedema, and in women with paroxysmal headache, sweating and palpitation.

Catecholamine metabolism is not altered in the pregnant state, and thus biochemical tests are the same as those in non-pregnant women, i.e. three 24-hour urine collections for the measurement of catecholamines and fractionated metanephrines. MRI is used for localization of tumours after confirmation of the diagnosis, as it avoids exposing the fetus to ionizing radiation.

Prenatal screening should be performed in high-risk women, for example those with a history or family history of multiple endocrine neoplasia type 2 or von Hippel–Lindau syndrome.

Treatment

Phenoxybenzamine (an alpha-blocker) is safe in pregnancy. It is started at a dose of 10 mg twice a day and is increased gradually to a maximum of 20 mg three times a day. Propranolol (a beta-blocker) should only be given after alpha-blockade (at a dose of 40 mg three times a day). Unopposed alpha-adrenergic activity may lead to vasoconstriction and a hypertensive crisis.

After 24 weeks of gestation, uterine size makes abdominal exploration and access to the tumour difficult, and surgery must be deferred until fetal maturity is reached. Removal of the tumour may then be combined with caesarean section. However, some surgeons perform the adrenalectomy 4–6 weeks after elective early caesarean section. Adequate adrenergic blockade must be ensured prior to surgery.

Diabetes mellitus in pregnancy

Gestational diabetes mellitus is defined as glucose intolerance with an onset or first recognition during pregnancy.

Gestational diabetes occurs in about 2.1% of pregnant women in the USA, usually in the second or third trimester.

During pregnancy, an increased placental secretion of diabetogenic hormones such as growth hormone, corticotrophin-releasing hormone (which stimulates ACTH and cortisol release), human placental lactogen (also known as chori-onic somatomammotrophin) and progesterone results in maternal insulin resistance. In addition, a post-receptor defect may also contribute to the decline in insulin action. Gestational diabetes occurs when a woman's pancreatic function cannot overcome both the insulin resistance created by these anti-insulin hormones and the increased fuel consumption necessary to provide for the growing mother and fetus.

Screening, diagnosis and further evaluation

Women with pregestational diabetes should ideally have received preconceptional counselling and advice about the management and potential complications of diabetes in pregnancy.

Pregnant women should be screened for gestational diabetes mellitus. Screening may be performed at 24–28 weeks of gestation or as early as the first prenatal visit if unrecognized pregestational diabetes is suspected.

A 75 g 2-hour (or a 100 g 3-hour) oral glucose tolerance test is performed to make a diagnosis of gestational diabetes. Gestational diabetes may be diagnosed if two or more of the following criteria (proposed by the Fourth International Workshop-Conference on Gestational Diabetes) are met:
- fasting serum glucose >5.3 mmol/L
- 1-hour serum glucose >10 mmol/L
- 2-hour serum glucose >8.6 mmol/L
- 3-hour serum glucose >7.8 mmol/L.

In addition to routine prenatal testing, the assessment of women with diabetes should include the measurement of glycated haemoglobin, urea, creatinine and electrolytes, TSH and free T_4, an ECG, a dilated and comprehensive eye examination by an ophthalmologist, and first-trimester ultrasound examination if pregnancy dating is uncertain.

Treatment

The care of women with diabetes during pregnancy requires a team approach. Women with gestational diabetes mellitus must be followed up in regular joint endocrinology/obstetrics specialist clinics. Patients must be reviewed by dietitians and diabetes specialist nurses for further advice regarding diet, insulin therapy, exercise and glucose monitoring.

A programme of medical nutritional therapy, self-monitoring of blood glucose, and insulin therapy, when needed, has been shown to improve perinatal outcome.

The initial approach is *medical nutritional therapy*. The calorie allocation is 12–40 kcal/kg current weight per day depending upon the extent to which current weight differs from ideal body weight. Calories should be composed of 40% carbohydrate, 40% fat and 20% protein, and divided over three meals and three snacks. In overweight and obese women, the snacks are often eliminated.

Breakfast should contain 10% of the total calories as insulin resistance is greatest in the morning. Lunch and dinner should each contain 30% of the total calories. The remaining (30% of total) calories are distributed, as needed, as snacks.

Patients should check their blood glucose upon awakening and 1 hour after each meal to evaluate the effectiveness of the medical nutritional therapy. A programme of moderate exercise is also recommended for women with no medical or obstetrical contraindications.

Insulin therapy must be initiated if adequate glycaemic control is not achieved with dietary therapy and exercise alone (i.e. when fasting blood glucose is >5 mmol/L or 1-hour postprandial blood glucose is ≥6.7 mmol/L on two or more occasions within a 2-week interval). Women should continue to monitor their blood glucose levels. The goal is a fasting blood glucose of less than 5 mmol/L and a 1-hour postprandial blood glucose of less than 6.7 mmol/L.

During labour and delivery, maternal blood glucose concentration should be maintained between 4 and 5 mmol/L.

Poorly controlled diabetes in the first trimester is associated with increased risks of miscarriage and congenital malformations. Fetal development is evaluated by obstetricians via sonographic examination and maternal serum multiple marker screening.

If there is good glycaemic control and there are no pregnancy or additional maternal complications, it is reasonable to wait for the spontaneous onset of labour. However, extending pregnancy beyond 40 weeks of gestation is not advised. Earlier delivery may be warranted in the presence of high-risk factors such as worsening retinopathy or nephropathy, poor control, pre-eclampsia or restricted fetal growth.

Induction should be avoided because of suspected fetal macrosomia. If the expected fetal weight is more than 4.5 kg, caesarean delivery is recommended to avoid possible trauma from shoulder dystocia.

Women with gestational diabetes are at increased risk of developing diabetes after pregnancy, and should have a 2-hour 75 g oral glucose tolerance test at least 2 weeks after delivery.

Exacerbation of retinopathy in pregnancy

Diabetic retinopathy may worsen during pregnancy. The Diabetes in Early Pregnancy study showed that the risk of progression of retinopathy is related to the severity of retinal involvement before pregnancy and the initial glycated haemoglobin values. Changes in hormones, growth factors and systemic haemodynamics, and lower retinal blood flow, may contribute to the exacerbation of retinopathy in pregnancy.

The modest increase in risk of worsening of retinopathy during pregnancy necessitates more frequent retinal evaluations during this time and for 1 year postpartum. Women should be screened during the first trimester and then every 3 months while pregnant.

Treatment recommendations are the same as for other patients. Laser therapy and vitreous surgery can be carried out safely during pregnancy if required. Women can be reassured that their long-term risk of retinopathy progression is not increased by pregnancy.

Key points:

- Normal pregnant women have increased serum 'total' T_4 and T_3 (due to raised thyroid-binding globulin levels), and a slight increase in serum free T_4 and T_3 levels and suppressed TSH levels in the first trimester (due to raised hCG levels).
- Pregnant women with subclinical hypothyroidism must be treated with levothyroxine.
- Overt hyperthyroidism should be treated with antithyroid drugs. Radio-iodine treatment is absolutely contraindicated in pregnancy.
- Women with macroprolactinomas must be treated with dopamine agonists to shrink the tumour substantially before they can attempt to become pregnant.
- The male partner of a woman with classic CAH must be screened for CAH.
- Phaeochromocytomas should be suspected in pregnant women with hypertension and no proteinuria or oedema.
- An oral glucose tolerance test is performed to make a diagnosis of gestational diabetes.
- Insulin therapy must be initiated if adequate glycaemic control is not achieved with dietary therapy and exercise alone.

Chapter 32

Neuroendocrine tumours

Neuroendocrine cells contain neurotransmitters, neuromodulators or neuropeptide hormones within secretory granules, from which they are released by exocytosis in response to an external stimulus. Unlike neurones, these cells do not have axons and do not make synapses. Neuroendocrine cells make up the diffuse neuroendocrine system, dispersed throughout the body. The *gastroentero-pancreatic neuroendocrine system* provides the richest source of regulatory peptides outside the brain.

It was originally thought that all neuroendocrine cells derived from neuroectoderm, but increasingly this has been found not to be the case for all neuroendocrine cells.

Neuroendocrine cells can be characterized by a number of molecular markers such as *chromogranin A* (a protein located alongside specific hormones in large dense-core vesicles) and the subtilase proprotein convertases 2 and 3.

Neuroendocrine tumours (NETs) originate from neuroendocrine cells within the gut (75%), pancreatic islet cells (5%), lung (15%) and other organs (e.g. parafollicular cells within the thyroid, giving rise to medullary thyroid carcinoma [MTC]). NETs may be classified according to their embryological origin into:

- foregut tumours (bronchi, stomach, duodenum, pancreas, gall bladder)
- midgut tumours (jejunum, ileum, appendix, right colon)
- hindgut tumours (left colon and rectum).

NETs may be functioning or non-functioning depending on whether a secreted hormone is detectable and associated symptoms are present.

The majority of NETs occur as non-familial (sporadic) isolated tumours. However, NETs may be part of familial syndromes such as multiple endocrine neoplasia type 1 (MEN 1), multiple endocrine neoplasia type 2 (MEN 2), neurofibromatosis type 1 (NF 1), von Hippel–Lindau syndrome (see Chapter 8) and Carney's complex (see Chapter 16).

The term *carcinoid* is used for NETs mostly derived from serotonin-producing enterochromaffin cells. In excess of 50% of NETs are of the 'carcinoid' type. About 70% of the carcinoid tumours occur in the gut, and 25% occur in the lung.

The classification of NETs into benign and malignant depends on tumour size, local spread, vascular invasion, metastases and nuclear atypia.

Aetiology

The aetiology of neuroendocrine disorders is poorly understood. Most NETs are sporadic, but epidemiological studies show a small increased familial risk for small intestinal and colon NETs.

Lecture Notes: Endocrinology and Diabetes. By A. Sam and K. Meeran. Published 2009 by Blackwell Publishing. ISBN 978-1-4051-5345-4.

It has been proposed that NETs may result from a series of genetic mutations leading to the activation of oncogenes and/or inactivation of tumour suppressor genes and failure of apoptosis. A number of genes are known to be involved in the formation of NETs, including *MEN1*, *RET*, *VHL*, *TSC1* and *TSC2*. Mutations in *MEN1* (a tumour suppressor gene) are the most common form of genetic predisposition to NETs.

Epidemiology

The incidence of NETs is about three per 100 000 per year. There is a slight predominance in women.

The annual incidence of pancreatic NETs is approximately 2–4 per million. However, post mortem data suggest a higher incidence. Insulinomas and gastrinomas are the most common among this rare group of tumours. The prevalence of NETs is relatively high because many NETs are slow growing and even malignant NETs are associated with prolonged survival.

The risk of a NET in an individual with one affected first-degree relative is about four times and with two affected first-degree relatives is over 12 times that in the general population.

MEN type 1 has a prevalence of about two per 100 000, and MEN type 2 has an estimated prevalence of 2.5 per 100 000 in the general population. The incidence of MEN 1 in gastroenteropancreatic NETs varies from virtually 0% in gut carcinoids to 5% in insulinomas and 25–30% in gastrinomas.

Clinical presentations

Gastroenteropancreatic tumours can be asymptomatic or may present with obstructive symptoms due to tumour bulk (pain, nausea, vomiting), symptoms of metastases (liver) or syndromes of hormone hypersecretion.

Carcinoid syndrome is usually a result of metastases to the liver with the subsequent release of hormones (serotonin, tachykinins and other vasoactive compounds) into the systemic circulation.

Carcinoid syndrome is characterized by flushing, diarrhoea and occasionally wheezing. Less commonly, patients may present with pellagra due to niacin deficiency (caused by the diversion of dietary tryptophan for the synthesis of large amounts of serotonin). Pellagra is characterized by dermatitis (rough scaly skin), glossitis, diarrhoea and dementia.

Muscle wasting may occur as a result of poor protein synthesis. Some patients may experience rhinorrhoea, lacrimation and episodic palpitations. About 70% of patients with carcinoid syndrome give a history of intermittent abdominal pain at the time of diagnosis. Patients with the 'atypical' carcinoid syndrome present with protracted purplish flushing, which affects the limbs as well as the upper trunk and frequently results in telangiectasia.

Carcinoid heart disease is seen if the syndrome has been present for some years. It is characterized by deposits of fibrous tissue on the endocardium of the valvular cusps and cardiac chambers. The right side of the heart is most often affected because the inactivation of humoral substances by the lung protects the left side of the heart.

Patients with bronchial carcinoid may present with evidence of bronchial obstruction, pneumonitis, pleuritic chest pain, dyspnoea, cough and haemoptysis in addition to a variety of other symptoms, including weakness, nausea, weight loss, night sweats, neuralgia and Cushing's syndrome.

The *carcinoid crisis* is characterised by profound flushing, bronchospasm, tachycardia and fluctuating blood pressure. It may be due to the release of mediators that lead to the production of high levels of serotonin and other vasoactive peptides. The carcinoid crisis may be precipitated by anaesthetic induction, intraoperative handling of the tumour or invasive therapeutic procedures such as embolization and radiofrequency ablation.

Presenting features of pancreatic NETs are summarized below:

- *Insulinoma*: symptoms and signs of hypoglycaemia: sweating, dizziness, tachycardia, weakness, confusion and unconsciousness. The symptoms are relieved by eating.
- *Gastrinoma* (Zollinger–Ellison syndrome): severe peptic ulceration and diarrhoea.
- *Glucagonoma:* necrolytic migratory erythema (a rash affecting the lower abdomen, buttocks,

perineum and groin), weight loss, diabetes mellitus, diarrhoea and stomatitis.

- *VIPoma* (Werner–Morrison syndrome): profuse watery diarrhoea with marked hypokalaemia.
- *Somatostatinoma*: cholelithiasis, weight loss, diarrhoea, steatorrhoea and diabetes mellitus.

It is important to search thoroughly for MEN 1, MEN 2 and NF 1 in all patients with NETs by obtaining a detailed family history and clinical examination. A familial syndrome should be suspected in all cases where there is a family history of a NET or a second endocrine tumour. A diagnosis of MEN 1, MEN 2 or NF 1 has important implications for the patient and the patient's relatives, who should be considered for genetic testing and screening for the associated tumours (see below).

Investigations

The diagnosis of gastroenteropancreatic NETs is based on clinical symptoms, hormone concentration, radiological and nuclear medicine imaging, and histological confirmation. The gold standard in diagnosis is detailed histology, and this should be obtained whenever possible. If histology is available from a previous primary site, biopsy of the secondaries may not be necessary.

Biochemical tests

If a patient presents with symptoms suspicious of a gastroenteropancreatic NET, biochemical tests should include:

- plasma *chromogranin A*
- 24-hour urinary *5-hydroxyindoleacetic acid* (5-HIAA)
- a *fasting gut hormone* profile including gastrin, glucagon, somatostatin, pancreatic polypeptide, vasoactive intestinal peptide and neurotensin. Blood should be taken in a 10 mL standard heparin bottle containing aprotinin (0.2 mL) and spun immediately before being frozen and sent to a reference laboratory. Multiple hormones may be secreted by some tumours.

All patients should be evaluated for second endocrine tumours and possibly for other gut

> **Box 32.1 Factors that affect urinary 5-hydroxyindoleacetic acid excretion**
>
> **Factors that may cause false-positive results**
> Bananas, avocados, aubergines, pineapples, plums, walnuts, caffeine
> Paracetamol, naproxen, fluorouracil, methysergide
>
> **Factors that may cause false-negative results**
> Aspirin, levodopa, methyldopa, phenothiazines

cancers. Baseline tests that may be appropriate include calcium, parathyroid hormone (PTH), PTH-related protein (if PTH is low), thyroid function tests, calcitonin, prolactin, alpha-fetoprotein, carcinoembryonic antigen (CEA) and beta-human chorionic gonadotrophin.

Chromogranin A is a large protein that is produced by all cells deriving from the neural crest. The function of chromogranin A is not known, but it is produced in very significant quantities by NET cells regardless of their secretory status.

5-HIAA is the main metabolite of serotonin. The 24-hour urinary 5-HIAA is raised in 70% of patients with midgut carcinoid and some patients with foregut carcinoid. Urinary excretion of 5-HIAA may be affected by certain foods and drugs if they are taken just before collection of the urine sample (Box 32.1). Tachykinins (neurokinin A and B) are raised in midgut carcinoids.

Specific endocrine tests should be requested depending on which syndrome is suspected.

Suspected insulinoma

In patients presenting with acute hypoglycaemia, serum should be taken quickly for blood glucose, *insulin* and *C-peptide* levels *prior* to giving glucose. Low C-peptide and high insulin levels indicate exogenous insulin. High C-peptide and insulin levels indicate endogenous insulin, for example either stimulated by surreptitious sulphonylurea ingestion or released by an insulinoma.

Patients with a history suggestive of hypoglycaemic episodes should be investigated with a 72-hour fast, allowing unlimited non-caloric fluids.

Box 32.2 Differential diagnosis of hypoglycaemia

Diabetic patients: insulin, oral hypoglycaemic agents
Drugs: alcohol, salicylates, quinine, pentamidine
Adrenal insufficiency
Hypopituitarism
Renal failure
Liver failure
Tumours: insulinomas, hepatomas, sarcomas, big-insulin-like growth factor 2

Elevated plasma insulin and C-peptide levels in the presence of hypoglycaemia (laboratory glucose <2.2 mmol/L) are diagnostic. A plasma glucose level of less than 2.2 mmol/L is achieved by 48 hours of fasting for over 95% of insulinomas. If no hypoglycaemia is achieved by the end of the fast, the sensitivity can be further increased by exercising the patient for 15 minutes. The fast is terminated after the exercise period, or prior to this if hypoglycaemia is achieved (but only after samples for insulin and C-peptide have been taken).

Patients with 'factitious hypoglycaemia' (due to exogenous insulin) do not have elevated C-peptide levels. All patients should also have simultaneous urine samples for *sulphonylurea analysis*, which must be shown to be negative for the diagnosis of insulinoma.

The differential diagnosis of fasting hypoglycaemia in summarized in Box 32. 2.

A rare cause of fasting hypoglycaemia is the secretion of an incompletely processed form of insulin-like growth factor 2 ('big-IGF-2') by mesenchymal tumours. These patients have suppressed insulin levels, low IGF-1 and a raised ratio of IGF-2 to IGF-1.

Suspected gastrinomas

Investigations for suspected gastrinomas include fasting gastrin level (raised basal serum gastrin) and gastric secretion studies (high gastric acid secretion).

To measure gastrin in a patient with a suspected gastrinoma, the patient must be off proton pump inhibitors for at least 2 weeks and off histamine 2-blockers for at least 3 days. Caution, however, is required if the clinical likelihood of a gastrinoma is high since there is a high risk of peptic ulcer perforation when medical therapy is stopped for the gastrin test. Even on proton pump inhibitors, very high gastrin levels (>250 pmol/L) are indicative of gastrinoma, and repeat testing off therapy should not be recommended.

Differential diagnoses, which include atrophic gastritis, hypercalcaemia and renal impairment, may be excluded by measuring basal acid output. Spontaneous basal acid outputs of 20–25 mmol per hour are almost diagnostic and over 10 mmol per hour are suggestive. If the test results are equivocal, the secretin test is helpful: a rise in gastrin of more than 100 pmol/L (instead of the normal fall) in response to intravenous secretin has a sensitivity of 80–85% for gastrinoma.

Imaging

The optimum imaging modality depends on whether it is to be used for detecting disease in a patient suspected of a NET or for assessing the extent of disease in a known case.

For detecting the primary tumour, a multimodality approach is best and may include computed tomography, magnetic resonance imaging, somatostatin receptor scintigraphy (SRS), endoscopic ultrasound (for pancreatic NETs, with a 94% sensitivity for detecting insulinomas) and visceral angiography (helpful for subcentimetre tumours, where a tumour blush is seen) plus calcium stimulation (see below). For assessing secondaries, SRS is the most sensitive modality. When a primary tumour has been resected, SRS may be indicated for follow-up. SRS has a sensitivity of up to 90% and a specificity of 80% (excluding insulinomas), and has a sensitivity of 10–50% for insulinomas.

With pancreatic tumours, the surgeon requires as much information as possible regarding location.

Selective angiography with secretagogue injection into the main pancreatic arteries allows angiographic and biochemical localization. In this procedure, the main pancreatic arteries (gastroduodenal, superior mesenteric, inferior pancreaticoduodenal, splenic) are cannulated separately and examined for a 'tumour blush'.

Calcium (acting as a secretagogue) is injected into each of these arteries individually, and venous samples are collected from the hepatic vein for biochemical analysis of the suspected hypersecreted hormone (e.g. gastrin, insulin). In the presence of a tumour, the hormone levels double after 30 seconds, whereas the normal effect is a reduction in levels. The hepatic artery is always cannulated at the end of the procedure. A rise in hormone levels detectable in the hepatic vein after calcium injection into the hepatic artery is diagnostic of liver metastases.

Treatment

All cases must be discussed and managed within a multidisciplinary team. The choice of treatment depends on the symptoms, stage of disease, degree of uptake of radionuclide and histological features of the tumour.

Surgery is the only curative treatment for NETs and should be offered to patients who are fit and have limited disease (i.e. primary tumour with or without positive regional lymph nodes).

For patients who are not fit for surgery, the aim of treatment is to improve and maintain an optimal quality of life. Treatment choices for non-resectable disease include somatostatin analogues, chemotherapy, radionuclides and ablation therapies. External beam radiotherapy may relieve bone pain from metastases.

Surgical treatment

Conduct of surgery is dependent on the method of presentation and stage of disease. Surgery should only be undertaken in specialist units. Patients presenting with suspected appendicitis, intestinal obstruction or other gastrointestinal emergencies are likely to require resections sufficient to correct the immediate problem. Once definitive histopathology has been obtained, a further more radical resection may have to be considered.

Where abdominal surgery is undertaken and long-term treatment with somatostatin analogues is likely, cholecystectomy should be considered (see the side-effects of somatostatin analogues, below).

Surgery also has a place in palliation when tumour bulk is too extensive for curative resections.

Liver metastases

Surgery should also be considered in those with liver metastases and potentially resectable disease. Cryosurgery, where a cryoprobe is inserted surgically into each metastasis, causing tumour necrosis, has been used in the palliation of liver metastases. Liver transplantation has been performed in selected patients with numerous liver metastases, with survival of about 50% after 1 year.

Preparation

A potential carcinoid crisis should be prevented by the intravenous infusion of octreotide at a dose of 50 µg per hour for 12 hours prior to and at least 48 hours after surgery. It is also important to avoid drugs that release histamine or activate the sympathetic nervous system. Other prophylactic measures for other NETs include glucose infusion for insulinomas, and proton pump inhibitors and intravenous octreotide for gastrinomas.

Medical treatment

Medical treatment has to be initiated for symptom control until curative surgical treatment is performed, or if surgery is not indicated. Box 32.3 summarizes the medical treatments for the various hypersecretion syndromes.

Somatostatin analogues

The only proven hormonal management of NETs is the administration of somatostatin analogues. Somatostatin receptors are present in 70–95% of NETs overall and in about 50% of insulinomas, and occur less often on poorly differentiated NETs and somatostatinomas. Somatostatin analogues inhibit the release of various peptide hormones in the gut and antagonize growth factor effects on tumour cells.

Patients may be stabilized with octreotide (short acting) for 10–28 days before converting them to long-acting somatostatin analogues. Octreotide is administered by subcutaneous injection starting at

---

Box 32.3 Medical treatments for neuroendocrine tumour syndromes

Carcinoid
Somatostatin analogue for SRS-positive carcinoid
Alpha-interferon for SRS-negative carcinoid
Histamine antagonists (H1 and H2), ondansetron, cyproheptadine, nicotinamide

Insulinoma
Frequent slow-release complex carbohydrate intake
Diazoxide for controlling hypoglycaemic symptoms; side-effects include fluid retention and hirsutism
Intravenous glucose for periods of fasting or acute hypoglycaemia
Intramuscular glucagon for the treatment of acute hypoglycaemia
Somatostatin analogue if SRS positive (usually malignant); these have variable effects on blood glucose, possibly due to the suppression of counterregulatory hormones such as glucagon

Gastrinoma
High-dose proton pump inhibitor (lifelong in patients with MEN 1, since there is a high recurrence rate with surgery)

Glucagonoma
Somatostatin analogue
Anticoagulation since associated with thrombophilia
Insulin for diabetes mellitus
Zinc therapy for skin lesions (necrolytic migratory erythema)

VIPoma
Somatostatin analogue (titrate the dose against vasoactive intestinal peptide levels, aiming for a normalization of levels)
Aggressive intravenous rehydration in acute attacks of diarrhoea
Potassium and bicarbonate in acute attacks

Somatostatinoma
Pancreatic enzyme supplementation
Insulin for diabetes mellitus

Non-functioning tumours
A somatostatin analogue if the SRS scan is positive and there is progressive disease

SRS, somatostatin receptor scintigraphy.

50–100 μg twice or three times a day to a maximum daily dose of 1500 μg. An inhibition of hormone production (biochemical response) is seen in 30–70% of patients, with symptomatic control in the majority of patients. Tumour growth may stabilize, and rarely shrinkage of tumour may be seen.

Analogues with sustained release from depot injections may be given every 2–4 weeks. Lanreotide (fortnightly injections), lanreotide Autogel and Sandostatin LAR (monthly injections) have been shown to significantly improve patients' quality of life. Lanreotide and octreotide bind preferentially to the subtype 2 somatostatin receptor and to a lesser extent to the subtype 5 somatostatin receptor.

The side-effects of somatostatin analogues include gall stones and gall bladder dysfunction, fat malabsorption, vitamin A and D malabsorption, headaches, diarrhoea, dizziness and hyperglycaemia. Monitoring circulating and, where relevant, urinary hormone levels should be undertaken during periods of treatment. Patients should also have regular relevant imaging.

Alpha-interferon

This is used in both secreting carcinoid tumours and other NETs on its own or added to long-acting somatostatin analogues if the patient is not responding to the maximum dosage of somato-statin analogues. Alpha-interferon may result in a 40–50% biochemical and 10–15% tumour response in carcinoid and neuroendocrine pancreatic tumours. Side-effects include flu-like symptoms, weight loss, fatigue, depression, hepatotoxicity and autoimmune disorders.

Chemotherapy

Chemotherapy may be used for inoperable or faster-growing metastatic pancreatic and bronchial tumours, and for poorly differentiated NETs. Various combinations of chemotherapy have been used, including streptozotocin and Adriamycin in well-differentiated pancreatic NETs, lomustine and 5-fluorouracil in advanced NETs, and etoposide and cisplatin in poorly differentiated and aggressive NETs. Toxicity rates are high.

Hepatic artery embolization

Hepatic artery embolization is indicated for patients with non-resectable multiple and hormone-secreting tumours with the intention of reducing tumour size and hormone output. Arterial embolization induces ischaemia of the tumour cells, thereby reducing their hormone output and causing liquefaction.

There are two types of embolization: particle embolization and chemoembolization. Particles used include polyvinyl alcohol and gel foam powder. For chemoembolization, agents such as doxorubicin and cisplatin are primarily used. Ischaemia of the tumour cells induced by embolization increases their sensitivity to chemotherapeutic substances.

Post-embolization syndrome (nausea, fever, abdominal pain) is the most common side-effect. Hormone therapy should be used prior to all embolizations: 50–100 μg octreotide per hour intravenously for 12 hours before and 48 hours after the procedure. Some units use hydrocortisone 100 mg intravenously and prophylactic antibiotics prior to the procedure, and pre-dosing with allopurinol to prevent a tumour lysis syndrome.

Targeted radionuclide therapy

This is a useful palliative option for symptomatic patients with inoperable or metastatic tumour. Beta-emitting radionuclides (^{131}I-MIBG, ^{90}Y-octreotide, ^{90}Y-lanreotide) are given to patients, with avid uptake of the corresponding gamma-emitting imaging radionuclide (^{123}I-MIBG, ^{111}In-octreotide) at all known tumour sites on diagnostic imaging.

Prognosis

Recent increases in the survival of individuals with NET have been documented. The overall 5-year survival of all NET cases is about 67%.

Survival depends on the histological type, degree of differentiation, mitotic rate, Ki-67 or MIB-1 index (indices of proliferative activity), tumour size (>3 cm), depth, location, presence of liver or lymph node metastases, and age over 50 years. Following complete resection of the primary tumour and liver metastases if present, the overall 5-year survival is 83%. In cases where this is not possible, survival ranges from 30% to 70% depending on the factors above and the treatment employed.

The best prognosis is in bronchial and appendicular carcinoids. The 5-year survival for typical lung carcinoids and carcinoid tumours of the appendix is 80–90%, whereas that for atypical lung tumours is 40–70%.

The overall 5-year survival for pancreatic NETs is 50–80%, with insulinomas and gastrinomas having up to 94% 5-year survival, although there is clearly a large variation depending on the stage at presentation and whether curative surgery is possible.

Multiple endocrine neoplasia

MEN is characterized by tumours involving two or more endocrine glands within a single patient. Although these syndromes are rare, recognition is important for both the treatment and evaluation of family members.

There are two major forms of MEN: type 1 (Wermer's syndrome) and type 2 (Sipple's syndrome). MEN syndromes are inherited as autosomal dominant disorders. Occasionally, MEN may arise sporadically. However, it is sometimes difficult to distinguish sporadic and familial forms as the parent with the disease may have died before developing any manifestations.

MEN type 1

MEN type 1 is characterized by a predisposition to:
• parathyroid adenomas
• enteropancreatic endocrine adenomas
• pituitary adenomas.

A consensus statement from an international group of endocrinologists defines MEN 1 as the presence of two of the above tumours. Familial MEN 1 is defined as an index MEN 1 case with at least one relative who has one of the above tumours.
• *Parathyroid adenomas* result in primary hyperparathyroidism and hypercalcaemia. This is the initial manifestation of the disorder in 90% of the patients and occurs in 95% of patients by age 50 years. About 1–2% of all cases of primary hyperparathyroidism are due to MEN 1.
• *Enteropancreatic endocrine adenomas* occur in 40% of individuals with MEN 1. The majority of patients with familial MEN 1 develop non-functioning pancreatic tumours; 40% develop gastrinomas and 10% develop insulinomas. Glucagonomas, VIPomas and somatostatinomas are rare. Pancreatic polypeptidomas are more common but remain asymptomatic.
• *Pituitary adenomas* occur in 30% of MEN 1 patients. Most (60%) are prolactinomas. Growth-hormone secreting tumours account for 20% of the pituitary tumours. Other types of pituitary adenoma that may occur in MEN 1 include non-functioning adenomas and corticotroph adenomas.

As tumours arise in patients with MEN 1, patients present with symptoms of hormone secretion (e.g. PTH, gastrin, insulin, prolactin, growth hormone) and tumour bulk (e.g. pituitary tumours compressing the optic chiasm, non-functioning pancreatic tumours with liver metastases).

Other tumours that may be associated with MEN 1 include facial angiofibromas (88%), collageno-mas (72%), carcinoid tumours (5–10%), adrenocortical tumours (5%) and lipomas (1%).

Aetiology

In MEN 1, germline inactivating mutations in the tumour suppressor gene *MEN1* (on chromosome 11) are found in 95% of patients. *MEN1* encodes a protein called menin. Menin suppresses gene transcription activated by *JunD* and controls cell proliferation.

Absence of detectable mutations in *MEN1* may reflect deficiencies of current technology or the fact that the inactivation process occurs via non-mutation mechanisms such as methylation of a region of the *MEN1* gene. Familial and somatic *MEN1* mutations differ in terms of the former usually presenting at an earlier age, with multiple organs affected and multiple tumours in one organ.

Screening

Indications for screening for MEN 1 are:
• two or more MEN 1-associated endocrine tumours
• one MEN 1-associated endocrine tumour and age less than 30 years
• any individual with a relative with MEN 1.

Screening involves genetic testing, thorough clinical history and examination, and biochemical tests.

Genetic testing for mutations in the *MEN1* gene is performed in index cases and asymptomatic relatives. Relatives who do not have the mutation can be reassured and do not require regular screening.

Clinical and biochemical screening is commenced annually from 5 years of age in MEN 1-affected families. Patients with known MEN 1 should have 6-monthly screening for additional tumours.

Clinical history and examination should look for symptoms and signs of the endocrine tumours associated with MEN 1:
• parathyroid adenomas: hypercalcaemia and nephrolithiasis
• gastrinomas: peptic ulcer disease

- insulinomas: symptoms and signs of sympathetic overactivity and neuroglycopenia
- pituitary adenomas: hypopituitarism, galactorrhoea and amenorrhoea in women, acromegaly, Cushing's disease and visual field loss
- subcutaneous lipomas, facial angiofibromas and collagenomas.

Biochemical tests should include serum *calcium* and *prolactin*. Measurement of gut hormones and specific endocrine function tests are indicated in those with symptoms and signs of MEN 1-associated tumours.

Management

The management of affected families is complex, requiring careful coordination between the medical team (endocrinologist, geneticist, surgeon, general practitioner) and the family. The management of MEN type 1 includes:

- subtotal parathyroidectomy for hyperparathyroidism
- surgical resection of pancreatic NETs where surgically feasible except for gastrinoma, for which recurrence is high after surgery in MEN 1 and for which some advocate non-surgical therapy
- the treatment of pituitary tumours in a similar way to sporadic cases.

MEN type 2

MEN 2 is the association of MTC with phaeochromocytoma. Three variants are recognized: MEN 2a, MEN 2b and MTC-only (Box 32.4).

Aetiology

MEN type 2 results from germline mutations in the *RET* proto-oncogene (on chromosome 10), which encodes a tyrosine kinase receptor. In all variants, there is a high (90%) penetrance of MTC. Around 98% of MEN 2 index cases have an identified *RET* mutation. *RET* mutations can be categorized as high, intermediate and low risk, referring to the potential risk for local and distant metastases at an early age. The likelihood of *RET* germline mutations in a patient with apparently sporadic MTC is 1–7%.

> **Box 32.4 Multiple endocrine neoplasia type 2 (MEN 2) syndromes**
>
> **MEN 2a (>75% of all MEN 2)**
> Medullary thyroid carcinoma (90%)
> Phaeochromocytoma (50%)
> Parathyroid adenomas (20–30%)
> Cutaneous lichen amyloidosis: pruritic, scaly, papular, pigmented skin lesions in the interscapular region or on the extensor surfaces of the extremities (rare)
>
> **MEN 2b**
> Medullary thyroid carcinoma (90%)
> Phaeochromocytoma
> Mucosal neuromas
> Intestinal autonomic ganglion dysfunction leading to multiple diverticulae and megacolon
> Marfanoid habitus
> Medullated corneal fibres
>
> **MTC-only**
> Medullary thyroid carcinoma

Screening

Indications for screening for MEN 2 are:
- MTC, or two or more MEN 2-associated endocrine tumours
- one MEN 2-associated endocrine tumour and age less than 30 years
- mucosal neuromas or somatic features of MEN 2b
- any individual with a relative with MEN 2.

Screening involves genetic testing, thorough clinical history and examination, and biochemical tests.

Genetic testing for mutations in the *RET* gene is indicated in index cases and asymptomatic (usually first-degree) relatives. Further clinical and biochemical screening is restricted to family members who have inherited the mutation.

Clinical and biochemical screening is performed every 3–6 months in patients known to have MEN 2 to identify the development of additional tumours, and every 6–12 months in unaffected carriers. Screening for phaeochromocytoma is started at age 5 years, and screening for primary hyperparathyroidism at age 10 years.

Clinical history and examination should look for symptoms and signs of endocrine tumours associated with MEN 2:

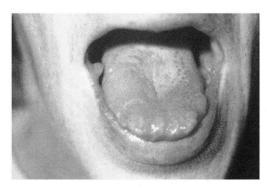

Figure 32.1 Mucosal neuromas on the tongue and lips in a patient with multiple endocrine neoplasia type 2b.

- MTC: lumps in the neck, dysphagia (16%) and diarrhoea (30%)
- phaeochromocytoma: headaches, palpitations, sweating and hypertension
- parathyroid adenomas: hypercalcaemia
- MEN 2b-related neuromas (Fig. 32.1) and somatic features.

Biochemical tests include serum calcitonin (basal and post-pentagastrin stimulation), 24-hour urinary catecholamines and/or metanephrines, and serum calcium and PTH.

Management

The management of affected families is complex, requiring careful coordination between the medical team (endocrinologist, geneticist, surgeon, general practitioner) and the family.

Total *thyroidectomy* should be performed for patients with MEN 2. Unfortunately, MTC tends not to be responsive to either chemotherapy or radiotherapy. Phaeochromocytomas, if present, should be removed before thyroidectomy. A number of strategies for adjuvant therapy after total thyroidectomy have been investigated, all with limited success.

Postoperatively, patients should be monitored with serum *calcitonin* measurements and neck ultrasound for evidence of recurrence. Calcitonin is measured at least yearly, and in intermediate- or high-risk patients every 6 months.

Serum CEA levels are also monitored by some experts. These often take several months to nor-malize postoperatively because CEA is a large gly-cosylated molecule. Calcitonin is a more sensitive test, but at a later stage of the disease, due to dedif-ferentiation, the ratio between calcitonin and CEA may change.

All *RET* mutation carriers should undergo pro-phylactic total thyroidectomy to prevent the almost certain development of MTC. Thyroidec-tomy should be performed before the age of 6 months in MEN 2b and before the age of 5 years in MEN 2a. MEN 2b has a more aggressive course than MEN 2a or familial MTC.

The preferred therapy for unilateral adrenal phaeochromocytoma is laparoscopic resection, following adequate preoperative alpha- and beta-adrenergic blockade. Bilateral adrenal and extra-adrenal phaeochromocytomas require open resection.

Hyperparathyroidism is milder than in MEN 1, but often more than one parathyroid gland is enlarged. The exact parathyroid procedure per-formed (e.g. subtotal, only enlarged glands) should be the same as in other disorders with multiple parathyroid tumours.

Key points:

- NETs originate from neuroendocrine cells within the gut, pancreatic islet cells, lung and other organs (e.g. parafollicular cells within the thyroid, giving rise to MTC).
- Gastroenteropancreatic tumours can be asymptom-atic or may present with obstructive symptoms due to tumour bulk (pain, nausea, vomiting), symptoms of metastases (liver) or syndromes of hormone hypersecretion.
- Carcinoid syndrome is characterized by flushing, diar-rhoea and occasionally wheezing.
- The initial investigation of gastroenteropancreatic NETs includes: plasma chromogranin A, 24-hour urinary 5-HIAA and a fasting gut hormone profile.
- Surgery is the only curative treatment for NETs.
- Medical treatment (e.g. somatostatin analogues) should be initiated for symptom control until curative surgical treatment is performed, or if surgery is not indicated.
- MEN type 1 is characterized by a predisposition to parathyroid adenomas, enteropancreatic endocrine ade-nomas and pituitary adenomas. MEN 2 is the association of MTC with phaeochromocytoma.

Chapter 33

Obesity

Appetite regulation

Appetite regulation is primarily controlled by peripheral hormones and neural signals that interact with the central nervous system (CNS) appetite circuits. The CNS receives afferent signals from the periphery, including the gut, pancreas and adipose tissue, about food intake and energy stores. This information is integrated, and appropriate cognitive and metabolic responses are initiated to control food intake and metabolism.

Afferent signals

Messages from the periphery reach the brain via:
• the circulation: for example, leptin, glucose and amino acids reach the brain by transport across the blood–brain barrier or directly in regions of the brain where this barrier is defective
• neural circuits, for example the *vagal afferents* from the gastrointestinal tract.
These signals are influenced by what is eaten.

Leptin is produced in adipocytes (fat cells) and signals to the brain about the quantity of stored fat. The primary role of leptin is to indicate whether fat stores are sufficient for survival and reproduction. It acts as a negative feedback signal to brain centres.

Lecture Notes: Endocrinology and Diabetes. By A. Sam and K. Meeran. Published 2009 by Blackwell Publishing. ISBN 978-1-4051-5345-4.

Leptin inhibits orexigenic neurones and stimulates anorexigenic neurones in the arcuate nucleus of the hypothalamus (see below).

Gut peptides such as cholecystokinin, enterostatin, peptide YY (PYY) 3–36 and glucagon-like peptide (GLP-1) reduce food intake. *Ghrelin*, a peptide produced in the stomach, increases food intake and stimulates growth hormone (GH) secretion. Serum levels of ghrelin increase in anticipation of a meal and are suppressed by food ingestion. Serum ghrelin levels increase after diet-induced weight loss, suggesting that it plays a role in the compensatory changes in appetite and energy expenditure that make the maintenance of diet-induced weight loss difficult.

CNS stimulators of food intake include melanin-concentrating hormone, GH-releasing hormone, orexin A and orexin B (also called hypocretins).

Other satiety signals include *gastric distension* and *nutrients* (e.g. glucose and lipids).

CNS areas involved in regulation of appetite

Several areas in the CNS are important in the regulation of appetite:
• The *nucleus of the tractus solitarius* receives and integrates vagal and other neural inputs.
• The *arcuate nucleus* (at the base of the hypothalamus) integrates leptin signals by changing the production and release of neuropeptide Y and

agouti-related peptide, which increase food intake, and alpha-melanocyte-stimulating hormone (α-MSH), which decreases food intake. There are reciprocal connections between the brainstem and hypothalamus.

- The *paraventricular nucleus* receives neural inputs from the arcuate nucleus.
- Damage to the *ventromedial hypothalamus* leads to increased food intake and obesity.
- Damage to the *lateral hypothalamus* leads to reduced food intake and lower body weight.

Noradrenaline, serotonin and several neuropeptides are involved as neurotransmitters or neuromodulators of this control system.

Efferent mediators

The sympathetic nervous system has a tonic role in maintaining energy expenditure.

Glucocorticoids increase food intake. In the absence of glucocorticoids, leptin deficiency or lesions of the ventromedial hypothalamus do not cause obesity. The permissive effect of glucocorticoids may be mediated via inhibition of the sympathetic nervous system.

Obesity

Obesity is associated with significant morbidity and mortality, and an excess risk of many disorders such as insulin resistance, diabetes mellitus, hypertension, dyslipidaemia, coronary heart disease, stroke, sleep apnoea and cancer.

The *body mass index* (BMI) is the most practical way to evaluate the degree of overweight. It is calculated from height and weight:

BMI = body weight (in kg)
÷ the square of the height (in metres)

The World Health Organization (WHO) has defined obesity as a BMI of $30 \, kg/m^2$ or more. Individuals with a BMI between 25 and 29.9 are 'overweight'.

Epidemiology

In most populations, the prevalence of overweight and obesity has steadily increased over the past 20 years. In the USA, the lifetime risks of becoming overweight or obese are about 50% and 25% respectively. In the United Kingdom, about 25% of adults are obese and about 50% are overweight.

Ethnicity influences the incidence of obesity. For example, black men tend to be less obese than white men. However, black women are more obese than white women. The prevalence of obesity in Hispanic men and women is higher than in white individuals.

Aetiology

Many factors may contribute to the development of obesity (Box 33.1).

Lifestyle and social factors

Sedentary lifestyle

A sedentary lifestyle reduces energy expenditure and promotes weight gain. In an affluent society, energy-sparing devices also reduce energy expenditure.

Sleep deprivation

Observational data suggest a possible association between sleep deprivation and obesity. Sleep restriction may be associated with a decrease in serum leptin (an anorexigenic hormone) and an increase in serum ghrelin (an orexigenic hormone).

Cessation of smoking

Weight gain is very common when people stop smoking. This may be mediated by nicotine withdrawal.

Box 33.1 Causes of obesity

Lifestyle and social factors
Dietary factors
Genetic factors
Drugs
Neuroendocrine disorders
Prenatal factors
Psychological factors

Social networks

A report of a social network constructed from the Framingham Offspring Study illustrated that an individual's chance of becoming obese was increased if he or she had a friend, sibling or spouse who became obese.

Dietary factors

Energy intake and the composition of the diet play an important role in the pathogenesis of obesity. Overeating relative to energy expenditure causes obesity. Most obese subjects have lost control of their eating (disinhibition). Epidemiological data suggest that a diet high in fat is associated with obesity.

Night-eating syndrome is a well-known pattern of disturbed eating in the obese. It is characterized by the consumption of at least 25% of energy between the evening meal and the next morning.

Infant feeding practices may also contribute to weight gain. Breast-feeding, when compared with formula feeding, may be associated with a lower risk of overweight.

Genetic factors

Studies of twins, adoptees and families suggest the existence of genetic factors in obesity. Genetic factors influence obesity in two ways:
- genes that are primary factors in the development of obesity, such as those relating to leptin deficiency
- susceptibility genes on which environmental factors act to cause obesity.

Obesity is a feature of at least 24 genetic disorders such as Prader–Willi (caused by a deletion of paternal DNA on the long arm of chromosome 15) and Bardet–Biedl (an autosomal recessive disorder) syndromes.

A small proportion of obesity is due to monogenic causes. Heterozygous mutations in the gene encoding the *melanocortin-4 receptor* (MC4R) are the most common monogenic cause of obesity in childhood. MC4R is the receptor for α-MSH, which is a potent inhibitor of food intake. Obesity due to leptin deficiency has been reported in some consanguineous families. Obesity resulting from leptin receptor deficiency has also been described. However, most obese subjects do not have any abnormalities in the leptin gene and have intact leptin receptors and high serum leptin levels.

The genes that contribute to the more common forms of obesity have been difficult to identify. A variant in the *FTO* (fat mass and obesity associated) *gene* on chromosome 16 increases the risk of obesity in the general population. Mutations in the gene for peroxisome proliferator-activated receptor gamma 2 (a transcription factor involved in adipocyte differentiation) accelerate the differentiation of adipocytes and are associated with obesity in some subjects.

Drugs

A number of drugs can cause weight gain, including atypical antipsychotics (e.g. clozapine, olanzapine), tricyclic antidepressants, antiepileptic drugs (e.g. valproate, carbamazepine), insulin (possibly through hypoglycaemia), sulphonylureas, thiazolidinediones and glucocorticoids.

Neuroendocrine disorders

Several neuroendocrine disorders may be associated with the development of obesity:
- *Hypothalamic obesity* is a rare syndrome in humans. Damage to certain hypothalamic nuclei, such as the ventromedial hypothalamus, by trauma, tumour, inflammatory disease or surgery may result in hyperphagia and obesity.
- In patients with *Cushing's syndrome*, a stimulation of food intake by excess glucocorticoids contributes to weight gain.
- In patients with *hypothyroidism*, the slowing of metabolic activity leads to weight gain.
- About half of patients with *polycystic ovary syndrome* are obese. The underlying aetiology is not fully understood.
- *GH deficiency* results in increased abdominal and visceral fat.

Prenatal factors

Maternal smoking and diabetes increase the risk of obesity in the offspring. Infants who are small, short or have a small head circumference are at higher risk of abdominal fatness and other comorbidities associated with obesity later in life.

Psychological factors

Seasonal affective disorder has been linked to weight gain.

Clinical evaluation

The clinical evaluation of overweight and obese individuals should include measurement of:
- height and weight, and calculation of BMI
- waist circumference in patients with a BMI less than 35 kg/m^2
- blood pressure
- lipid profile (serum triglyceride, high-density and low-density lipoprotein-cholesterol)
- fasting blood glucose.

The medical history should include age at onset of weight gain, change in dietary patterns, history of exercise and questions regarding the possible aetiology, including medications, history of smoking cessation and features of endocrine disorders such as hypothyroidism, polycystic ovary syndrome and Cushing's syndrome.

Treatment

Diet and lifestyle

Obese patients should receive counselling on diet, lifestyle and exercise. Overweight patients who have an increased waist circumference (>102 cm in men or >88 cm in women) or comorbidities, deserve the same consideration for obesity intervention as obese patients. Readiness to change is an essential feature of those who are successful in losing weight.

Approximately 22 kcal per day is required to maintain 1 kg of body weight in a normal adult (i.e. 2200 kcal per day for an individual weighing 100 kg). All subjects should lose weight if they comply with a diet of 800–1200 kcal per day. Those who claim to eat less than 1200 kcal per day yet fail to lose weight are recording their food intake erroneously and should reduce what they claim to eat by half.

A weight loss of 5% or more by 6 months is realistic. Fewer than 50% of subjects will lose 10% or more of their initial body weight before reaching a plateau.

Physical exercise and behaviour modification are essential components of treatment and are important for long-term maintenance of a lower body weight.

Achieving and maintaining weight loss is made difficult by the reduction in energy expenditure that is associated with weight loss. Serum ghrelin levels increase following diet-induced weight loss. Ghrelin stimulates appetite and may play a role in the difficulty with maintaining weight loss.

Pharmacological therapy

Pharmacological therapy should be considered for patients who have failed to achieve their weight loss goals through diet and exercise alone. It is important for patients to understand that current drug therapy does not cure obesity. Patients must be advised that when the maximal therapeutic effect is achieved, weight loss ceases. When drug therapy is discontinued, weight is regained.

The goals for weight loss must be realistic, and a return to normal body weight is unrealistic. Success may be assessed by the degree of weight loss and improvement in associated risk factors. During the first month of drug therapy, weight should be reduced by more than 2 kg. Weight should fall more than 5% below baseline by 3–6 months and remain at this level to be considered effective. A weight loss of 5–10% can significantly reduce the risk factors for diabetes and cardiovascular disease in higher-risk patients.

Orlistat inhibits pancreatic lipases and prevents the hydrolysis of ingested fat to fatty acids and glycerol, resulting in increased faecal fat excretion. Orlistat (120 mg three times a day before meals) may be started as first-line pharmacological therapy in obese patients with elevated blood pressure, dyslipidaemia or cardiovascular disease. Orlistat has beneficial effects on lipid profile and an excellent cardiovascular safety profile.

The main side-effects of orlistat therapy are gastrointestinal, including intestinal cramps, flatus, faecal incontinence and oily spotting. The side-effects may occur at frequency rates of 15–30%. However, these subside as patients learn how to avoid high-fat diets and stick to the recommended intake of no more than 30% fat. The absorption of vitamins A and E and beta-carotene may be slightly reduced, and it may be advisable to give vitamin supplements to patients treated with this drug. Orlistat does not seem to affect the absorption of other drugs except for ciclosporin.

Sibutramine (5–15 mg a day) may be given to otherwise healthy obese patients because of its efficacy and easy tolerability. Sibutramine is a specific inhibitor of noradrenaline, serotonin and to a lesser extent dopamine reuptake into nerve terminals. Sibutramine inhibits food intake, but its thermogenic effect in humans is controversial. It should be avoided in patients with a history of any cardiac disease or stroke, individuals receiving monoamine oxidase inhibitors or selective serotonin reuptake inhibitors (due to a risk of serotonin syndrome) and patients taking drugs that affect the cytochrome P450 enzyme system, such as erythromycin and ketoconazole (as sibutramine is metabolized by this system).

Patients with type 2 diabetes should be started on metformin in addition to lifestyle modifications. If further weight reduction is needed, orlistat should be considered. Glucagon-like peptide-1 agonists such as exenatide have been shown to reduce food intake as well as improving glycaemic control (see Chapter 35).

Improvements in risk factors such as blood pressure, lipid profile and hyperglycaemia after weight loss are important criteria in the determination of whether to continue therapy. The maximal duration of published treatment results is 2 years for sibutramine and 4 years for orlistat. Treatment guidelines suggest up to 2 years of treatment.

Bariatric surgery

Indication

Bariatric surgery should be considered for patients with a BMI of 40 kg/m^2 or more who are well informed and motivated, have an acceptable risk for surgery and have failed previous non-surgical weight loss strategies. Patients with a BMI of greater than 35 kg/m^2 and obesity-related comorbidities (e.g. hypertension, diabetes mellitus, dyslipidaemia, sleep apnoea, joint disease) should also be considered for bariatric surgery. Weight loss surgery should only be performed in the context of a multidisciplinary programme, with extensive expertise in bariatric surgery.

Contraindications

Contraindications to bariatric surgery include patients with untreated major depression or psychosis, binge eating disorders, drug or alcohol abuse, severe coagulopathy, severe cardiac disease with an excessive anaesthetic risk or inability to comply with lifelong vitamin replacement. Bariatric surgery in those above 65 or under 18 is controversial.

Outcomes

All bariatric procedures are effective in achieving weight loss and improving the associated comorbidities in the morbidly obese. The mean overall percentage of excess weight lost is about 60%, varying according to the specific bariatric procedure performed. Bariatric procedures have been shown to improve diabetes (in around 85–90% of cases), hyperlipidaemia (in approximately 75%), hypertension (in around 75–80%) and obstructive sleep apnoea (in around 85%). The reduction in comorbidities appears to translate into a reduction in mortality. The Swedish Obese Subjects (SOS) trial showed that bariatric surgery for severe obesity is associated with long-term weight loss and decreased overall mortality.

Surgical procedures

Surgical therapies are based on two mechanisms:
- *Restrictive procedures* result in a restriction of caloric intake via a small stomach reservoir. Examples of this type of surgery include vertical banded gastroplasty and laparoscopic adjustable gastric banding (Fig. 33.1). The latter procedure has become popular due to its simplicity of technique,

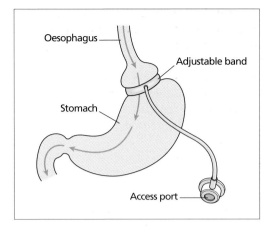

Figure 33.1 Adjustable gastric banding: a silicone band is placed around the entrance to the stomach. The band is connected to a tube that extends to a port underneath the skin. The entrance to the stomach can be narrowed or widened by injection or removal of saline through the port. The patient feels full after eating less as the passage of food from the upper pouch to the rest of the stomach is delayed.

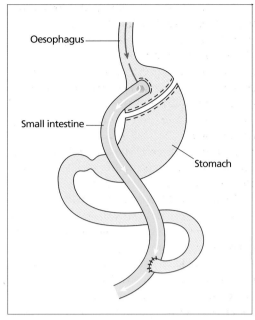

Figure 33.2 Roux-en-Y gastric bypass.

adjustability, reversibility and exceedingly small mortality.

• *Malabsorptive procedures* result in a malabsorption of nutrients via a shortened functional small bowel length. These procedures are highly effective in weight loss but carry metabolic complications. Examples of this type of surgery include jejunoileal bypass, biliopancreatic diversion and biliopancreatic diversion with duodenal switch.

• *Mixed restrictive and malabsorptive procedures*: roux-en-Y gastric bypass (RYGB; Fig. 33.2) causes weight loss by both restrictive and malabsorptive mechanisms. RYGB has been shown to be better than purely restrictive procedures in long-term weight reduction.

The most widely performed procedures are the RYGB and adjustable gastric banding. The rate of weight loss appears to be more gradual after adjustable gastric banding compared with gastric bypass.

The changes in gut hormones following gastric bypass may also contribute to the weight loss achieved through this procedure. It seems that gastric bypass provides a secretory stimulus to the distal endocrine L-cells, resulting in an increase in the gut hormones such as PYY and the entero-

glucagon family of peptides. It is likely that gut hormones play a role in the reduced hunger and increased satiety experienced by those who undergo bariatric surgery.

Complications

Early complications are typically managed by the surgical team and include bleeding, staple line leak, bowel perforation and obstruction, and wound infections. Medical complications include pulmonary embolism, myocardial infarction, pneumonia and urinary tract infection. The overall 30-day postoperative mortality is 0.1% for restrictive procedures, 0.5% for gastric bypass and 1.1% for biliopancreatic diversion or duodenal switch.

After bariatric surgery, patients experience changes in medical comorbidities and eating, and significant psychological changes.

Prolonged vomiting is a common complication and may be due to food intolerances, overeating or the development of stomal stenosis, marginal ulcers in gastric bypass patients, or overtightening of the band. Dumping syndrome occurs in approximately 50% of patients after RYGB and is characterized by symptoms of nausea, shaking, sweating and diarrhoea immediately after eating foods containing high quantities of glucose. Patients should be advised to avoid foods that provoke symptoms.

Female patients must be advised to avoid pregnancy for 12–18 months after surgical weight loss procedures.

Postoperative diet and vitamin/mineral supplements

Bariatric surgery programmes provide patients with a specific series of dietary transitions postoperatively. Patients are at risk of nutritional deficiencies after bariatric surgery. Therefore, they should receive a daily multivitamin, calcium and vitamin D supplementation (800 IU daily), and vitamin B_{12} (1 mg intramuscularly every month). Patients at risk of iron deficiency (e.g. menstruating women, those intolerant to iron-containing foods) should take iron supplements prophylactically.

Follow-up and monitoring

Patients should be evaluated every 4–6 weeks until rapid weight loss decreases (usually about 6 months). Patients should then be evaluated annually.

At each visit in the first 6 months:
- Protein and food intake and patterns of eating should be reviewed, and individuals should be assessed for the development of psychological or eating disorders.
- Blood pressure and weight should be measured.
- Full blood count, urea, creatinine and electrolytes, liver function tests, glucose, albumin and

serum should be measured. In addition, serum magnesium, phosphate, vitamin B_{12} and iron studies should be measured in patients who are losing more than 9 kg (20 lb) per month.
- Medications for hypertension and diabetes frequently need to be reduced or stopped.
- In women of childbearing potential, pregnancy testing should be done in case of cessation of menses.

Serum full blood count, electrolytes, albumin, calcium, iron studies, vitamin B_{12}, folate and 25-hydroxyvitamin D should be measured at each annual visit.

Key points:

- Peripheral signals such as gut peptides, nutrients and leptin from adipose tissue signal to the hypothalamus and the brainstem via the circulation and vagal afferents. This information is integrated, and appropriate cognitive and metabolic responses are initiated to control food intake and metabolism.
- The WHO has defined obesity as a BMI of 30 kg/m² or more. Individuals with a BMI between 25 and 29.9 are 'overweight'.
- Obesity is associated with significant morbidity and mortality.
- Many factors contribute to the development of obesity, including lifestyle and social factors, dietary habits, genetic factors, drugs and neuroendocrine disorders.
- The clinical evaluation of obese patients should include measurement of BMI, waist circumference, blood pressure, lipid profile and fasting blood glucose.
- The treatment of obesity includes counselling on diet, lifestyle and exercise, pharmacological therapy (e.g. orlistat or sibutramine) and bariatric surgery.

Lecture Notes: Endocrinology and Diabetes. By A. Sam and K. Meeran. Published 2009 by Blackwell Publishing. ISBN 978-1-4051-5345-4.

Chapter 34

Insulin and diabetes mellitus: classification, pathogenesis and diagnosis

Insulin

Insulin is a 51-amino acid peptide hormone synthesized and secreted by *beta (β) cells* in the pancreatic *islets of Langerhans*.

Proinsulin is the prohormone precursor to insulin. Cleavage of an internal fragment from proinsulin generates the *C-peptide* and mature *insulin*, consisting of the A chain and B chain connected by disulfide bonds (Fig. 34.1).

In addition to beta cells, the pancreatic islets also contain alpha cells (located at the periphery of the islets) secreting glucagon, and delta cells secreting somatostatin.

Postprandially, the glucose load elicits a rise in insulin and a fall in glucagon.

Insulin release

The key regulator of insulin release is glucose. However, amino acids, gastrointestinal peptides (e.g. glucagon-like peptide 1) and neurotransmitters also influence insulin secretion. Glucose is transported into pancreatic beta cells by the GLUT2 transporter. Glucose is phosphorylated to glucose-6-phosphate by the enzyme *glucokinase*. Further metabolism of glucose-6-phosphate generates ATP,

which inhibits the activity of an ATP-sensitive potassium channel. This results in depolarization of the beta cell membrane, opening of voltage-gated calcium channels and insulin release.

Mechanism of action of insulin

Binding of insulin to its receptor on the cell membrane of the target cells results in autophosphorylation of the receptor via the receptor's intrinsic tyrosine kinase activity. The phosphorylated receptor in turn phosphorylates the insulin receptor substrate 1 and 2.

The activated insulin receptor substrates bind to a number of docking proteins (e.g. GRB2), which in turn bind to other cellular proteins (e.g. SOS) to initiate a cascade of phosphorylation and dephosphorylation reactions resulting in the transcription of insulin-regulated genes.

Insulin receptor-mediated activation of the mitogen-activated protein kinase pathway has been implicated in insulin's effects on growth (see below).

Metabolic effects of insulin

Insulin lowers blood glucose levels by:
- *inhibition of gluconeogenesis* in the liver and kidney, directly and indirectly via a decreased availability of gluconeogenic precursors: free fatty acids and amino acids. Insulin inhibits the

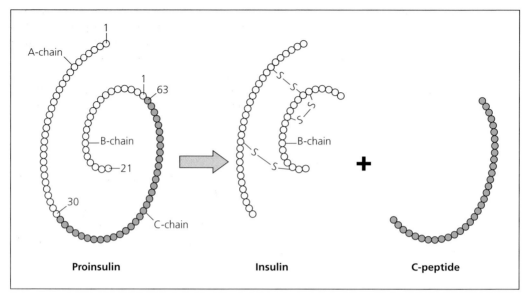

Figure 34.1 Proinsulin, insulin and C-peptide.

lipolysis of stored triglycerides by inhibiting hormone-sensitive lipase and increases triglyceride storage. Insulin also inhibits protein breakdown and increases protein synthesis.

- *inhibition of glycogenolysis* via inhibition of glycogen phosphorylase and stimulation of glycogen synthase
- *increased glucose uptake* into adipocytes and skeletal muscle cells by activation of phosphoinositide 3 kinase and translocation of the glucose transporter GLUT4 from the cytoplasm to the cell membrane
- *increased glycolysis* (glucose breakdown) in adipocytes and skeletal muscle cells by increasing the activity of hexokinase and 6-phosphofructokinase.

Insulin also has paracrine effects on the neighbouring islet cells. Insulin reduces glucagon secretion by the alpha cells. This in turn increases the metabolic effects of insulin since glucagon normally stimulates glycogenolysis and gluconeogenesis by the liver and kidney.

Other actions of insulin

In addition to its metabolic effects, insulin can also affect steroidogenesis, vascular function, fibrinolysis, growth regulation and cancer (e.g. colorectal,

ovarian and breast cancer). The latter effect may be mediated through both anabolic effects on protein and lipid metabolism, and interactions with other mediators of growth e.g. insulin-like growth factors 1 and 2 and their receptors. Insulin resistance and hyperinsulinaemia (e.g. in polycystic ovary syndrome) may stimulate ovarian androgen secretion by stimulating luteinizing hormone release or increasing ovarian luteinizing hormone receptors.

Diabetes mellitus

Diabetes mellitus comprises a group of common metabolic disorders that share the phenotype of *hyperglycaemia* (see 'Diagnosis of diabetes mellitus', below).

Presentation

Patients with diabetes may present with:
- fatigue
- polyuria, polydipsia and nocturia
- recent weight loss (less frequently in type 2 than in type 1 diabetes)
- diabetic ketoacidosis or hyperosmolar hyperglycaemic state (see Chapter 36)

- microvascular complications (retinopathy, nephropathy, neuropathy)
- macrovascular complications (ischaemic heart disease, stroke, peripheral vascular disease)
- recurrent infections.

Many patients with type 2 diabetes are asymptomatic at presentation and are identified by screening.

Classification and pathogenesis of diabetes mellitus

Type 1 diabetes

Type 1 diabetes mellitus is caused by destruction of the pancreatic insulin-producing beta cells, resulting in absolute insulin deficiency. The beta cell destruction is caused by an autoimmune process in 90% of patients with type 1 diabetes. This process progresses over a latent period (many months or years) during which the individual is asymptomatic and euglycaemic. This reflects the large number of functioning beta cells that must be lost before hyperglycaemia occurs.

A number of pancreatic beta cell autoantigens may play a role in the initiation or progression of autoimmune islet injury. These include glutamic acid decarboxylase (GAD), insulin and insulinoma-associated protein (IA-2). The cation efflux zinc transporter (ZnT8) has recently been recognized as another candidate type 1 diabetes autoantigen. However, it is not clear which of these autoantigens is involved in the initiation of the injury, and which is released only after the injury.

Type 1 diabetes is likely to occur in genetically susceptible subjects and is probably triggered by environmental agents.

Polymorphisms of a number of genes may influence the risk of type 1 diabetes. These include the gene encoding preproinsulin and a number of genes related to immune system function such as those for HLA-DQ alpha, HLA-DQ beta and HLA-DR (encoding class II major histocompatibility complex molecules, which present antigens to T lymphocytes), PTPN22 (lymphoid protein tyrosine phosphatase, a suppressor of T cell activation) and cytotoxic T lymphocyte antigen (CTLA-4).

Several environmental factors have been suggested to trigger the autoimmune process in type 1 diabetes. However, none has been conclusively linked to diabetes. Factors include pregnancy-related and perinatal influences, viruses (e.g. coxsackie, rubella) and dietary factors (e.g. bovine milk proteins, cereals and omega-3 fatty acids).

Type 2 diabetes

Type 2 diabetes is characterized by increased *peripheral resistance to insulin* action, *impaired insulin secretion* and increased hepatic glucose output. Both genetic and environmental factors contribute to the development of insulin resistance and relative insulin deficiency in type 2 diabetes.

A genetic influence on the development of type 2 diabetes is supported by the following observations:

- Monozygotic twins have a 90% concordance rate.
- 40% of patients with type 2 diabetes have at least one parent with type 2 diabetes.
- The lifetime risk for a first-degree relative of a patient with type 2 diabetes is 5–10 times higher than for those without a family history of diabetes.

Monogenic causes of type 2 diabetes represent a very small fraction of cases (Box 34.1). It is likely that multiple genetic anomalies at different loci confer varying degrees of predisposition to type 2 diabetes. Several inherited polymorphisms have been identified which individually contribute only small degrees of risk for diabetes (see below).

The gene for the protease calpain 10 may confer major susceptibility to type 2 diabetes in Mexican-American individuals.

Peripheral insulin resistance

Obesity causes peripheral resistance to insulin-mediated glucose uptake and may also decrease the sensitivity of the beta cells to glucose. Upper body or male-type obesity has a much greater association with insulin resistance than lower body or female-type obesity. The mechanism by

Box 34.1 Causes of diabetes mellitus

Type 1 diabetes
Type 1A: immune mediated
Type 1B: idiopathic

Type 2 diabetes

Genetic defects of beta cell function
MODY 1: mutations in hepatocyte nuclear transcription factor 4-alpha
MODY 2: mutations in glucokinase
MODY 3: mutations in hepatocyte nuclear transcription factor 1-alpha
MODY 4: mutations in insulin promoter factor 1
MODY 5: mutations in hepatocyte nuclear transcription factor 1-beta
MODY 6: mutations in neurogenic differentiation 1
Mutations in mitochondrial DNA (maternally transmitted)

Genetic defects in insulin action resulting in insulin resistance
Type A insulin resistance: caused by insulin receptor mutations in some, but by an unknown signalling defect in most
Donohue syndrome (leprechaunism): caused by insulin receptor mutations; associated with intrauterine growth retardation
    and dysmorphic features, e.g. protuberant and low-set ears, flaring nostrils and thick lips. Death occurs in childhood
Rabson–Mendenhall syndrome (caused by insulin receptor mutations; associated with coarse and senile-appearing
    facies, premature and abnormal dentition, abdominal distension, enlarged genitalia and a hypertrophic pineal gland)
Lipodystrophic syndromes: congenital or acquired disorders characterized by a complete or partial lack of adipose tissue
    (lipoatrophy)

Pancreatic diseases
Chronic pancreatitis
Cystic fibrosis
Hereditary haemochromatosis
Pancreatic cancer
Fibrocalculous pancreatopathy
Surgical removal of the pancreas

Endocrinopathies (excess secretion of hormones that antagonize the metabolic effects of insulin)
Cushing's syndrome (excess cortisol)
Acromegaly (excess growth hormone)
Phaeochromocytoma (excess catecholamines)
Glucagonoma (excess glucagon)
Somatostatinoma (excess somatostatin)

Drug-induced diabetes
Glucocorticoids, atypical antipsychotic agents, protease inhibitors, beta-blockers, thiazide diuretics, ciclosporin, nicotinic acid

Infections
Congenital rubella, coxsackie virus, cytomegalovirus

Gestational diabetes

Uncommon forms of immune-mediated diabetes
Stiff man syndrome (associated with muscle stiffness and anti-glutamic acid decarboxylase antibodies)
Insulin receptor autoantibodies

Genetic syndromes associated with diabetes
Down's syndrome, Klinefelter's syndrome, Turner's syndrome, Wolfram's syndrome, Prader–Willi syndrome, Lawrence–
    Moon–Biedl syndrome, Huntington's chorea, Friedreich's ataxia, myotonic dystrophy, porphyria

MODY, maturity-onset diabetes of the young

which obesity induces insulin resistance is poorly understood. The c-Jun amino-terminal kinase (JNK) pathway may be an important mediator of the relationship between obesity and insulin resistance as JNK activity is increased in obesity and can interfere with insulin action.

Plasma *free fatty acid* concentrations are high in obese patients. A high plasma free fatty acid concentration can impair insulin-stimulated glucose uptake in skeletal muscle.

Insulin resistance may, at least in part, be related to *adipokines*, including leptin, adiponectin, tumour necrosis factor-alpha (TNF-α) and resistin, secreted by adipocytes. Leptin deficiency and leptin resistance are associated with obesity and insulin resistance. Adiponectin deficiency may contribute to the development of insulin resistance and subsequent type 2 diabetes. Increased release of TNF-α from adipocytes may also play a role in the impairment of insulin action.

Polymorphisms in the gene for peroxisome proliferator-activated receptor (PPAR) gamma-2, a transcription factor that has a key role in adipocyte differentiation, may contribute to the variability in insulin sensitivity in the general population.

Impaired insulin secretion

The reasons for the decline in insulin secretory capacity in type 2 diabetes are not clear. Chronic hyperglycaemia can have a toxic effect on beta cells (*glucotoxicity*). An elevation of free fatty acid levels may also worsen pancreatic beta cell function (*lipotoxicity*).

Animal models have suggested that GLUT2 (a beta cell glucose transporter) and Abca1 (ATP-binding cassette transporter, a cellular cholesterol transporter) may play a role in impaired insulin secretion and the development of type 2 diabetes. There is evidence that processing of proinsulin to insulin in the beta cells may be impaired in type 2 diabetes.

Islet amyloid polypeptide (amylin) is stored in insulin secretory granules in the pancreatic beta cells. Many patients with type 2 diabetes have increased amounts of amylin in their pancreas. However, it is not clear whether this has a causative

role or is a consequence of the defect in insulin secretion.

Single nucleotide polymorphisms in the gene for TCF7L2 (transcription factor 7-like 2) significantly increase the risk of type 2 diabetes. This variant genotype is associated with decreased insulin secretion from beta cells in response to glucose.

Maturity-onset diabetes of the young

Maturity onset diabetes of the young (MODY) is a rare cause of type 2 diabetes resulting from mutations transmitted in an autosomal dominant manner. These mutations are very rare in ordinary type 2 diabetes.

MODY type 1, MODY 3 and MODY 5 are due to mutations in the genes encoding hepatocyte nuclear transcription factors 4-alpha, 1-alpha and 1-beta, respectively. The mechanism by which these mutations result in diabetes is not well understood. In addition to liver, these transcription factors are also expressed in other tissues such as kidney. As a result, patients may also have renal cysts and renal absorption abnormalities.

MODY 2 is caused by mutations in the glucokinase gene. Glucokinase phosphorylates glucose to glucose-6-phosphate and acts as the glucose sensor within the pancreatic beta cells. As a result, higher glucose levels are required to elicit insulin secretory responses in patients with MODY 2.

MODY 4 is caused by mutations in the insulin promoter factor 1, a transcription factor that regulates pancreatic development and insulin gene transcription.

MODY 6 is caused by mutations of the gene encoding the protein neurogenic differentiation 1 (NeuroD1). NeuroD1 is a transcription factor that promotes transcription of the insulin gene as well as some genes involved in formation of beta cells and parts of the nervous system.

Other causes of diabetes

Other rare causes of diabetes mellitus are listed in Box 34.1. Gestational diabetes is discussed in Chapter 31.

Syndromes of insulin resistance

Several rare syndromes of severe insulin resistance have been identified, many of which are associated with mutations of the insulin receptor gene (Box 34.1). These syndromes are characterized by hyperinsulinaemia and sometimes other abnormalities, such as acanthosis nigricans and signs of hyperandrogenism (hirsutism, acne and oligomenorrhoea in women). Impaired glucose tolerance or overt diabetes occurs if compensatory increases in insulin secretion are inadequate.

Epidemiology of diabetes mellitus

Type 2 diabetes accounts for over 80% of cases of diabetes in Europe and North America. Type 1 diabetes is responsible for another 5–10%, with the remainder being due to other causes (Box 34.1). The prevalence of both type 1 and type 2 diabetes is increasing worldwide.

Type 1 diabetes mellitus

Type 1 diabetes is one of the most common chronic diseases in childhood, with a prevalence of 0.25% in the United Kingdom. There is considerable geographical variation in the incidence of type 1 diabetes. For example, the incidence of type 1 diabetes in Scandinavia (e.g. 35 per 100000 per year in Finland) is much higher than that in the Pacific Rim (e.g. 2 per 100000 per year in Japan and China). The United States and Northern Europe have an intermediate incidence (8–17 per 100000 per year).

Type 2 diabetes mellitus

The prevalence of type 2 diabetes in the UK is 5–10%. The prevalence of type 2 diabetes varies remarkably between ethnic groups living in the same environment. People of Asian, African and Hispanic descent are at greater risk of developing type 2 diabetes. The incidence of type 2 diabetes has increased dramatically over the last 20 years. The rise in type 2 diabetes has occurred in parallel with an increasing prevalence of obesity worldwide.

Diagnosis of diabetes mellitus

A person is diagnosed with diabetes mellitus if he or she has one or more of the following criteria:
• symptoms of diabetes and a random plasma glucose ≥11.1 mmol/L
• fasting plasma glucose ≥7.0 mmol/L (after an overnight fast of at least 8 hours)
• 2-hour plasma glucose levels ≥11.1 mmol/L after a 75 g oral glucose tolerance test.

In the absence of unequivocal hyperglycaemia and acute metabolic decompensation, these criteria should be confirmed by repeat testing on another day.

Prediabetes

Prediabetes can be diagnosed based upon a fasting blood glucose test or an oral glucose tolerance test:
• *Impaired fasting glucose* is defined as a fasting plasma glucose between 5.6 and 6.9 mmol/L.
• *Impaired glucose tolerance* is defined as a plasma glucose level of 7.8–11.0 mmol/L measured 2 hours after a 75 g oral glucose tolerance test.

Individuals with impaired fasting glucose or impaired glucose tolerance are at considerable risk for developing type 2 diabetes (40% risk over the next 5 years). Impaired glucose tolerance is very common and affects about 11% of people between the ages of 20 and 74 years.

Distinguishing type 1 and 2 diabetes mellitus

The need for insulin treatment does not distinguish between type 1 and type 2 diabetes as many patients with type 2 diabetes also require insulin for glucose control. Patients with type 1 diabetes are more likely to have the following features:
• age of onset ≤30 years
• body mass index <25 kg/m^2
• acute symptoms
• a personal or family history of autoimmune disease.

However, none of these criteria is absolute and specific for type 1 diabetes. Autoimmune-mediated destruction of the beta cells can occur at any age. It is estimated that 5–10% of those who develop diabetes after age 30 have type 1 diabetes, known as *latent autoimmune diabetes in adults* (LADA; see below). Furthermore, type 2 diabetes may occur in overweight children and adolescents.

Although an acute presentation with diabetic ketoacidosis is a typical feature of type 1 diabetes, it can also occur in type 2 diabetes in certain circumstances, such as severe infection or other illnesses. Patients with *ketosis-prone type 2 diabetes* present with diabetic ketoacidosis as their first manifestation of type 2 diabetes. These patients are usually obese and typically of African, Hispanic or Caribbean descent. The mean age for diagnosis is 40 years. The cause of the ketoacidosis in these cases is unknown. These patients are initially treated with insulin. However, 50–70% achieve diabetic remission 3 months after presentation. Hyperglycaemia often relapses by 2 years.

When it is difficult to distinguish between type 1 and type 2 diabetes, testing for *islet cell antibodies* and *anti-GAD* antibodies may be helpful in establishing the diagnosis of autoimmune type 1 diabetes. Genetic tests to exclude the diagnosis of MODY are also useful if the diagnosis is in doubt.

If type 1 diabetes is suspected on clinical grounds or if islet cell or GAD antibodies are positive, the patient should be presumed to have type 1 diabetes and treated with insulin replacement therapy. Insulin should also be started in any patient who is catabolic (i.e. presents with *weight loss* or *dehydration* in the setting of hyperglycaemia) or who has *increased ketogenesis* (ketonuria or ketoacidosis).

LADA is defined as adult-onset diabetes with circulating islet antibodies but not requiring insulin therapy initially. Patients with LADA have a high risk of progression to insulin dependency.

Key points:

- Insulin is a peptide hormone synthesized and secreted by the beta cells in the pancreatic islets of Langerhans.
- Insulin release is stimulated by a rise in plasma glucose. Insulin lowers postprandial blood glucose by an inhibition of gluconeogenesis and glycogenolysis, increased glucose uptake into adipocytes and skeletal muscle cells and increased glycolysis.
- Patients with diabetes may present with fatigue, polyuria, polydipsia, weight loss, diabetic ketoacidosis, a hyperosmolar hyperglycaemic state, recurrent infections and microvascular or macrovascular complications.
- Type 1 diabetes mellitus results from destruction of the pancreatic insulin-producing beta cells, usually due to an autoimmune process.
- Type 2 diabetes results from peripheral insulin resistance and impaired insulin secretion.
- Type 2 diabetes accounts for over 80% of cases of diabetes in Europe and North America. Type 1 diabetes is responsible for another 5–10%, with the remainder being due to other causes such as genetic mutations affecting beta cell function, pancreatic diseases, endocrinopathies and drugs such as glucocorticoids.
- Diabetes mellitus can be diagnosed based on one or more of the following criteria:
  – symptoms of diabetes and a random plasma glucose ≥11.1 mmol/L
  – fasting plasma glucose ≥7.0 mmol/L (after an overnight fast of at least 8 hours)
  – 2-hour plasma glucose ≥11.1 mmol/L after a 75 g oral glucose tolerance test.

Chapter 35

Treatment of diabetes mellitus

The treatment of a patient with diabetes mellitus has four main components:
- patient education
- glycaemic control
- screening for and treatment of complications
- screening for and treatment of cardiovascular risk factors.

Patient education

Being diagnosed with type 2 diabetes can be an overwhelming experience, and patients commonly have questions about why it has developed.

A good general approach is first to explore the patient's understanding of diabetes. All newly diagnosed patients should receive verbal and written information about their diagnosis, possible complications, the need for regular follow-up, treatment options and lifestyle adjustments. Women of reproductive age should be made aware of the importance of tight glycaemic control before and during pregnancy.

Patients should be provided with resources for medical as well as psychological support, such as group classes, meetings with a *diabetic specialist nurse* and dietitian and other educational resources such as books, charities (e.g. Diabetes UK), websites or magazines.

It must be emphasized to the patient that people who have diabetes can lead active lives and enjoy the foods and activities that they previously enjoyed.

Glycaemic control in type 1 diabetes

All patients with type 1 diabetes must be treated with *insulin*. *Diet* and *exercise* are important components of non-pharmacological therapy in patients with type 1 diabetes.

The Diabetes Control and Complications Trial (DCCT) showed that intensive insulin therapy to achieve lower levels of glycaemia reduces the risk of microvascular complications (retinopathy, nephropathy, neuropathy). Intensive insulin therapy also decreased fatal and non-fatal cardiovascular events in the Epidemiology of Diabetes Interventions and Complications (EDIC) follow-up study to the DCCT.

Glycated haemoglobin and the goal of glycaemic control

Glycated haemoglobin (HbA$_{1c}$) is formed in a non-enzymatic pathway by irreversible attachment of glucose to haemoglobin. HbA$_{1c}$ correlates with mean blood glucose over the previous 8–12 weeks.

HbA$_{1c}$ values are influenced by red cell survival. HbA$_{1c}$ values may be falsely high when red cell turnover is low (e.g. in iron, vitamin B$_{12}$ or folate

Lecture Notes: Endocrinology and Diabetes. By A. Sam and K. Meeran. Published 2009 by Blackwell Publishing. ISBN 978-1-4051-5345-4.

deficiency). On the other hand, HbA_{1c} values may be falsely low when red cell turnover is rapid (e.g. in sickle cell disease). Fructosamine (glycated albumin) may be used to estimate glycaemic control in these circumstances. The turnover of serum albumin is about 28 days, and therefore serum fructosamine values reflect mean blood glucose values over the previous 1–2 weeks. Fructosamine values may be falsely low when albumin turnover is rapid (e.g. in protein-losing enteropathy or nephrotic syndrome).

The goal of glycaemic control is to achieve normal or near-normal glycaemia with an HbA_{1c} under 7%. However, the benefits of intensive insulin therapy have to be weighed against the risk of severe hypoglycaemia associated with intensive therapy for each patient. Less stringent goals may be appropriate for older patients and patients with a history of severe hypoglycaemia, limited life expectancies or comorbid conditions.

HbA_{1c} must be obtained at least twice yearly in patients who are meeting glycaemic goals, and every 3 months in patients who are not meeting glycaemic goals and in those whose treatment has changed.

A new standard for HbA_{1c} has been prepared by the International Federation of Clinical Chemistry and Laboratory Medicine (IFCC), and in the near future, manufacturers will supply IFCC standardized values for their calibrators. The units for reporting HbA_{1c} will be changed to *mmol per mol* of haemoglobin without glucose attached. Thus, HbA_{1c} reported by laboratories will be traceable to the IFCC reference method, allowing a global comparison of HbA_{1c} results. The equivalent of the current HbA_{1c} target of 7% is 53 mmol/mol in the new units. A guide to the new values expressed as mmol/mol is:

HbA_{1c} (%)	HbA_{1c} (mmol/mol)
6.0	42
6.5	48
7.0	53
7.5	59
8.0	64
9.0	75

Insulin types

The first successful insulin preparations came from cow and pig pancreata (bovine and porcine insulin). These are effective but may cause allergic reactions in some patients. This problem has been minimized with the advent of synthetic human insulin manufactured using recombinant DNA technology.

Soluble (regular) insulin is a short-acting form of insulin and should be injected 30 minutes before meals.

In *rapid-acting insulin analogues (lispro, aspart, glulisine)*, the normal amino acid sequence has been altered to reduce the tendency of the insulin to form hexamers by self-association. This keeps the insulin in dimeric and monomeric forms, which results in faster absorption, more rapid onset and a shorter duration of action. Rapid-acting insulin analogues can be injected shortly before a meal. Hypoglycaemia occurs less frequently with rapid-acting insulin analogues than with soluble insulin.

Inhaled insulin may be used (if available) in patients who have a very strong and lasting fear of injections, or persistent problems with injection sites. It is inhaled 10 minutes before eating a meal. Patients must have pulmonary function tests at baseline, after 6 months of therapy and annually thereafter. Inhaled insulin must not be given to patients with any lung disease or a decline of 20% or more in forced expiratory volume in 1 second from baseline.

Isophane insulin is an *intermediate-acting* insulin formed by the addition of protamine to soluble insulin. It is also known as neutral protamine Hagedorn (NPH) as Hans Christian Hagedorn discovered that the effects of insulin could be prolonged by the addition of protamine (Table 35.1).

Of the *long-acting insulin analogues*, glargine is kept in hexamer form for a longer period due to alterations in its amino acid sequence. This results in a slower onset and longer duration of action. *Detemir* has a fatty acyl side chain that binds to albumin subcutaneously and in plasma. This delays dissociation and the release of the insulin into the circulation.

Table 35.1 Types of insulin

	Onset of action	Time to peak effect	Duration of action
Lispro, aspart, glulisine	5–15 minutes	45–75 minutes	2–4 hours
Soluble	~30 minutes	2–4 hours	5–8 hours
Isophane	~2 hours	6–10 hours	18–28 hours
Glargine	~2 hours	No peak	20 to >24 hours
Detemir	~2 hours	No peak	6–24 hours

Table 35.1 summarizes the pharmacokinetics of most commonly used insulin preparations.

Insulin regimens

Intensive therapy involves the administration of a *basal* level of insulin (isophane, glargine, detemir) and premeal *boluses* of a rapid-acting insulin preparation (lispro, aspart, glulisine). The administration of a basal long-acting insulin and boluses of rapid acting insulin with meals intends to mimic the normal insulin secretion profile of the pancreas. The basal insulin suppresses lipolysis and hepatic glucose production. The boluses of insulin minimize the postprandial rise in blood glucose.

For intensive insulin regimens, patients must be committed and be supported by an experienced diabetic team. Motivated patients can attend 'DAFNE' (Dose Adjustment for Normal Eating) courses to learn how to calculate their carbohydrate intake and adjust their insulin doses accordingly.

The use of premixed insulins (see 'Insulin treatment in type 2 diabetes') is not recommended for patients with type 1 diabetes. This is because intensive therapy in patients with type 1 diabetes requires frequent adjustments of the premeal bolus of the rapid-acting insulin.

Basal insulin is delivered by daily or twice daily injections of a long-acting insulin preparation, or by continuous subcutaneous infusion of a rapid-acting insulin preparation via a pump ('continuous subcutaneous insulin infusion'). HbA$_{1c}$ values are similar in studies comparing isophane insulin with glargine. However, patients using glargine have fewer hypoglycaemic episodes. Insulin detemir must be given twice daily as it has a shorter duration of action than glargine.

Insulin injection devices, technique and sites

Insulin is injected subcutaneously using single-use *syringes* with needles, *insulin pens* with needles or an *insulin pump* (Fig. 35.1).

Insulin pumps may give slightly better glycaemic control. However, they are costly and cumbersome for some patients, and ketoacidosis may occur if the pump malfunctions. Patients choosing this regimen must have 24-hour access to expert advice.

Insulin pens may be *prefilled* (disposable) or *reusable*. Prefilled pens (e.g. FlexPen, InnoLet, OptiSet) are discarded when the insulin cartridge is spent. Reusable pens (e.g. OptiPen, NovoPen, Autopen, HumaPen) contain a replaceable insulin cartridge that is loaded into and removed from the pen by the patient.

Injection technique is the same with insulin syringes and with pens. Patients should learn the proper insulin injection technique from a diabetes specialist nurse. An area of the body in which about 2.5 cm of subcutaneous fat can be pinched between two fingers should be used. The needle (e.g. Micro-Fine 27G, Ultra-Fine 29G) is inserted perpendicular to the pinched skin up to the hilt. The length of the needle used depends on whether the patient is thin/child (5 mm), normal weight (8 mm) or overweight (12.7 mm). The needle is held in place for several seconds after insulin injection to avoid insulin leakage after withdrawal of the needle. Patients should be advised on the safe disposal of syringes and needles.

Potential sites for insulin injection are the upper arms, abdominal wall, upper legs and buttocks (Fig. 35.2). Insulin is absorbed fastest from the

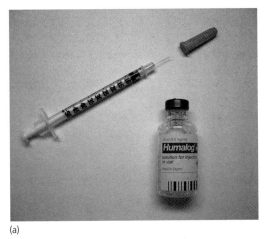

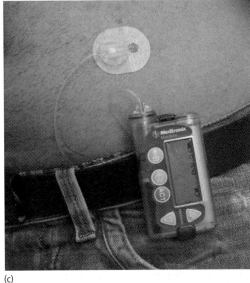

(a)

(c)

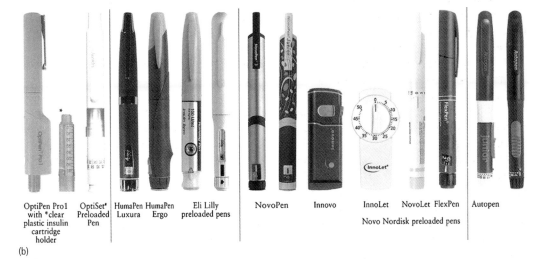

| OptiPen Pro1 with *clear plastic insulin cartridge holder | OptiSet* Preloaded Pen | HumaPen Luxura | HumaPen Ergo | Eli Lilly preloaded pens | NovoPen | Innovo | InnoLet | NovoLet | FlexPen | Autopen |

Novo Nordisk preloaded pens

(b)

Figure 35.1 (a) Insulin vial and syringe. (b) Insulin pens. (c) Insulin pump.

abdominal wall, slowest from the leg and buttock, and at an intermediate rate from the arm.

The long-acting insulin preparations are best injected into the leg or buttock (from which absorption is slow). The rapid-acting insulin preparations are best injected into the abdominal wall (from which insulin is absorbed more rapidly).

The injection sites must be rotated to avoid the risk of *lipohypertrophy* (Fig. 35.3).

Insulin dose

Insulin requirement depends on body weight, age and pubertal stage. Newly diagnosed children usually require an initial total daily insulin dose of 0.5–1.0 U/kg. Prepubertal children often require lower doses, and pubertal children may need higher doses. Patients in ketoacidosis and those receiving glucocorticoids also require higher doses.

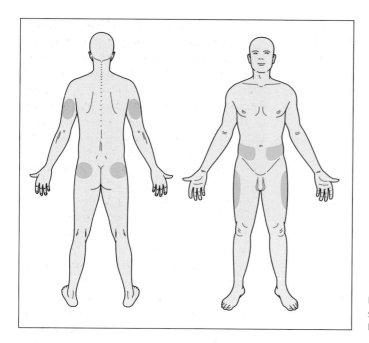

Figure 35.2 Insulin may be injected subcutaneously into the shaded areas. Injection sites should be rotated.

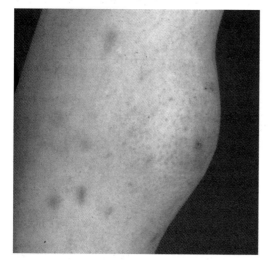

Figure 35.3 Lipohypertrophy caused by repeated insulin injections into the same site.

The basal insulin dose comprises about 50% of the total daily dose. The remaining 50% of insulin is given as rapid-acting insulin divided into three doses, administered before each meal. The boluses are adjusted according to the carbohydrate content of the meals and the current blood glucose level.

A period of decreasing insulin requirement may be seen in children and adolescents a few weeks after the diagnosis and initiation of insulin. This *'honeymoon phase'* is due to a secretion of some endogenous insulin from the remaining functional beta cells and may last several months or occasionally years. Blood glucose must be closely monitored during this period. Hypoglycaemic episodes may occur if the insulin dose is not adjusted appropriately.

Side-effects

The main side-effects of intensive insulin therapy are *hypoglycaemia* and *weight gain*. Patients and their families should be educated to recognize and deal with hypoglycaemic episodes. The treatment of hypoglycaemia is discussed in Chapter 36.

Weight gain can limit patient compliance. Patients must pay attention to caloric intake and exercise to avoid the weight gain that commonly accompanies intensive insulin therapy.

Monitoring of control

Patients must monitor their blood glucose using a *glucometer* 4–7 times daily (before meals, midmorning, mid-afternoon, before bedtime and occasionally at 3 a.m.). HbA$_{1c}$ should be checked regularly to confirm chronic glucose control (see above). Patients should be seen at least every 3 months, and must have access to as-needed telephone or e-mail consultations for insulin regimen adjustments.

Glycaemic control in type 2 diabetes

The *United Kingdom Prospective Diabetes Study* (UKPDS) showed that intensive therapy to achieve lower levels of glycaemia in patients with type 2 diabetes reduces the risk of microvascular complications (retinopathy, nephropathy, neuropathy). The 10-year post-trial monitoring data from the UKPDS show that early intensive glucose control reduces the risk of myocardial infarction and all-cause mortality as well as continuing to reduce the risk of microvascular complications.

The aim is to achieve normal or near-normal glycaemia with an HbA$_{1c}$ goal of below 7%. However, less stringent goals may be appropriate for older patients and patients with a history of severe hypoglycaemia, limited life expectancy or comorbid conditions.

In both the *Action to Control Cardiovascular Risk in Diabetes* (ACCORD) trial and the *Action in Diabetes and Vascular Disease: Preterax and Diamicron MR Controlled Evaluation* (ADVANCE) trials, intensive glycaemic control to achieve HbA$_{1c}$ levels below 6.5% in patients with longstanding diabetes did not reduce cardiovascular events over the time period studied (3.5–5 years). Data from the ACCORD study suggest that, in patients with a long history of diabetes and at high risk of cardiovascular disease, reducing HbA$_{1c}$ to near-normal may be unsafe (associated with a higher number of total and cardiovascular deaths, and a more common occurrence of severe hypoglycaemia). Therefore a target HbA$_{1c}$ of 7–7.9% may be safer for these patients.

HbA$_{1c}$ must be obtained at least twice yearly in patients who are meeting glycaemic goals, and every 3 months in patients who are not meeting glycaemic goals and in those whose treatment has changed.

Dietary modification and *exercise* are major components of non-pharmacological therapy in type 2 diabetes. Changes in lifestyle also slow the progression of impaired glucose tolerance to overt diabetes. However, a sudden initiation of vigorous exercise in sedentary patients can precipitate myocardial infarction. Therefore prior to starting an exercise programme, patients over age 35 years who have had diabetes for more than 10 years should be thoroughly examined, and an exercise stress test should be considered.

Patients should exercise regularly (at least three times per week) and preferably at the same time in relation to meals (and insulin injections). The American Diabetes Association recommends at least 150 minutes of moderate-intensity aerobic activity distributed over at least 3 days each week. Patients with proliferative retinopathy should avoid weight-lifting due to the increased risk of intraocular haemorrhage. Patients with neuropathy should avoid long-distance running or prolonged downhill skiing. These activities may precipitate stress fractures and pressure ulcers in the feet.

An overview of pharmacological therapy for glycaemic control in type 2 diabetes is summarized in Fig. 35.4.

Metformin

Metformin should be started at the time of diagnosis in patients with type 2 diabetes (if there are no specific contraindications), along with advice regarding lifestyle modification. Metformin may be started at 500 mg once daily with meals. It is titrated up over 1–2 months to the maximally effective dose (850 mg three times a day) as tolerated. A longer-acting formulation is available in some countries and can be given once per day.

Mechanism of action and efficacy

Metformin decreases hepatic glucose output, inhibits lipolysis (reduces serum free fatty acid levels and hence substrate availability for gluconeogenesis) and increases insulin-mediated glucose utilization in the peripheral tissues (muscle

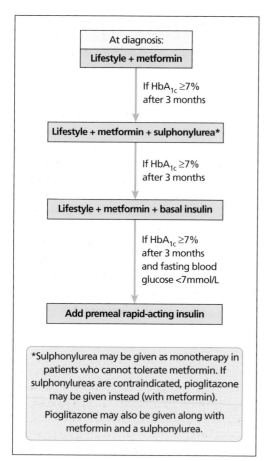

At diagnosis:

Lifestyle + metformin

If HbA$_{1c}$ ≥7%
after 3 months

Lifestyle + metformin + sulphonylurea*

If HbA$_{1c}$ ≥7%
after 3 months

Lifestyle + metformin + basal insulin

If HbA$_{1c}$ ≥7%
after 3 months
and fasting blood
glucose <7 mmol/L

Add premeal rapid-acting insulin

*Sulphonylurea may be given as monotherapy in patients who cannot tolerate metformin. If sulphonylureas are contraindicated, pioglitazone may be given instead (with metformin).

Pioglitazone may also be given along with metformin and a sulphonylurea.

Figure 35.4 Overview of pharmacological therapy for glycaemic control in type 2 diabetes.

and liver). Metformin lowers serum lipid and blood glucose possibly by working through LKB1 (a protein-threonine kinase), which phosphorylates and activates the enzyme adenosine monophosphate-activated protein kinase.

Metformin is not associated with weight gain and typically reduces HbA$_{1c}$ levels by about 1.5%. It is less likely to cause hypoglycaemia than sulphonylureas and insulin. It can cause a decrease in serum triglyceride (triacylglycerol) levels, a small decrease in serum low-density lipoprotein (LDL) cholesterol, and a very modest increase in serum high-density lipoprotein (HDL) cholesterol. In overweight and obese individuals with diabetes, metformin may reduce all-cause mortality and rate

of myocardial infarction. Metformin has been suggested to reduce the risk of macrovascular complications, independently of its effects on glycaemic control.

Side-effects

Gastrointestinal side-effects (e.g. nausea, anorexia, abdominal discomfort, diarrhoea, a metallic taste in the mouth) are common with metformin.

A rare but serious side-effect of metformin is lactic acidosis. Thus metformin should not be administered in conditions predisposing to lactic acidosis, for example reduced tissue perfusion, infection, cardiac failure, renal impairment (creatinine >125 μmol/L in women, >135 μmol/L in men), liver disease or alcohol abuse. The use of serum creatinine alone to assess renal function may not be accurate in elderly patients or others with reduced muscle mass. An estimated glomerular filtration rate of less than 60 mL per minute would be the equivalent of the above serum creatinine cut-off levels in these patients.

Those who are about to receive intravenous iodinated contrast material or undergo a surgical procedure (with potential compromise of the circulation) should stop taking metformin immediately prior to and for 48 hours after the procedure. This is to avoid the potential for high plasma metformin levels (and lactic acidosis) if the patient develops contrast-induced acute renal failure.

If lifestyle modification and metformin do not achieve or sustain the glycaemic goals (i.e. HbA$_{1c}$ <7%) within 2–3 months, a sulphonylurea should be started (if not contraindicated).

Sulphonylureas

Sulphonylureas are indicated in:
- patients who are not a candidate for metformin or who cannot tolerate metformin
- patients in whom metformin therapy alone is not controlling the glycaemia.

The choice of sulphonylurea primarily depends on cost and availability. The dose is gradually increased if adequate glycaemic control is not attained (initially after 2–4 weeks). Shorter-acting sulphonylureas (e.g. glipizide, gliclazide) are preferred in elderly patients.

Mechanism of action

Sulphonylureas bind to and inhibit the ATP-dependent potassium channel in the pancreatic beta cells, resulting in a depolarization of the beta cell membrane, calcium influx and a stimulation of insulin secretion. Sulphonylureas are useful only in patients with some beta cell function.

Side-effects

The most common side-effect of sulphonylureas is *hypoglycaemia*. This is more common with long-acting sulphonylureas (e.g. glyburide, chlorpropamide). Patients should be advised about the situations in which hypoglycaemia is most likely to occur. These include after exercise or a missed meal, with a high drug dose, in malnourishment or alcohol abuse, and with impaired renal or cardiac function, gastrointestinal disease, concurrent treatment with salicylates, sulphonamides, fibrates or warfarin, and after being in hospital.

Other less common side-effects that can occur with all sulphonylureas include nausea, skin reactions (including photosensitivity) and abnormal liver function tests. Some studies suggest that sulphonylureas may be associated with poorer outcomes after a myocardial infarction.

Thiazolidinediones

The two thiazolidinediones used for treatment of type 2 diabetes are pioglitazone and rosiglitazone. However, rosiglitazone has been linked to an increased risk of myocardial infarction and is no longer recommended in the updated American Diabetes Association algorithm for managing type 2 diabetes.

Pioglitazone may be considered when sulphonylureas are contraindicated or when hypoglycaemia is particularly undesirable, such as in those holding hazardous jobs. Thiazolidinediones may reduce HbA$_{1c}$ levels by about 1.5% when used as monotherapy. The addition of pioglitazone to metformin and/or sulphonylureas should be considered only for individuals without risk factors for heart failure or fracture (see 'Side-effects' below).

Mechanism of action

Thiazolidinediones act mainly by increasing insulin sensitivity and the peripheral uptake and utilization of glucose in muscle and fat. They bind to and activate peroxisome proliferator-activated receptors (PPARs), which regulate gene expression. Rosiglitazone is a pure PPAR-gamma agonist. Pioglitazone has PPAR-gamma with some PPAR-alpha agonist activity. Thiazolidinediones may improve insulin responsiveness by facilitating glucose transport in skeletal muscle and regulation of expression of adipose tissue adipokines. They may also decrease hepatic glucose production and improve pancreatic beta cell dysfunction.

Side-effects

Thiazolidinediones may cause weight gain and *fluid retention*, and increase the risk of *heart failure*. Rosiglitazone has been linked to an increased risk of myocardial infarction. An increased incidence of bone *fractures* (in the upper arm, hand and foot) has been observed in female patients treated with rosiglitazone. Therefore the risk of fracture should be considered prior to initiation and during use.

Meglitinides

The meglitinides (repaglinide, nateglinide) are short-acting drugs that act by regulating ATP-dependent potassium channels in pancreatic beta cells, thereby increasing insulin secretion. The clinical efficacy of meglitinide monotherapy is similar to that of the sulphonylureas. Meglitinides can be used alone or in combination with metformin. They are taken before each meal, and the dose should be skipped if the meal is missed. Hypoglycaemia is the most common adverse effect. Repaglinide is principally metabolized by the liver, and less than 10% is renally excreted. Therefore dose adjustments may not be necessary in patients with renal insufficiency.

GLP-1 analogues, DPP-IV inhibitors and pramlintide

Oral glucose has a greater stimulatory effect on insulin secretion than intravenous glucose. This *'incretin'* effect is mediated by several gastrointestinal peptides, particularly *glucagon-like peptide-1* (GLP-1). GLP-1 is produced from the proglucagon gene in the L cells of the small intestine and is secreted in response to nutrients. GLP-1 stimulates glucose-dependent insulin release, inhibits glucagon release, slows gastric emptying and reduces food intake. GLP-1 has a short half-life due to N-terminal degradation by the enzyme *dipeptidyl peptidase IV* (DPP-IV).

GLP-1 analogues (e.g. exenatide) and DPP-IV inhibitors (e.g. sitagliptin) have recently been added to the armamentarium of drugs used to treat type 2 diabetes. However, the exact role for these drugs among the myriad of other drugs used for diabetes management is unclear.

Exenatide requires two daily subcutaneous injections and can be considered for patients with type 2 diabetes who are inadequately controlled on maximal doses of one or two oral agents. An advantage of exenatide is *weight loss*. Exenatide may be considered for patients in whom hypoglycaemia is particularly undesirable, such as those holding hazardous jobs. Exenatide is started at an initial dose of 5 µg twice daily (within 60 minutes prior to a meal). The dose may be increased to 10 µg twice daily after 1 month based on response. Caution is suggested in giving exenatide to patients with confirmed gastroparesis.

Sitagliptin can be considered as monotherapy in patients who have contraindications or an intolerance to metformin, sulphonylureas or thiazolidinediones (e.g. those with chronic kidney disease). Sitagliptin may also be used as add-on drug therapy for patients who do not achieve adequate glycaemic control on metformin, a thiazolidinedione or a sulphonylurea.

Pramlintide is a synthetic analogue of human amylin. It slows gastric emptying, reduces postprandial rises in blood glucose and improves HbA$_{1c}$ in patients with type 1 and type 2 diabetes. The exact role for pramlintide among the myriad of other drugs for diabetes management and its long-term outcomes are unclear. Pramlintide may be considered in patients with type 1 or type 2 diabetes inadequately controlled with insulin therapy alone, particularly in those who gain weight despite lifestyle intervention. It requires subcutaneous injections with each meal in type 1 diabetes, and at least twice daily in type 2 diabetes. Patients should be educated and carefully monitored to avoid severe hypoglycaemia.

Insulin treatment in type 2 diabetes

In most patients with type 2 diabetes, blood glucose levels and HbA$_{1c}$ rise over time due to worsening beta cell dysfunction, decreased insulin release and more severe insulin resistance. Insulin should be started in patients who do not achieve optimal diabetes control despite a maximal tolerated dose of oral antidiabetic treatment.

Insulin may be administered as first-line therapy to patients presenting with HbA$_{1c}$ of over 10%, weight loss or ketonuria despite adequate calorie intake. Insulin is also initiated in patients in whom it is difficult to distinguish type 1 from type 2 diabetes.

Insulin therapy may be started with a bedtime injection of an intermediate-acting insulin (e.g. isophane) or bedtime or morning long-acting insulin (e.g. detemir, glargine). Insulin can be initiated at a dose of 10 U, or 0.2 U/kg.

Patients should check their *fasting blood glucose* levels usually daily, and increase their insulin dose, typically by 2 U every 3 days, until fasting blood glucose levels are consistently in the target range (4–7 mmol/L). If fasting blood glucose is more than 10 mmol/L, the dose can be increased in larger increments (e.g. by 4 U every 3 days). If HbA$_{1c}$ is 7% or more after 2–3 months, and fasting blood glucose is in the target range, additional *premeal boluses* of rapid-acting insulin are required to control postprandial hyperglycaemia:

- If pre-lunch blood glucose is out of range: add rapid-acting insulin at breakfast.
- If pre-dinner blood glucose is out of range: add rapid-acting insulin at lunch.
- If pre-bed blood glucose is out of range: add rapid-acting insulin at dinner.

A rapid-acting insulin preparation can usually be started at a dose of about 4 U and is adjusted by 2 U every 3 days until blood glucose is in range. Patients should check their postprandial blood glucose (2 hours after meals) and adjust their premeal insulin boluses accordingly.

If hypoglycaemia occurs, or fasting blood glucose is less than 3.9 mmol/L, the bedtime insulin dose should be reduced by 4 U or 10% (whichever is greater).

Some patients with type 2 diabetes who require premeal insulin in addition to basal insulin prefer *premixed insulins* for convenience. Premixed (biphasic) insulins contain a mixture of short-acting insulin (e.g. 30% regular insulin or insulin analogues) and intermediate-acting insulin (e.g. 70% isophane insulin).

Patients with type 2 diabetes often need large daily doses of insulin (>65 U per day, and usually much more) to achieve acceptable glycaemic control.

Details of the different types of insulin, side-effects, insulin regimens, devices, injection technique and sites were discussed earlier in this chapter (see 'Glycaemic control in type 1 diabetes').

Insulin and exercise

The effect of exercise on blood glucose depends on whether the person is hypoinsulinaemic or hyper-insulinaemic at the time of exercise.

In normal individuals, the exercising muscles take up glucose from the circulation. As the blood glucose concentration starts to fall, insulin secretion decreases and the levels of counterregulatory hormones (glucagon, catecholamines, growth hormone, cortisol) rise. Exercise may cause hypoglycaemia in diabetic patients with adequate serum insulin levels. This is because exogenous insulin cannot be shut off, and maintains muscle glucose uptake and inhibits hepatic glucose output. In addition, the increased temperature and blood flow associated with exercise may enhance insulin absorption from subcutaneous depots.

Blood glucose must be measured and documented before, during and after exercise. Patients may need to reduce the insulin dose that affects that time of the day, and the injection may be given 60–90 minutes before exercise. Insulin should be injected in a site not close to the exercised muscles to prevent increased insulin absorption (e.g. the arm is a suitable site if the patient is cycling).

Patients may need to take extra food (15–30 g of quickly absorbed carbohydrate, e.g. hard candies or juice) 15–30 minutes before exercise and approximately every 30 minutes during exercise. Late hypoglycaemia due to a replenishment of depleted glycogen stores can usually be avoided by eating slowly absorbed carbohydrates (e.g. dried fruit) immediately after exercise.

In contrast, exercise can cause paradoxical hyperglycaemia if the blood glucose concentration is over 14 mmol/L before exercise and should therefore be delayed until blood glucose levels are better controlled. The lack of insulin impairs glucose uptake by the muscles and cannot prevent the increase in hepatic glucose output caused by the counterregulatory hormones secreted during exercise.

In patients with type 2 diabetes on oral hypoglycaemic drugs, exercise tends to lower blood glucose levels. This effect may depend on the timing of the patient's last meal. Exercise may result in hypoglycaemia if it is carried out after eating.

Treatment of obesity

Pharmacotherapy for weight loss may be used in obese patients with type 2 diabetes. However, the weight loss may not be effectively sustained due to side-effects of the drugs. *Bariatric surgery* results in the largest degree of sustained weight loss and improvements in blood glucose control (see Chapter 33).

Screening for and treatment of complications

Retinopathy

Patients with diabetes should have regular eye examinations, ideally with *digital retinal photography*. The incidence of diabetic retinopathy increases over time in patients with both type 1 and type 2 diabetes. The progression of retinopathy can be slowed by *laser photocoagulation* therapy.

Nephropathy

The progression of nephropathy can be slowed by the administration of an angiotensin-converting enzyme (ACE) inhibitor or angiotensin II receptor blocker (ARB).

Microalbuminuria is the earliest clinical finding in diabetic nephropathy. It is defined as urinary albumin excretion rate of between 30 and 300 mg per day (20–200 µg per minute). Microalbuminuria may be diagnosed by measuring the *albumin-to-creatinine ratio* in a spot urine sample. Abnormal results (urinary albumin-to-creatinine ratio >2.5 mg/mmol in men, >3.5 mg/mmol in women) should be repeated at least two or three times over a 3–6-month period to exclude false-positive results (e.g. transient microalbuminuria due to exercise, fever, heart failure or poor glycaemic control).

All patients with type 2 diabetes should be screened for microalbuminuria from the time of diagnosis as they may have had diabetes for several years before diagnosis. Screening can be deferred for 5 years after the onset of disease in type 1 diabetes since microalbuminuria is uncommon before this time.

ACE inhibitors both lower urinary protein excretion and slow the rate of disease progression. Patients with microalbuminuria or overt nephropathy should receive an ACE inhibitor or an ARB even if they are normotensive. The maintenance of strict glycaemic control is also essential. Dietary protein restriction may be beneficial in patients with established nephropathy.

Diabetic foot problems

Foot problems due to ischaemia and/or neuropathy are a common and important source of morbidity in diabetic patients. Patients should have regular (at least annual) screening examinations by their doctor for neuropathic and vascular involvement of the lower extremities. They must

also be advised to inspect their feet regularly at home.

Examination of the feet in the diabetic clinic should include:
- *inspection* for integrity of the skin (especially between the toes and under the metatarsal heads), and the presence of erythema, warmth and callus
- checking for neuropathy (vibration sensation, *10 g monofilament testing*)
- screening for peripheral arterial disease by *palpation of the pedal pulses* and asking about a history of claudication. An ankle–brachial pressure index should be obtained if peripheral arterial disease is suspected.

Patients with any foot abnormality should be referred to clinicians with expertise in diabetic foot care. All patients should be advised to:
- wash and check their feet daily (patients must test the water temperature before stepping into a bath)
- avoid going barefoot at home
- trim their toenails to shape of the toe, remove sharp edges with a nail file and avoid cutting the cuticles
- avoid tight shoes
- change their socks daily.

Screening for and treatment of cardiovascular risk factors

Patients with diabetes are at increased risk of developing cardiovascular disease and of dying when cardiovascular disease is present. At the time of diagnosis of type 2 diabetes, many patients already have risk factors for macrovascular disease (e.g. hypertension, obesity, dyslipidaemia, smoking) and many have evidence of atherosclerosis (e.g. peripheral vascular disease, history of ischaemic heart disease, ischaemic changes on ECG).

Cardiovascular risk factor modification in patients with diabetes should include:
- blood pressure control
- screening for and treatment of dyslipidaemia
- smoking cessation
- aspirin.

The Steno-2 study showed that an intensified intervention aimed at multiple risk factors in patients with type 2 diabetes and microalbuminuria reduces the risk of cardiovascular and microvascular events by about 50%. The intensive therapy regimen in this trial included smoking cessation, tight glycaemic control, blood pressure control, exercise, reduced dietary fat and lipid-lowering therapy.

Blood pressure control

Extracellular fluid volume expansion (due to reabsorption of the excess filtered glucose in the proximal tubules along with sodium), hyperinsulinaemia (in type 2 diabetes), increased arterial stiffness and diabetic nephropathy may contribute to the development of hypertension in diabetes.

Early and effective treatment of high blood pressure prevents cardiovascular disease and minimizes the rate of progression of diabetic nephropathy and retinopathy. Blood pressure must be measured at every routine diabetes visit. The recommended goal blood pressure for most diabetic patients is less than 130/80 mmHg, but even lower values may be beneficial in patients with diabetic nephropathy.

Non-pharmacological treatments should include advice regarding weight reduction, increased consumption of fresh fruits and vegetables, a low-fat intake, exercise, sodium restriction and avoidance of smoking and excess alcohol intake.

Most diabetologists usually initiate therapy with an *ACE inhibitor* or an *ARB* as these protect against the development of progressive nephropathy. Other antihypertensive agents, for example thiazide diuretics, may be added if the goal blood pressure is not achieved with the maximally tolerated dose of an ACE inhibitor or ARB.

Although there are concerns about the masking of hypoglycaemic symptoms and possible exacerbation of peripheral vascular disease, beta-blockers are commonly used to treat hypertension in patients with diabetes. Some beta-blockers may cause a modest worsening of glycaemic control. If a beta-blocker is given, carvedilol (a combined non-selective beta- and alpha-1-adrenergic antagonist) may be the drug of choice. The Glycemic Effects in Diabetes Mellitus: Carvedilol-Metoprolol Comparison in Hypertensives (GEMINI) trial showed that the use of carvedilol in the presence of an ACE inhibitor or ARB does not exacerbate glycaemic control.

Screening for and treatment of dyslipidaemia

Hypercholesterolaemia increases the risk of cardiovascular disease. Screening for dyslipidaemia should be done at least annually, and more often if needed to achieve goals.

Both the Cholesterol and Recurrent Events (CARE) trial and the Heart Protection Study showed significant improvement in outcomes with statin therapy even at LDL-cholesterol values below 3.0 mmol/L. The Collaborative AtoRvastatin Diabetes Study (CARDS) found similar benefits of statin therapy in patients with an LDL-cholesterol above or below 3.1 mmol/L. Patients should be treated with a statin to reduce the LDL-cholesterol levels to below 2 mmol/L (and total cholesterol <4 mmol/L). If target levels cannot be achieved with statins alone, it is uncertain whether the addition of other agents such as ezetimibe (which inhibits cholesterol absorption) provides additional clinical benefit.

Triglyceride levels below 1.7 mmol/L and HDL levels above 1.0 mmol/L are preferable. When triglycerides are moderately elevated, treatment should include weight reduction strategies, increased physical activity and a statin. When triglycerides are very high (>10 mmol/L), an omega-3 fatty acid compound or a fibrate may be given to prevent pancreatitis. Combination of a statin and a fibrate increases the risk of myositis, particularly in patients with renal impairment or hypothyroidism. Combination therapy should therefore be used with caution with monitoring of liver function tests and serum creatinine kinase.

Smoking cessation

A meta-analysis of several of the cardiovascular risk reduction trials showed that *smoking cessation* had a much greater benefit on survival than most other interventions. Pharmacological therapy (e.g.

bupropion, nicotine replacement therapy) should be combined with behavioural interventions (e.g. brief clinician counselling in the office).

Aspirin

The benefit of aspirin therapy in patients with macrovascular disease is widely accepted. Aspirin (75 mg per day) is recommended for secondary prevention in patients with diabetes and a history of ischaemic heart disease, stroke, transient ischemic attack or peripheral vascular disease.

Aspirin is commonly prescribed in patients with diabetes and an additional cardiovascular risk factor (age >40 years, hypertension, smoking, obesity, microalbuminuria, hyperlipidaemia, family history of coronary artery disease). However, contrary to published guidelines, aspirin may not offer primary preventive benefits against cardiovascular disease in high-risk diabetic patients. In the Prevention of Progression of Arterial Disease and Diabetes (POPADAD) trial, aspirin did not reduce the development of cardiovascular events in patients with diabetes mellitus and asymptomatic peripheral arterial disease.

Aspirin is not recommended for patients under the age of 30 years because of lack of evidence of benefit, and it is contraindicated in those under the age of 21 years due to the increased risk of Reye's syndrome. Patients who cannot take aspirin may benefit from clopidogrel, although this is not well proven.

Pancreatic islet cell transplantation

Pancreatic islets isolated from cadaver pancreases may be infused into the portal vein or liver via a percutaneous catheter. This procedure should at present be performed only within the context of a controlled research study. Although the outcome has improved with the Edmonton protocol (using glucocorticoid-free immunosuppression and an adequate islet mass), insulin independence occurs in only 10% of patients at 5 years.

Even a small residual islet function can markedly decrease hypoglycaemic events for unexplained reasons. Thus the main indication for pancreatic islet cell transplantation is *problematic hypoglycaemia unawareness*.

The main complications include those related to the procedure (e.g. haemorrhage, portal vein thrombosis) and those caused by immunosuppression (e.g. mouth ulcers, diarrhoea, anaemia).

Key points:

- The four main components of treatment of a patient with diabetes mellitus are patient education, glycaemic control, screening for and treatment of complications, and screening for and treatment of cardiovascular risk factors.
- Diet and exercise are important components of non-pharmacological therapy in patients with diabetes.
- Intensive insulin therapy to achieve lower levels of glycaemia reduces the risk of microvascular complications (retinopathy, nephropathy, neuropathy) in both type 1 and type 2 diabetes.
- All patients with type 1 diabetes must be treated with insulin.
- All patients with type 2 diabetes should received metformin (if not contraindicated) and advice regarding lifestyle modification at diagnosis.
- The goal of glycaemic control is to achieve normal or near-normal glycaemia with an HbA_{1c} under 7%. However, less stringent goals may be appropriate for older patients and patients with a history of severe hypoglycaemia, limited life expectancies or comorbid conditions.
- The main side-effects of intensive insulin therapy are hypoglycaemia and weight gain.
- Cardiovascular risk factor modification in patients with diabetes should include blood pressure control, screening for and treatment of dyslipidaemia, smoking cessation and aspirin.

Chapter 36

Diabetic emergencies

Diabetic ketoacidosis

The triad of diabetic ketoacidosis (DKA) consists of *hyperglycaemia, high anion gap metabolic acidosis* and *ketonaemia*. DKA is characteristically associated with type 1 diabetes. However, it has become increasingly common in patients with type 2 diabetes.

Aetiology and pathogenesis

The precipitating factors for DKA are summarized in Box 36.1. DKA may be the first presentation of type 1 diabetes. DKA may occasionally be the first presentation of type 2 diabetes, especially in Afro-Caribbean individuals ('ketosis-prone type 2 diabetes').

In patients with known diabetes, inadequate insulin treatment or non-compliance is a common precipitating factor for DKA. DKA may also be precipitated by stresses that increase the secretion of the counterregulatory hormones glucagon, catecholamines, cortisol and growth hormone. Infection, such as pneumonia, gastroenteritis and urinary tract infection, can be found in about 30–40% of patients with DKA.

Insulin deficiency causes impaired glucose utilization, as well as increased gluconeogenesis and

> **Box 36.1 Precipitating factors for diabetic ketoacidosis**
>
> Infection (30–40%)
> New-onset diabetes (25%)
> Inadequate insulin treatment or non-compliance (20%)
> Myocardial infarction
> Stroke
> Acute pancreatitis
> Trauma
> Drugs: clozapine/olanzapine, cocaine, lithium, terbutaline

glycogenolysis, resulting in *hyperglycaemia*. The elevated plasma glucose increases the filtered load of glucose in the renal tubules. As the maximal renal tubular reabsorptive capacity is exceeded, glucose is excreted in the urine (*glycosuria*). The osmotic force exerted by unreabsorbed glucose holds water in the tubules, thereby preventing its reabsorption and increasing urine output (*osmotic diuresis*). This leads to dehydration and loss of electrolytes.

Insulin deficiency and increased catecholamines and growth hormone increase lipolysis, thereby increasing free fatty acid delivery to the liver. Normally, free fatty acids are converted to triglycerides in the liver. However, in DKA, hyperglucagonaemia alters hepatic metabolism to favour ketogenesis. Glucagon excess decreases the production of malonyl coenzyme A, thereby increasing the activity of the mitochondrial enzyme carnitine palmitoyltransferase I. Carnitine palmitoyltransferase I mediates the transport of free fatty acyl coenzyme

Lecture Notes: Endocrinology and Diabetes. By A. Sam and K. Meeran. Published 2009 by Blackwell Publishing. ISBN 978-1-4051-5345-4.

A into the mitochondria, where conversion to ketones occurs.

Three ketone bodies are produced in DKA: two ketoacids (beta-hydroxybutyric acid and acetoacetic acid) and one neutral ketone (acetone). Acetoacetic acid is the initial ketone formed. It may then be reduced to beta-hydroxybutyric acid, or non-enzymatically decarboxylated to acetone. Ketones provide an alternate source of energy when glucose utilization is impaired.

Hyperglycaemic crises are proinflammatory states that lead to the generation of reactive oxygen species, which are indicators of oxidative stress.

Clinical presentations

Patients with DKA may present with:
- polyuria and polydipsia resulting in dehydration
- abdominal pain and vomiting (which exacerbates the dehydration). Abdominal pain requires further evaluation if it does not resolve with treatment of the acidosis
- fatigue, weakness and weight loss
- confusion; coma (10% of patients).

Clinical examination includes assessment of cardiorespiratory status, volume status and mental status to look for:
- evidence of dehydration: tachycardia, postural hypotension, reduced tissue turgor and confusion
- Kussmaul's respiration (deep sighing respiration secondary to acidosis) and ketotic breath.

A medical history and clinical examination may identify a precipitating event such as infection (e.g. pneumonia, urinary tract infection) or discontinuation of or inadequate insulin therapy in known diabetics.

Investigations

The investigations in patients presenting with DKA are summarized in Box 36.2. The diagnosis of DKA requires:
- plasma glucose >11 mmol/L (and usually <44 mmol/L)
- positive urinary ketones, or plasma ketones >3 mmol/L

> **Box 36.2 Investigations in diabetic ketoacidosis**
>
> Urinary or plasma ketones
> Blood glucose
> Venous blood gas analysis: pH, PCO_2, bicarbonate, chloride, lactate
> Urea, creatinine and electrolytes: sodium, potassium, phosphate, magnesium
> Full blood count
> Septic screen: C-reactive protein, blood culture, chest radiograph, urinalysis and urine culture
> ECG

- acidosis (pH ≤7.30, bicarbonate <15 mmol/L). The acidosis in DKA is a *metabolic acidosis* (associated with low bicarbonate levels and a reduction of partial pressure of carbon dioxide [PCO_2] due to compensatory hyperventilation) with a *high anion gap* (>12 mmol/L).

The plasma anion gap is calculated from the difference between the primary measured cations and the primary measured anions, i.e. serum $[Na^+ + K^+]$ – serum $[Cl^- + HCO_3^-]$.

In normal subjects, the anion gap is primarily determined by the negative charges on the plasma proteins, particularly albumin. The anion gap is elevated in those forms of metabolic acidosis in which there is buffering of the excess acid by bicarbonate (resulting in a reduction of bicarbonate) and replacement of the bicarbonate by an unmeasured anion (e.g. ketoacid anions in DKA).

Blood glucose levels as low as 10 mmol/L and severe acidaemia may be seen in patients who have recently taken insulin, as this alone is insufficient to correct the acidosis in the presence of dehydration.

Urine ketone detection systems generally detect acetoacetic acid and acetone, but not beta-hydroxybutyric acid. Sulfhydryl drugs, such as captopril, penicillamine and mesna, interact with the nitroprusside reagent and can cause a false-positive ketone test. In patients treated with these drugs, direct measurement of beta-hydroxybutyric acid is recommended. *Capillary ketone meters* measure the level of beta-hydroxybutyric acid, which is the principal ketone produced in DKA.

A septic screen should be performed to look for an underlying infection. An electrocardiogram (ECG) should be done to exclude acute coronary syndrome as a precipitating factor.

The white cell count may be elevated due to an underlying infection. However, an elevated white cell count (usually less than 25×10^9/L) is also commonly seen in the absence of infection. This may occur as a result of hypercortisolaemia and increased catecholamine secretion.

Serum amylase and lipase levels are elevated in 15–25% of patients with DKA and, in most cases, do not reflect acute pancreatitis. However, acute pancreatitis may occur in about 10% of patients with DKA (often in association with hypertriglyceridaemia). The diagnosis of pancreatitis in patients with DKA should be based upon the clinical findings and a computed tomography (CT) scan.

Differential diagnosis

Ketoacidosis may also be caused by alcohol abuse or fasting. Other causes of a high anion gap metabolic acidosis include lactic acidosis (due to tissue hypoperfusion caused by hypovolaemia, cardiac failure or sepsis), renal failure and drugs such as aspirin, methanol and ethylene glycol.

Treatment

Patients should ideally be managed and closely monitored in a high-dependency or intensive therapy unit. Treatment of DKA includes:
- resuscitation (airway, breathing, circulation)
- insulin
- fluids
- potassium.

Broad-spectrum antibiotics are given if infection is suspected.

Patients should remain nil by mouth for at least 6 hours as gastroparesis is common. In patients with impaired conscious level, a nasogastric tube is inserted to prevent vomiting and aspiration.

Two intravenous cannulae should be sited, one in each arm: one for 0.9% saline and one for insulin and later 5% dextrose. A urinary catheter is inserted in patients with oliguria or elevated serum creatinine. A central line may be inserted in those with a history of cardiac disease or autonomic neuropathy and in those who are elderly.

All patients should have thromboprophylaxis with low molecular weight heparin.

Insulin replacement

The only indication for delaying insulin is a serum potassium less than 3.3 mmol/L, as insulin will worsen the hypokalaemia by driving potassium into the cells. Patients with an initial serum potassium of less than 3.3 mmol/L should receive fluid and potassium replacement prior to insulin.

Fifty units of soluble insulin are added to 50 mL 0.9% saline. Insulin infusion is started at a *fixed* rate of 0.1 U/kg per hour (approximately 6–7 U per hour). The response to insulin infusion is reviewed after 1 hour. If blood glucose level is not dropping by 5 mmol per hour and capillary ketones by 1 mmol per hour, the infusion rate is increased by 1 per hour.

The fixed-rate insulin is continued until capillary ketones are below 0.3 mmol/L, venous pH is above 7.3 and venous bicarbonate is above 18 mmol/L. At this point, if the patient is eating and drinking regularly, a subcutaneous insulin regimen is started, and the intravenous insulin pump is discontinued 1–2 hours afterwards. If the patient is not eating and drinking, an intravenous sliding scale is used (Table 36.1).

Ketonuria may persist for more than 36 hours due to the slower removal of acetone, in part via

Table 36.1 Insulin sliding scale

Blood glucose (mmol/L)	Insulin infusion (U/hour)
0–4.0	0.5
4.1–7.0	1
7.1–11.0	2
11.1–15.0	3
15.1–20	4
>20.0	6

50 U of soluble insulin is added to 50 mL 0.9% saline in a syringe and the intravenous infusion is administered via a pump. The rate of insulin infusion is adjusted according to the hourly capillary blood glucose measurements.

the lungs. However, as acetone is biochemically neutral, these patients do not have persistent ketoacidosis.

Individuals who normally take long-acting insulin (e.g. glargine or detemir) should continue their usual dose from the day of admission.

Fluid replacement

The average fluid loss in DKA is 100 mL/kg; *0.9% saline* is used to replace the fluid deficit.

If the patient is hypotensive, 500 mL of intravenous 0.9% saline is given over 15–20 minutes. This may be repeated (up to three times) until the systolic blood pressure is over 100 mmHg. This is followed by:
- 1 L of 0.9% saline 2-hourly × 3 (potassium chloride is added to the second bag of fluid and all subsequent bags; see below)
- 1 L of 0.9% saline 3-hourly × 3 (plus potassium replacement; see below).

When the blood glucose reaches 15 mmol/L, intravenous *5% dextrose* is given concurrently with 0.9% saline (through an intravenous cannula in the other arm):
- When the blood glucose is 7–15 mmol/L: 1 L of 5% dextrose (plus 20 mmol potassium chloride) is administered over 8 hours.
- When the blood glucose is below 7 mmol/L: 500 mL of 10% dextrose (plus 10 mmol potassium chloride) is administered over 4 hours.

The above regimen should be modified for patients with cardiac disease.

Potassium replacement

In patients with DKA, both renal and gastrointestinal losses contribute to the potassium depletion. The increase in renal potassium excretion is primarily related to the glycosuria-induced osmotic diuresis and to hypovolaemia-induced hyperaldosteronism. However, despite this deficit, the serum potassium concentration is often high at presentation as insulin deficiency leads to potassium movement out of the cells and into the extracellular fluid.

Treatment with insulin lowers the potassium concentration and may cause severe hypokalaemia

Table 36.2 Potassium replacement

Potassium level	Replacement per litre fluid
>5.5 mmol/L	Nil
2.5–5.5 mmol/L	40 mmol/L
<2.5 mmol/L	60–80 mmol/L

as potassium shifts into the cells under the action of insulin. Therefore careful monitoring and administration of potassium are essential.

Potassium chloride is not given in the first litre of fluid or if the serum potassium is over 5.5 mmol/L. All subsequent fluids for the next 24 hours should contain potassium chloride, unless urine output is below 30 mL per hour or serum potassium is over 5.5 mmol/L. The amount of potassium added to the fluids is adjusted according to plasma potassium levels (Table 36.2).

Bicarbonate

The use of bicarbonate is controversial and there is no evidence that it improves outcome in DKA. There are three potential concerns with alkali therapy:
- a reduced acidaemic stimulus to hyperventilation, which leads to a rise in PCO_2. The carbon dioxide can rapidly cross the blood–brain barrier resulting in a paradoxical fall in cerebral pH
- a reduced rate of recovery of the ketosis
- post-treatment metabolic alkalosis, since the metabolism of ketoacid anions with insulin results in the generation of bicarbonate and spontaneous correction of most of the metabolic acidosis.

Bicarbonate may be considered in patients with an arterial pH lower than 7, in whom decreased cardiac contractility and vasodilatation can further impair tissue perfusion. If the arterial pH is 6.9–7.0, 50 mmol of sodium bicarbonate and 10 mmol of potassium chloride may be given in 200 mL of water over 2 hours. If the arterial pH is below 6.90, 100 mmol of sodium bicarbonate and 20 mmol of potassium chloride may be given in 400 mL water over 2 hours. The venous pH should be monitored every 2 hours, and bicarbonate dosed as above, until the pH rises above 7.0.

Phosphate and magnesium

Randomized trials of phosphate replacement in DKA in adults have failed to show any clinical benefit. Phosphate administration may induce hypocalcaemia and hypomagnesaemia. The main indication for phosphate therapy is a serum phosphate concentration less than 0.30 mmol/L. Intravenous phosphate (monobasic potassium phosphate) is infused at a maximum rate of 9 mmol every 12 hours. When phosphate is given, serum calcium and magnesium levels should be monitored.

Serum magnesium may fall during insulin therapy. If magnesium levels fall below 0.5 mmol/L, 4–8 mmol (2 mL of 50%) magnesium sulphate is administered over 15–30 minutes in 50 mL 0.9% saline.

Monitoring

Close monitoring of the following is critical.

For the *first 15 hours*:
- Blood glucose, capillary ketones and urine output are monitored hourly
- Urea and electrolytes are monitored 4-hourly.
- Venous blood gas is monitored at 0, 2, 4, 8 and 12 hours and before stopping the fixed-rate intravenous insulin regimen.

15–30 hours:
- Plasma glucose is monitored hourly.
- Capillary ketones are monitored every 2 hours.
- Serum potassium is monitored 12-hourly.
- Plasma phosphate and magnesium are monitored daily.

An arterial line is inserted in the intensive care unit to monitor pH, bicarbonate and potassium levels. If an arterial line is not inserted, patients should have venous samples for measurement of pH and bicarbonate rather than repeated arterial blood gases, which are uncomfortable.

Almost all patients with DKA (except those with advanced renal failure) develop a normal anion gap acidosis during treatment. Insulin converts ketoacid anions back into bicarbonate. However, as some of the ketoacid anions (i.e. bicarbonate precursors) are excreted in the urine with sodium or potassium, the anion gap is reduced, but the acidosis persists.

Cerebral oedema

Cerebral oedema occurs in 0.3–1% of children with DKA and has a high mortality rate of 20–25%. Younger children and those with newly diagnosed DKA, elevated serum urea, more profound acidosis or neurological symptoms are at greatest risk for cerebral oedema. Cerebral oedema generally develops during treatment for DKA due to sudden shifts in plasma osmolality. However, up to 20% of cases of cerebral oedema occur before the initiation of treatment.

All children should be carefully monitored for early signs of cerebral oedema throughout the course of treatment for DKA. Specific signs of increased intracranial pressure and radiological changes detected by head CT often occur too late for effective intervention. Cerebral oedema should be suspected in patients with headache, recurrent vomiting, age-inappropriate incontinence, irritability, lethargy and altered level of consciousness.

If cerebral oedema is suspected, treatment should be started promptly by reducing the rate of fluid administration and administering intravenous mannitol (0.25–1.0 g/kg) or hypertonic 3% saline.

Hyperosmolar hyperglycaemic state

Hyperosmolar hyperglycaemic state (HHS) and DKA are part of a spectrum representing the metabolic consequences of insulin deficiency, glucagon excess and counterregulatory hormonal responses to stressful triggers in diabetic patients.

In HHS, there is little or no ketoacid accumulation, the serum glucose concentration often exceeds 50 mmol/L, the plasma osmolality may reach 380 mosmol/kg, and neurological abnormalities are frequently present.

Insulin levels in HHS are insufficient to allow appropriate glucose utilization but are adequate to prevent lipolysis and subsequent ketogenesis. HHS is also known as hyperosmolar non-ketotic acidosis (HONK). Lower levels of counterregulatory hormones and free fatty acids have been found in HHS than in DKA.

HHS usually occurs in elderly patients with type 2 diabetes. It has a substantially higher mortality than DKA (up to 15% in some clinical series).

Clinical presentations

Patients with HHS present with:
- an insidious onset of polyuria and polydipsia (patients with DKA generally excrete glucose more effectively than older patients with HHS)
- severe dehydration
- neurological symptoms when the effective serum osmolality is over 320 mosmol/kg. Coma is usually associated with an osmolality of above 440 mosmol/kg (25–50% of cases).

The history and clinical examination may reveal symptoms and signs of the underlying precipitating factors (Box 36.3).

Investigations

Investigations in patients with HHS are similar to those with DKA (see Box 36.2).

The *serum glucose* concentration often exceeds 50 mmol/L.

The *serum sodium* level reflects the balance between the dilution of sodium due to osmotic water movement out of the cells, and the concentration of sodium due to glycosuria-induced osmotic diuresis resulting in loss of water in excess of sodium. Reversing the hyperglycaemia with

---

Box 36.3 Precipitating factors for a hyperosmolar hyperglycaemic state

Poor compliance with treatment
Previously undiagnosed diabetes
Infection (e.g. urinary tract, pneumonia)
Myocardial infarction
Stroke, subdural haematoma
Pulmonary embolism
Acute pancreatitis, intestinal obstruction
Hypothermia
Drugs: diuretics, beta-blockers, antihistamines, steroids
Total parenteral nutrition
Trauma

---

insulin will cause water to move from the extracellular fluid into the cells and increases the serum sodium concentration. Therefore a patient with a normal initial serum sodium concentration will probably become hypernatraemic during therapy.

The *effective plasma osmolality* can be estimated from either of the following equations:

$$2 \times (Na^+ + K^+) + glucose\,(all\ in\,mmol/L),\ or$$

$$Measured\ plasma\ osmolality - urea\,(in\ mmol/L)$$

The multiple 2 in the first equation accounts for the osmotic contribution of the anions (i.e. chloride and bicarbonate) accompanying sodium and potassium. Note that in the calculation of effective plasma osmolality, the urea concentration is not taken into account because urea is freely permeable and its accumulation does not induce major changes in the osmotic gradient across the cell membrane.

The presence of stupor or coma in diabetic patients with an effective serum osmolality below 320 mosmol/kg warrants prompt investigation with head CT and lumbar puncture for causes other than HHS.

Treatment

Patients with HHS are severely dehydrated and may require 8–10 L of fluid in the first 48 hours. *Rehydration* is started with 1 L of 0.9% saline over the first hour, then 1 L 2-hourly for 4 hours, and then 1 L 6-hourly until the person is rehydrated. If the sodium level is over 160 mmol/L, 0.45% saline may be considered for the first 3 L.

Potassium 20–30 mmol is given in each litre of intravenous fluid to keep the serum potassium concentration between 4 and 5 mmol/L.

Patients with HHS tend to be more sensitive to the effects of insulin. Intravenous *insulin* is usually given at a rate of 2–3 U per hour and should not exceed 4 U per hour.

The underlying cause must be treated (e.g. antibiotics for suspected infection). Patients with HHS are at increased risk of venous and arterial thromboses, and *thromboprophylaxis* with low molecular weight heparin (e.g. enoxaparin or dalteparin) is essential. Fluid balance, urea and electrolytes, plasma glucose and osmolality must be carefully monitored.

When the blood glucose reaches 15 mmol/L and the patient is able to eat:

- intravenous insulin can be tapered/stopped
- 0.9% saline is switched to 5% dextrose
- subcutaneous insulin or oral hypoglycaemic agents are started
- blood glucose monitoring is continued.

Reducing the serum glucose acutely below 14 mmol/L may promote the development of cerebral oedema. Once the intravenous insulin infusion has been stopped, blood glucose levels may start to rise if the individual has an underlying infection (which may have precipitated the HHS). Sliding scale insulin may need to be started as for any poorly controlled diabetic patient with sepsis.

Hypoglycaemia

Hypoglycaemia (low serum glucose concentration) is a common complication of treatment with insulin or oral hypoglycaemic agents (particularly long-acting sulphonylureas, e.g. glibenclamide). Hypoglycaemia is more common in patients with type 1 diabetes mellitus.

The responses to hypoglycaemia in normal subjects include the ability to suppress insulin release and an increased release of counterregulatory hormones (glucagon and adrenaline), which raise plasma glucose concentrations by stimulating gluconeogenesis and antagonizing the insulin-induced increase in glucose utilization.

In diabetic patients, the protective responses to hypoglycaemia are impaired: insulin is supplied exogenously and its release cannot be turned off. In addition, the glucagon and adrenaline response to hypoglycaemia becomes impaired later in the course of diabetes.

Recurrent hypoglycaemia itself also may contribute to the impaired counterregulatory response. The compensatory increase in cortisol production during the first hypoglycaemic episode may play a role in minimizing the protective hormonal responses during subsequent episodes.

Patients who have diabetes following a total pancreatectomy have more frequent and severe episodes of hypoglycaemia because they lack glucagon-producing (alpha) cells as well as beta cells.

Clinical presentations

Hypoglycaemia causes symptoms of sympathetic overactivity (when the plasma glucose is <3.6 mmol/L) and symptoms of neuroglycopenia if the serum glucose concentration falls further (<2.6 mmol/L):

- The symptoms and signs of *sympathetic overactivity* include sweating, anxiety, tremor, tachycardia, palpitations, pallor, nausea and hunger.
- The symptoms and signs of *neuroglycopenia* include dizziness, headache, visual disturbances, focal neurological defect (stroke-like syndromes), difficulty speaking, inability to concentrate, abnormal behavior, confusion, drowsiness and ultimately loss of consciousness or seizures (blood glucose <1.5 mmol/L).

Patients whose diabetes is well controlled (glycated haemoglobin [HbA_{1c}] <8%) may have few warning symptoms when their plasma glucose concentration falls. These patients may develop neuroglycopenia before sympathetic activation and complain of 'loss of warning' (*hypoglycaemic unawareness*). Hypoglycaemic episodes may lead to an upregulation of glucose transporters in the brain, resulting in the maintenance of glucose uptake and therefore the prevention of warning symptoms of hypoglycaemia.

Another factor that may contribute to hypoglycaemia unawareness is diabetic autonomic neuropathy. Beta-blockers can also blunt the warning symptoms of sympathetic activation.

Patients with poorly controlled diabetes (HbA_{1c} >12%) may develop sympathetic signs of hypoglycaemia when their blood glucose values fall to about 5.6 mmol/L. One mechanism by which this might occur is downregulation of glucose transporters in the brain in chronically hyperglycaemic patients.

Investigations

Glucometers are inaccurate at low blood glucose levels, and capillary blood glucose measurement must be confirmed by laboratory glucose measurements.

Urea and electrolytes must be measured as recurrent hypoglycaemia may be due to diabetic nephropathy. Diabetic nephropathy decreases insulin requirements as insulin is partly degraded by the kidney. Sulphonylureas are renally excreted.

Treatment

If the patient is conscious and cooperative, he or she should receive 50 g of oral glucose (e.g. in the form of Lucozade, milk, sugar or three dextrose tablets. Capillary blood glucose should be checked again in 10 minutes, and if it is still below 4 mmol/L more fast-acting glucose should be given. This should be followed with a starchy snack. Patients should not drive for 45 minutes.

If the individual has a reduced level of consciousness, 50 mL of 50% glucose should be given intravenously. If there is no intravenous access, 1 mg of glucagon should be administered intramuscularly. Capillary blood glucose should be measured in 10 minutes. Patients should have a carbohydrate-rich snack when they are able to eat.

Patients should regain consciousness or become coherent within 10 minutes, although complete cognitive and neurological recovery may lag by 30–45 minutes. Subsequent regular doses of insulin should not be omitted but may need to be reduced. Bedtime snacks are the traditional strategy for preventing nocturnal hypoglycaemia.

If hypoglycaemia is secondary to a sulphonylurea or long-acting insulin, patients should be admitted for intravenous infusion of 10% dextrose and blood glucose monitoring.

In those with a history of excess alcohol intake, intravenous thiamine (1–2 mg/kg) should be given prior to dextrose to reduce the risk of precipitating Wernicke's encephalopathy.

In those with hypoglycaemic unawareness, avoidance of hypoglycaemia for about 6 months can improve autonomic symptoms and restore hypoglycaemic awareness, even though counter-regulatory responses do not normalize.

Key points:

- The triad of DKA consists of hyperglycaemia, high anion gap metabolic acidosis and ketonaemia.
- Precipitating factors for DKA and HHS include infection, new-onset diabetes, inadequate insulin treatment or non-compliance, myocardial infarction and stroke.
- Investigations in DKA include urinary or plasma ketones, blood glucose, venous gas analysis (pH, PCO_2, bicarbonate, chloride, lactate), urea and electrolytes, full blood count, a septic screen and ECG.
- Close monitoring of blood glucose, capillary ketones, urine output, urea and electrolytes and venous blood gas is critical.
- In HHS, there is little or no ketoacid accumulation, plasma glucose often exceeds 50 mmol/L, and plasma osmolality may reach 380 mosmol/kg.
- Treatment of DKA and HHS includes insulin, fluids and potassium replacement, treatment of the underlying condition, and thromboprophylaxis with low molecular weight heparins.
- Hypoglycaemia in a patient with a reduced level of consciousness should be treated with 50 mL of 50% glucose intravenously or 1 mg of intramuscular glucagon if there is no intravenous access.

Chapter 37

Diabetic retinopathy

Diabetic retinopathy is a progressive ophthalmic microvascular complication of diabetes. Diabetic retinopathy is a major cause of morbidity in patients with diabetes mellitus.

Epidemiology

Diabetic retinopathy is the leading cause of blindness among the UK's working age population. The Wisconsin Epidemiologic Study of Diabetic Retinopathy showed that the prevalence of retinopathy increases progressively with increasing duration of disease in both type 1 and type 2 diabetes mellitus:

- In *type 1* diabetes, retinopathy starts to occur about 3–5 years after diagnosis. Retinopathy is present in almost all patients at 20 years.
- In *type 2* diabetes, some patients have retinopathy at the time of diagnosis, reflecting the insidious onset of hyperglycaemia in type 2 diabetes. Retinopathy is present in 50–80% of patients at 20 years.

Aetiology

The primary cause of diabetic retinopathy is thought to be chronic hyperglycaemia. The Diabetes Control and Complications Trial (DCCT) and

Lecture Notes: Endocrinology and Diabetes. By A. Sam and K. Meeran. Published 2009 by Blackwell Publishing. ISBN 978-1-4051-5345-4.

the United Kingdom Prospective Diabetes Study (UKPDS) found that glycaemic control reduces the incidence of retinopathy in type 1 and type 2 diabetes respectively.

The main hypotheses for the pathogenesis of diabetic retinopathy include:
- impaired autoregulation of retinal blood flow
- accumulation of sorbitol within the retinal cells
- accumulation of advanced glycosylation endproducts (AGEs) in the extracellular fluid.

Impaired autoregulation of retinal blood flow

Retinal blood flow autoregulation (i.e. maintenance of a constant blood flow despite an increase in the mean arterial pressure of less than 40% above baseline) is impaired in the presence of hyperglycaemia. The ensuing increase in retinal blood flow in diabetic patients may cause increased shear stress on the retinal blood vessels, resulting in vascular leakage and the production of vasoactive substances.

Accumulation of sorbitol within retinal cells

Glucose is metabolized to sorbitol within the retinal cells by the enzyme aldose reductase. The role of sorbitol in the pathogenesis of diabetic retinopathy is uncertain. During sorbitol production, consumption of NADPH can result in oxidative stress. Sorbitol accumulation can lead to alterations in the activity of protein kinase C, which may mediate the activity of vascular endothelial growth factor (VEGF) and regulate vascular permeability.

Advanced glycosylation end-products

Non-enzymatic combination between some of the excess glucose and amino acids in proteins results in the formation of AGEs. AGEs may cross-link with collagen and initiate microvascular complications. In addition, the interaction between AGEs and their receptor (RAGE) may generate new reactive oxygen species and cause vascular inflammation.

Other factors

Growth factors such as insulin-like growth factor-1 (IGF-1) and VEGF, and erythropoietin, may increase vascular permeability and promote the growth of new blood vessels. Basic fibroblast growth factor may also contribute to the progression of the retinal disease. Carbonic anhydrase appears to play a role in retinal vascular permeability in patients with proliferative retinopathy. Genetic factors may affect the severity of retinopathy. In the DCCT, severe retinopathy was three times more frequent among the relatives of the retinopathy-positive patients.

Clinical presentations

The majority of patients who develop diabetic retinopathy have no symptoms until the late stages, when it may be too late for effective treatment.

Rarely, patients may present with sudden loss of vision due to retinal detachment or a vitreous haemorrhage, decreased visual acuity due to macular oedema, floaters during the resolution of vitreous bleeds or odd colours in the peripheral vision due to cataracts.

The various identifiable stages of diabetic retinopathy are described as:
- *background* retinopathy
- *preproliferative* retinopathy
- *proliferative* retinopathy.

> **Box 37.1 National Screening Committee Grading Criteria for Diabetic Retinopathy**
>
> **R0—none**
>
> **R1—background**
> Microaneurysms
> Retinal haemorrhages
> Hard exudates
>
> **R2—preproliferative**
> Cotton wool spots
> Venous beading, loops, reduplication, intraretinal microvascular abnormalities (IRMAs)
> Multiple deep, round or blot haemorrhages
>
> **R3—proliferative**
> New vessels on disc (NVD)
> New vessels elsewhere (NVE)
> Preretinal or vitreous haemorrhage
> Preretinal fibrosis +/– retinal detachment
>
> **M0—no maculopathy**
>
> **M1—maculopathy**
> Exudates within one disc diameter of the centre of the fovea
> Microaneurysms or haemorrhage within one disc diameter of the centre of the fovea associated with visual acuity ≤6/12
> Retinal thickening within one disc diameter of the centre of the fovea (if stereo available)
>
> **P—evidence of previous photocoagulation**

The UK National Screening Committee (NSC) has produced grading criteria describing various levels of disease (Box 37.1).

Background retinopathy (R1)

The early changes in diabetic retinopathy include death of the retinal pericytes, thickening of the retinal basement membrane and impairment of its function. Pericytes are mesenchymal-like cells that support the walls of small blood vessels.

These changes are associated with the formation of retinal capillary *microaneurysms* (outpouchings of retinal capillaries with weakened walls partly due to pericyte loss) and increased vascular permeability, resulting in the leakage of lipid and protein-

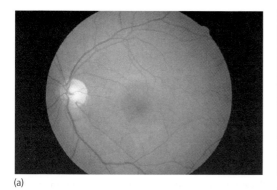

(a)

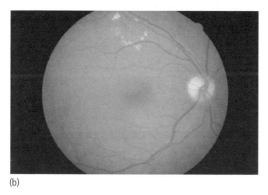

(b)

Figure 37.1 (a) Normal retina with no retinopathy (NSC grade R0). (b) Background retinopathy with microaneurysms, haemorrhages and hard exudates (NSC grade R1).

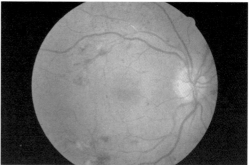

Figure 37.2 Preproliferative retinopathy (NSC grade R2) with cotton wool spots, intraretinal microvascular abnormalities and multiple blot haemorrhages.

are dilated capillaries that occur in response to retinal ischaemia.

Proliferative retinopathy (R3)

Progressive microvascular occlusion and retinal ischaemia results in an increased release of vaso-proliferative substances such as IGF-1 and VEGF, which promote the formation of new vessels (*neovascularization*). New vessels (Fig. 37.3) can arise from arteries or veins. The new vessels form a lace-like pattern with a fine mesh of fibrous tissue connecting them. There are two main risks associated with new vessel formation:

• *Pre-retinal or vitreous haemorrhage:* the new vessels are fragile and therefore prone to rupture.
• *Retinal detachment:* as new vessels mature, the fibrous component becomes more prominent, resulting in contraction.

New vessel proliferation can also occur on the surface of the iris and in the anterior chamber. The latter change can cause glaucoma by blocking the outflow of the aqueous humour.

aceous material (*hard exudates*) (Fig. 37.1). Capillary leakage often spreads in a circinate pattern.

The initial stage of cell death may be followed by cycles of renewal and further cell death. The intraluminal proliferation of cells, as well as changes in platelet function, erythrocyte aggregation and high plasma fibrinogen levels, can cause vascular occlusion and rupture. This can result in small flame-shaped and blot haemorrhages proximal to the occlusion.

Preproliferative retinopathy (R2)

Intraretinal infarcts (*cotton wool spots* or *soft exudates*) may occur distal to microvascular occlusions (Fig. 37.2). Proliferation of the endothelial cells of retinal veins results in venous calibre abnormalities, such as venous beading, loops and dilation. Intraretinal microvascular abnormalities (IRMAs)

Maculopathy (M1)

Maculopathy is characterized by exudates or retinal thickening within one disc diameter of the centre of the fovea, or microaneurysms or haemorrhage within one disc diameter of the centre of the fovea associated with a best visual acuity of 6/12 or less (Fig. 37.4).

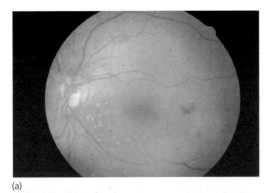

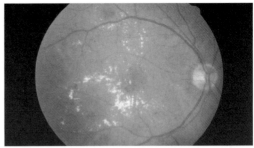

Figure 37.4 Diabetic maculopathy with haemorrhages and circinate exudates (NSC grade R2 M1).

(a)

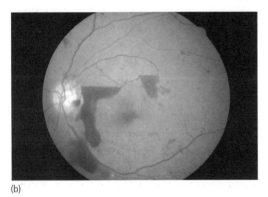

(b)

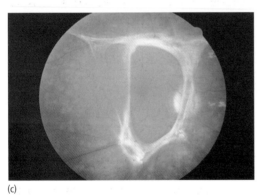

(c)

Figure 37.3 (a) Proliferative retinopathy (NSC grade R3) with new vessels at the optic disc. (b) Proliferative retinopathy with preretinal and vitreous haemorrhages (NSC grade R3). (c) Proliferative retinopathy with fibrous proliferation (NSC grade R3).

Macular oedema

Macular oedema is characterized by retinal thickening due to leaky blood vessels and can develop at any stage of retinopathy. It typically presents with a gradual-onset blurring of near and distant vision. Macular oedema is difficult to detect on routine examination. Patients with suspected macular oedema should be referred to an ophthalmologist for a slit lamp examination (to detect thickening) and fluorescein angiography (to detect local leakage associated with oedema).

Exacerbation of retinopathy in pregnancy

Diabetic retinopathy may worsen during pregnancy. The Diabetes in Early Pregnancy (DIEP) study showed that the risk of progression of retinopathy is related to the severity of retinal involvement before pregnancy and the initial glycated haemoglobin (HbA$_{1c}$) values. Changes in hormones, growth factors and systemic haemodynamics, and lower retinal blood flow, may contribute to the exacerbation of retinopathy in pregnancy.

Transient exacerbation of retinopathy with intensive insulin therapy

Data from the DCCT and other trials suggest that intensive insulin therapy may be associated with a transient worsening of retinopathy during the first year. This may result from closure of the small retinal blood vessels due to reduced plasma volume caused by the correction of hyperglycaemia. Increased IGF-1 levels may also contribute to the exacerbation of retinopathy.

Screening

It is important to screen diabetic patients regularly with digital retinal photography for the development of retinopathy. Patients with NSC grades R0 and R1 need annual screening. Those with NSC grade R3 should be seen by hospital eye service/specialists immediately. Those with NSC grade R2 or M1 should be seen by hospital eye service/specialists urgently (within 4 weeks).

Treatment

Treatment of diabetic retinopathy is directed both at reducing the risk and progression of retinopathy, and at the treatment of established disease.

Reducing risk and progression of retinopathy

Glycaemic control

Strict *glycaemic control* is effective in primary prevention in patients without retinopathy, and in slowing the rate of progression of retinopathy in patients with mild-to-moderate non-proliferative retinopathy. However, it is of little or no benefit in patients with advanced retinopathy. Despite the general efficacy of glycaemic control, there is often transient worsening of the retinopathy during the first year of intensive glycaemic management (see above).

The DCCT found that intensive insulin therapy reduced the incidence of new cases of retinopathy in type 1 diabetics by 76% compared with conventional therapy. Progressive retinopathy was uncommon in patients with an HbA_{1c} below 7%. The UKPDS showed that each 1% point reduction in HbA_{1c} in patients with type 2 diabetes was associated with a 37% reduction in the development of retinopathy.

Blood pressure control

Control of hypertension slows the rate of progression of diabetic retinopathy. The UKPDS showed that patients with lower blood pressures had a reduced deterioration in retinopathy and visual acuity.

Lisinopril (an angiotensin-converting enzyme inhibitor) has been reported to reduce the progression of retinopathy in normotensive patients with type 1 diabetes. The mechanism by which angiotensin-converting enzyme inhibitors might inhibit the progression of retinopathy is unclear.

Multifactorial risk reduction

The Steno-2 trial showed that intensive risk factor reduction in patients with type 2 diabetes and microalbuminuria (using behavioural therapy, advice regarding diet, exercise and smoking cessation, and the administration of multiple medications to achieve several aggressive therapeutic goals) reduced the development or progression of retinopathy.

Antiplatelet agents

The Early Treatment of Diabetic Retinopathy Study reported that aspirin has no beneficial effect on the development or progression of proliferative retinopathy, vitreous bleeding or visual loss. However, there were no ocular contraindications to its use in persons with diabetes who required aspirin for the treatment of cardiovascular disease or for other medical indications.

Fibrates

The Fenofibrate Intervention and Event Lowering in Diabetes (FIELD) study demonstrated a 30% relative reduction in the need for first retinal laser therapy in patients with type 2 diabetes treated with fenofibrate. A reduction in progression of diabetic retinopathy was observed in those with retinopathy at baseline. However, further clinical and experimental studies are needed before fenofibrate can be launched as a new tool in the management of diabetic retinopathy.

Treatment of established retinopathy

Photocoagulation

Laser photocoagulation (Fig. 37.5) is the primary treatment for advanced retinopathy and reduces

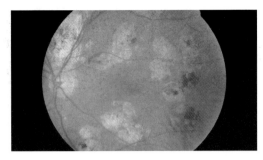

Figure 37.5 Evidence of previous laser photocoagulation (NSC grade P).

the risk of developing visual loss. Early photocoagulation is not usually recommended except for focal laser therapy used to treat macular oedema. This therapy reduces the risk of visual loss. With aggressive monitoring and treatment, good visual acuity can be maintained.

Intravitreal steroids

Intravitreal triamcinolone injection may be used for macular oedema and may improve visual acuity. The treatment response in diabetic macular oedema may be transient, and repeated injections are often necessary.

Vitrectomy

Vitrectomy can also be used to preserve useful vision in advanced cases. Removal of the opaque vitreous humour followed by photocoagulation to the retina can restore some functional vision. The timing of such interventions is critical.

Growth factor inhibitors

As mentioned above, VEGF increases retinal vascular permeability. The effects of VEGF are mediated, in part, by protein kinase C. Subcutaneous pegaptanib, a VEGF inhibitor, has been used in diabetic patients with macular oedema in a phase II randomized controlled trial. It has been reported to improve visual acuity, decrease retinal thickness and need for photocoagulation, and possibly cause some regression in retinal neovascularization. A preliminary study of intravitreal bevacizumab (a monoclonal antibody against VEGF) in patients with proliferative diabetic retinopathy has demonstrated a reduction of angiographic fluorescein leakage.

Initial clinical trials of orally administered ruboxistaurin (a protein kinase C beta inhibitor) in severe non-proliferative diabetic retinopathy found that although it reduced the risk of moderate visual loss, it did not prevent the progression of retinopathy. Larger studies are required to determine the potential clinical implications of this agent.

Pregnancy

The modest increase in risk of worsening of retinopathy during pregnancy necessitates more frequent retinal evaluations during this time and for 1 year postpartum. Women should be screened during the first trimester and then every 3 months while pregnant. Treatment recommendations are the same as for other patients. Laser therapy and vitreous surgery can be carried out safely during pregnancy if required. Women can be reassured that their long-term risk of retinopathy progression is not increased by pregnancy.

Key points:

- Diabetic retinopathy is a progressive ophthalmic microvascular complication of diabetes.
- Glycaemic control reduces the incidence of retinopathy in both type 1 and type 2 diabetes.
- Control of hypertension slows the rate of progression of diabetic retinopathy.
- The majority of patients who develop diabetic retinopathy have no symptoms until the late stages. Therefore it is important to screen patients with diabetes regularly for the development of retinopathy.
- The various identifiable stages of diabetic retinopathy are described as background retinopathy, preproliferative retinopathy and proliferative retinopathy.
- Patients with proliferative retinopathy should be seen by hospital eye service/specialists immediately. Patients with preproliferative retinopathy and those with maculopathy should be seen urgently by hospital eye service/specialists.
- Laser photocoagulation is the primary treatment for advanced retinopathy and reduces the risk of developing visual loss.

Chapter 38

Diabetic nephropathy

Diabetic nephropathy (kidney disease) occurs in both type 1 and type 2 diabetes mellitus.

The natural history of diabetic nephropathy is characterized by a fairly predictable sequence of events (Fig. 38.1). Glomerular hyperperfusion, increased glomerular filtration and increased kidney size (renal hypertrophy) occur in the first years after the onset of diabetes.

The earliest clinical finding of diabetic nephropathy is *microalbuminuria*. Microalbuminuria is defined as the persistent excretion of small amounts of albumin (30–300 mg per day) into the urine. Microalbuminuria is an important predictor of progression to *proteinuria* (>300 mg per day). Once proteinuria appears, there is a steady decline in the glomerular filtration rate (GFR). Patients with microalbuminuria or reduced GFR are at increased risk of *end-stage renal disease* and premature cardiovascular morbidity and mortality.

The major histological changes in the glomeruli in diabetic nephropathy include:
- *expansion of the mesangium* (glomerular supporting tissues)
- *glomerular basement membrane thickening*
- *glomerular sclerosis*.

Diabetic glomerular sclerosis may be diffuse or nodular. The latter is known as the *Kimmelstiel–Wilson lesion*. Nodular glomerular sclerosis is usually associated with hyaline deposits in the glomerular arterioles, reflecting the insinuation of plasma proteins such as albumin, fibrin, immunoglobulins and complement into the vascular wall.

Patients with type 1 diabetes and nephropathy almost always have retinopathy. However, the converse is not true. Most patients with advanced retinopathy have little or no renal disease as assessed by renal biopsy and protein excretion. The relationship between diabetic nephropathy and retinopathy is less predictable in type 2 diabetes.

Type IV renal tubular acidosis (hyporeninaemic hypoaldosteronism) also occurs in diabetes mellitus. Patients develop a propensity to hyperkalaemia.

Diabetic patients are predisposed to radiocontrast-induced nephrotoxicity. Patients with diabetes mellitus undergoing radiological investigations with contrast dye should be well hydrated before and after the procedure, and the serum creatinine should be monitored for several days after imaging. Treatment with acetylcysteine (600 mg twice a day) on the day before and the day of the radiocontrast administration appears to protect high-risk patients from nephrotoxicity.

Pathogenesis

Figure 38.2b shows a simplified model for the pathogenesis of diabetic nephropathy. The mechanisms by which diabetes leads to nephropathy

Lecture Notes: Endocrinology and Diabetes. By A. Sam and K. Meeran. Published 2009 by Blackwell Publishing. ISBN 978-1-4051-5345-4.

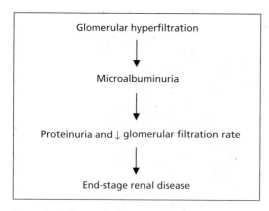

Glomerular hyperfiltration

↓

Microalbuminuria

↓

Proteinuria and ↓ glomerular filtration rate

↓

End-stage renal disease

Figure 38.1 Sequence of events in diabetic nephropathy.

involve advanced glycosylation end-products (AGEs), cytokines, growth factors, angiotensin II and haemodynamic factors.

Hyperglycaemia results in increased *reactive oxygen species* (by increased activation of mitochondrial electron transport) and *AGEs* (generated by non-enzymatic combination of the excess glucose with amino acids in proteins). These in turn activate a number of signalling pathways involving *protein kinase C, mitogen-activated protein kinase* (MAPK) and *transforming growth factor-beta* (TGF-β), resulting in the accumulation of extracellular matrix proteins (e.g. collagen type IV and fibronectin) in the mesangial space, and 'glomerulosclerosis' (fibrosis in the renal glomeruli). Diabetes is associated with a reduced expression of renal bone morphogenic protein-7 (BMP-7), which appears to counter the profibrogenic actions of TGF-β.

Haemodynamic factors including systemic hypertension and *glomerular hypertension* contribute to the pathogenesis of diabetic nephropathy. Diabetes is associated with impaired renal autoregulation. As a result, increased systemic blood pressure does not produce the expected afferent arteriolar vasoconstriction and leads to intraglomerular hypertension. Glomerular hypertension, the resultant mesangial cell stretch and *angiotensin II* also stimulate glomerulosclerosis.

Other factors that may play a role in the development of diabetic nephropathy include increased plasma *prorenin* activity (which activates MAPK),

increased expression of *heparanase* (causing a loss of negatively charged heparan sulfates and increased glomerular basement membrane permeability to albumin) and a reduced expression of renal *nephrin* (a transmembrane protein expressed by podocytes).

In addition to mesangial cells, glomerular endothelial cells, podocytes and tubular epithelial cells are also targets of hyperglycaemic injury. There is substantial crosstalk between endothelial cells, podocytes and mesangial cells. *Endothelial dysfunction* and *podocyte damage* may result in diabetic glomerulosclerosis.

The likelihood of developing diabetic nephropathy is markedly increased in patients with a diabetic sibling or parent who has diabetic nephropathy. A number of factors, such as increasing age, race, obesity, smoking and oral contraceptive use, may increase the risk of developing diabetic nephropathy.

Epidemiology

Diabetic nephropathy is the most common cause of end-stage renal disease in the UK and the USA.

Type 1 diabetes

After 10 years of type 1 diabetes, 20–30% of patients will have microalbuminuria. Less than 50% of patients with microalbuminuria will progress to proteinuria over an average period of 5–10 years. In total, 50% of patients with proteinuria reach end-stage renal disease after 10 years. Those patients who have no proteinuria after 20–25 years have a risk of developing overt renal disease of only about 1% per year.

Microalbuminuria may regress or remain stable with improved glycaemic and blood pressure control and the use of angiotensin-converting enzyme (ACE) inhibitors.

Type 2 diabetes

At 10 years following diagnosis, 25% of patients have microalbuminuria. The time from the onset of diabetes to proteinuria (around 15 years) and

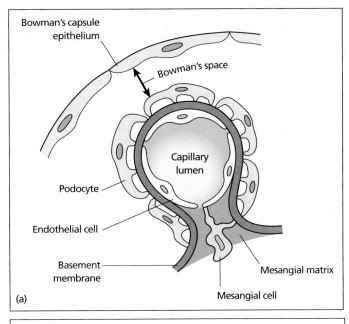

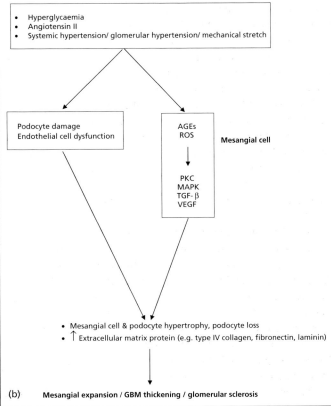

Figure 38.2 (a) Glomerular cells. (b) Simplified model of pathogenesis of diabetic nephropathy. AGEs, advanced glycosylation end-products; GBM, glomerular basement membrane; MAPK, mitogen-activated protein kinases; ROS, reactive oxygen species; PKC, protein kinase C; TGF-β, transforming growth factor-β; VEGF, vascular endothelial growth factor.

from the time from onset of proteinuria to end-stage renal disease (around 10 years) is similar in type 1 and type 2 disease.

Microalbuminuria may be present in about 8% of patients with type 2 diabetes at diagnosis. This may be due to an initial delay in the diagnosis of type 2 diabetes. The incidence and severity of diabetic nephropathy are increased in African-Americans, Mexican-Americans and Pima Indians.

Diagnosis

Microalbuminuria is not detected by a simple urine dipstick. As part of the diabetic follow-up, a spot urine sample must be sent to the laboratory for measurement of urine albumin and creatinine concentrations. The latter compensates for variations in urine concentration in spot-check samples. Microalbuminuria is defined as an *albumin-to-creatinine ratio* (ACR) above 2.5 g/mol in men or above 3.5 g/mol in women.

If microalbuminuria is detected, conditions that transiently increase albumin extraction must be excluded and the test should be repeated. Urinary tract infection, fever, exercise, menstruation, semen, cardiac failure and poor glycaemic control can cause transient microalbuminuria. A persistent elevation in albumin excretion should be demonstrated for establishing the diagnosis of microalbuminuria. If two of the three spot urine tests are positive, treatment should be started.

If the spot urine dipstick detects proteinuria (>300 mg per day), a 24-hour urine collection may be requested to quantify the proteinuria.

Serum creatinine is regularly monitored in diabetic patients. However, it is an inaccurate reflection of the GFR. The *estimated GFR* (eGFR) should be calculated by the MDRD (Modification of Diet in Renal Disease study) equation using serum creatinine, age, sex and race.

In diabetic patients with raised serum creatinine, other causes of kidney disease should be excluded. Blood tests for autoimmune renal disease (erythrocyte sedimentation rate, antinuclear antibodies, antineutrophil cytoplasmic antibodies, anti-double-stranded DNA antibodies, anti-glomerular basement membrane antibodies, complement),

myeloma (serum protein electrophoresis) and prostate-specific antigen, urine microscopy and a renal ultrasound should be performed.

When eGFR falls below 60 mL/min/1.73 m^2, the full blood count, calcium, phosphate and parathyroid hormone (PTH) should be monitored every 6 months. If the PTH is elevated, 25-hydroxyvitamin D should be measured.

Indications for referral to nephrologists include:
- eGFR less than 45 mL/min/1.73 m^2
- doubt about the diagnosis
- blood pressure control not achieved
- active urine sediment (i.e. urine containing red cells and cellular casts)
- anaemia
- phosphate over 1.8 mmol/L or PTH more than twice the upper limit of normal.

The clinical clues suggesting glomerular disease other than diabetes include:
- an acute onset of renal disease or onset of proteinuria less than 5 years from the onset of diabetes. However, this is more difficult to ascertain in type 2 diabetes as the true onset of disease is not known
- an active urine sediment
- the absence of diabetic retinopathy or neuropathy in type 1 diabetes
- signs and/or symptoms of other systemic diseases
- a significant decrease in the GFR (>30%) within 2–3 months of starting ACE inhibitors or angiotensin II receptor blockers (ARBs).

Treatment

The risk of progression of diabetic nephropathy may be reduced by:
- ACE inhibitors and ARBs
- Blood pressure control
- Control of glycaemia
- Diet: protein restriction.

ACE inhibitors and ARBs

ACE inhibitors reduce blood pressure as well as glomerular pressure. They also antagonize the profibrotic effects of angiotensin II (see 'Pathogenesis', above). ACE inhibitors decrease microalbuminuria and reduce the risk of progression of proteinuria in both type 1 and type 2 diabetes. A drug-specific benefit in diabetic nephropathy independent of blood pressure control has been shown for ARBs in type 2 diabetes.

The dose of ACE inhibitor should be titrated up until either the microalbuminuria disappears or the maximum dose is reached. If the use of ACE inhibitors is limited by their side-effects (e.g. hyperkalaemia or cough), ARBs can be used as alternatives. ARBs (e.g. irbesartan, losartan) may also be added in patients whose hypertension or proteinuria is not controlled with ACE inhibitors. Combining ARBs with maximal doses of ACE inhibitors may further reduce blood pressure and proteinuria. Serum potassium must be monitored. A mild chronic increase in potassium (up to 5.5 mmol/L) is acceptable.

Blood pressure control

The effectiveness of strict *blood pressure control* in slowing the decline in renal function has been shown in several studies. In patients with nephropathy due to type 1 diabetes, higher blood pressures are associated with a worsening of microalbuminuria. In the United Kingdom Prospective Diabetes Study (UKPDS), tighter blood pressure control was associated with a reduced risk of microalbuminuria in type 2 diabetes.

Blood pressure should be maintained at less than 130/80 mmHg in diabetic patients without proteinuria. The target blood pressure in patients with microalbuminuria or overt nephropathy is slightly lower (125/75 mmHg).

Glycaemic control

Improved *glycaemic control* has been shown to reduce the rate of development and progression of nephropathy. The Diabetes Control and Complications Trial (DCCT) showed that tight glycaemic control in type 1 diabetes reduces the risk of development and progression of microalbuminuria by approximately 40% and 54% respectively. In the UKPDS, tight glycaemic control resulted in a 33% relative risk reduction for the development of microalbuminuria in type 2 diabetes.

Insulin requirements may decrease during the phase of declining renal function, as the kidney is a site of insulin degradation. Metformin and sulphonylureas are contraindicated in advanced renal failure.

Other treatments

In a meta-analysis of smaller studies, *protein restriction* has been shown to reduce the decline in GFR. A consensus panel of the American Diabetes Association suggests a restriction of protein intake to 0.8 g/kg per day in patients with microalbuminuria or to less than 0.8 g/kg per day in overt nephropathy.

The leading cause of death in diabetic patients on dialysis is hyperlipidaemia, and this should be treated aggressively with statins. Stopping smoking is also likely to be of renal benefit.

Patients with end-stage renal disease require dialysis. Haemodialysis in diabetic patients is associated with more frequent complications such as hypotension (caused by autonomic neuropathy) and more difficult vascular access. Following the onset of end-stage renal disease, survival is shorter in patients with diabetes compared with those without diabetes but with similar clinical features.

> **Key points:**
>
> - The earliest clinical finding of diabetic nephropathy is microalbuminuria.
> - Microalbuminuria is an important predictor of progression to proteinuria, reduced GFR and end-stage renal disease.
> - The mechanisms by which diabetes leads to nephropathy involve AGEs, reactive oxygen species, signalling pathways involving protein kinase C, MAPK, growth factors, angiotensin II and haemodynamic factors.
> - The average time from the onset of diabetes to proteinuria is 15 years, and the average time from the onset of proteinuria to end-stage renal disease is 10 years.
> - As part of the diabetic follow-up, a spot urine sample must be sent to the laboratory for measurement of urine ACR. Microalbuminuria is defined as an ACR above 2.5 g/mol in men or above 3.5 g/mol in women.
> - Strict blood pressure and glycaemic control, ACE inhibitors, ARBs and protein restriction reduce the risk of progression of diabetic nephropathy.

Chapter 39

Diabetic neuropathy

In diabetic neuropathy, both myelinated and unmyelinated nerve fibres are lost. The development of diabetic neuropathy correlates with the duration of diabetes and glycaemic control. In diabetic neuropathy, the distal sensory and autonomic fibres are preferentially affected.

Epidemiology

The prevalence of neuropathy is estimated to be around 34% in type 1 diabetes and 26% in type 2 diabetes. Clinically detectable neuropathy occurred in 10% of patients with type 1 diabetes after 5 years of enrolment in the Diabetes Control and Complications Trial (DCCT). The incidence of neuropathy in type 2 diabetes is about 6% per year.

Pathogenesis

Metabolic and vascular factors and impaired nerve repair mechanisms are likely to contribute to the pathogenesis of diabetic neuropathy.

Metabolic risk factors

Metabolic factors that have been implicated in the pathogenesis of diabetic neuropathy include the following:

Lecture Notes: Endocrinology and Diabetes. By A. Sam and K. Meeran. Published 2009 by Blackwell Publishing. ISBN 978-1-4051-5345-4.

- *Advanced glycosylation end-products (AGEs):* AGEs are formed by non-enzymatic combination of some of the excess glucose with amino acids in proteins. Advanced glycosylation of essential nerve proteins has been implicated in the pathogenesis of diabetic neuropathy.
- *Sorbitol:* glucose that enters cells is metabolized in part by the enzyme aldose reductase to sorbitol. This process is more pronounced with chronic hyperglycaemia. The accumulation of intracellular sorbitol in tissues such as peripheral nerves results in a rise in cell osmolality, a decrease in intracellular myoinositol and Na–K-ATPase activity, and a slowing of nerve conduction velocities.
- *Oxidative stress:* hyperglycaemia results in the accumulation and stabilization of reactive oxygen species, which may damage peripheral nerves.

Vascular risk factors

Morphological abnormalities of the vasa nervorum (small arterioles supplying the nerves) are present early in the course of diabetic polyneuropathy, and parallel the severity of the nerve fibre loss.

The prospective EURODIAB study showed that the incidence of neuropathy in type 1 diabetes is associated with potentially modifiable cardiovascular risk factors, including a raised triglyceride level, raised body mass index, smoking and hypertension.

Thrombomodulin and tissue plasminogen activator levels are reduced in peripheral nerve microvessels from diabetic patients. This suggests that an impairment of antithrombotic mechanisms may play a role in the pathogenesis of diabetic polyneuropathy.

Impairment of peripheral nerve repair

Loss of neurotrophic peptides that mediate nerve repair and regeneration may contribute to the pathogenesis of diabetic neuropathy. These peptides include nerve growth factor, brain-derived neurotrophic factor, neurotrophin-3, the insulin-like growth factors and vascular endothelial growth factor.

Clinical presentations

Diabetic neuropathy may manifest as:
- distal symmetrical polyneuropathy
- polyradiculopathy
- mononeuropathy
- autonomic neuropathy.

Distal symmetrical polyneuropathy

Distal symmetrical polyneuropathy is the most common form of diabetic neuropathy. Patients may present with distal (glove and stocking distribution) sensory loss or paraesthesia, i.e. a sensation of numbness, tingling, burning or sharpness that starts in the feet and spreads proximally. Some patients develop neuropathic pain, typically involving the lower extremities, usually at rest and worst at night. This is occasionally preceded by improvements in glycaemic control. Painful diabetic neuropathy may be acute (lasting less than 12 months) or chronic.

Signs of distal symmetrical polyneuropathy include loss of pinprick, temperature, vibration and joint position sensation, and diminished ankle reflexes.

Polyradiculopathy

Diabetic *polyradiculopathy* is characterized by severe pain in the distribution of one or more nerve roots. Diabetic polyradiculopathy usually resolves over 6–12 months. Pain over the chest or abdomen may be due to intercostal or truncal radiculopathy. Sensory symptoms may be accompanied by muscle weakness. Patients with involvement of the lumbar plexus may present with thigh or hip pain and weakness of the hip flexors or extensors (*diabetic amyotrophy*).

Mononeuropathy

Diabetic patients may present with motor weakness and pain in the distribution of a single cranial or peripheral nerve (e.g. cranial nerves III, IV, VI or VII, median, ulnar or peroneal nerve). Mononeuropathy is less common than polyneuropathy. The most common presentation of mononeuropathy in diabetic patients is ptosis and ophthalmoplegia due to *IIIrd cranial nerve palsy*. Patients may also present with simultaneous involvement of more than one nerve (mononeuropathy multiplex).

Autonomic neuropathy

Longstanding diabetes may lead to autonomic dysfunction involving the cholinergic, noradrenergic and peptidergic (e.g. substance P, pancreatic polypeptide) systems. Autonomic neuropathy usually involves multiple systems:
- *Cardiovascular*: there may be resting tachycardia, *postural hypotension*, neuropathic oedema (due to loss of sympathetic vascular innervation and increased peripheral blood flow through arteriovenous shunts).
- *Gastrointestinal*: delayed gastric emptying (*gastroparesis*) may present with anorexia, nausea, vomiting, early satiety and bloating. Altered small and large bowel motility (autonomic enteropathy) may present with diarrhoea and/or constipation.
- *Genitourinary*: bladder dysfunction (inability to sense a full bladder, failure to void completely, incontinence, recurrent urinary tract infection), erectile dysfunction, retrograde ejaculation and female sexual dysfunction (reduced libido, reduced vaginal lubrication and dyspareunia) can occur.
- *Hypoglycaemia unawareness* arises when reduced adrenaline release results in a loss of the adrenergic symptoms of hypoglycaemia.

• Hyperhidrosis (upper extremities), anhidrosis (lower extremities, resulting in dry skin and cracking of the feet and an increased risk of foot ulcers).

Diagnosis

Diabetic neuropathy should be suspected in all patients with type 2 diabetes and in any patient with type 1 diabetes of more than 5 years' duration.

Pinprick, temperature, vibration (using a 128 Hz tuning fork) and pressure sensation (using a 10 g monofilament) must be examined to assess sensory function.

The clinical features of diabetic neuropathy are similar to those of other neuropathies (Box 39.1). Other possible aetiologies should be excluded before a diagnosis of diabetic neuropathy is made.

In the Rochester Diabetic Study, the most sensitive tests for the diagnosis of diabetic neuropathy were nerve conduction studies and autonomic testing by using heart rate change (R–R interval on the electrocardiogram) during the Valsalva manoeuvre.

When *gastroparesis* is suspected, an upper endoscopy or a barium meal should be performed to exclude mechanical obstruction and mucosal disease. These tests may also show retained food after an overnight fast. A barium follow-through examination is necessary in patients with colicky abdominal pain to exclude a small bowel lesion.

The best study to document gastroparesis is nuclear medicine scintigraphy after the ingestion of a radio-labelled meal. Gastric retention of more than 70% at 2 hours and more than 10% at 4 hours is abnormal. In patients with type 1 diabetes and enteropathy, coeliac disease must be excluded.

Diagnostic evaluation of diabetic *bladder dysfunction* includes cystometry and urodynamic studies.

Treatment

Chronic painful diabetic neuropathy is difficult to treat. With tighter glycaemic control, clinically detectable neuropathy is reduced in both type 1 (DCCT findings) and type 2 diabetes. Although tighter glycaemic control improves nerve conduction velocity, existing symptoms may not improve. Hypoglycaemic unawareness due to autonomic neuropathy may limit efforts to optimize glycaemic control.

Pain control

Tricyclic antidepressants (e.g. amitriptyline) are useful in the treatment of painful neuropathy. However, their use may be limited by side-effects such as sedation. Nortriptyline and desipramine are associated with lower levels of sedation.

Duloxetine is also effective in reducing pain scores. Side-effects include somnolence and constipation. Other agents used for painful neuropathy include pregabalin, oxycodone, tramadol, gabapentin, carbamazepine, phenytoin, lamotrigine, venlafaxine and capsaicin cream. Difficult cases should be referred to pain management teams.

Aldose reductase inhibitors reduce the accumulation of sorbitol in nerve cells. However, despite some benefits for motor neuropathy, they do not offer significant symptomatic relief for sensory or autonomic neuropathy.

Surgical decompression should be considered for patients with carpal tunnel syndrome.

Postural hypotension

Exacerbating drugs (e.g. tranquillizers, antidepressants, diuretics) should be discontinued if possible. Dorsiflexion of the feet before standing, standing slowly in 'stages' and tensing the legs by crossing them while standing, may be helpful. Body stockings and gravity suits (used to increase peripheral

---

Box 39.1 Differential diagnosis of diabetic neuropathy

Uraemia
Vitamin B_{12}/folate deficiency
Hypothyroidism
Amyloidosis, acute intermittent porphyria
Toxins: alcohol, medications (e.g. chemotherapy), heavy metals (lead, mercury)
Inflammation: chronic inflammatory demyelinating polyneuropathy, connective tissue diseases/vasculitis
Infection: HIV, leprosy
Paraneoplastic syndromes
Hereditary sensory and motor neuropathy

vascular tone) may also be used but have limited success.

Medical treatment of postural hypotension consists of increasing the plasma volume with the mineralocorticoid *fludrocortisone* (100–400 μg per day), a high-salt diet and adequate hydration. However, this regimen can cause hypertension or peripheral oedema. Treatment of anaemia, if present, may also be helpful.

Other treatments that have been tried with variable success include atrial tachypacing, midodrine (alpha-adrenoreceptor agonist), fluoxetine and desmopressin. The somatostatin analogue octreotide may be tried (50 μg three times a day, subcutaneously) in refractory and symptomatic postural or postprandial hypotension.

Neuropathic oedema

Sympathomimetic drugs such as midodrine and ephedrine can reduce arteriovenous shunting and may have a beneficial effect on neuropathic oedema. Non-pharmacological treatments include foot elevation when sitting and support stockings.

Careful foot care is essential to prevent foot infection and ulceration. Patients with diabetic neuropathy should be referred to a podiatrist. The patient must be advised to carefully inspect his or her feet daily.

Gastroparesis

Symptoms of gastroparesis may be minimized by more frequent, smaller meals that are easier to digest (liquid) and are low in fat and fibre. Optimizing glycaemic control may improve gastric function. Prokinetics such as metoclopramide (5–10 mg three times a day), domperidone (10–20 mg three times daily), erythromycin (125–250 mg three times daily) and cisapride (10–20 mg three times a day) in countries in which it remains available may be administered 10–15 minutes before meals. Metoclopramide and domperidone are dopamine antagonists. Erythromycin interacts with the motilin receptor.

Patients who are unable to maintain their nutritional status or adequate hydration orally may require jejunal feeding tubes.

Autonomic enteropathy

Treatment of diabetic autonomic enteropathy includes loperamide (for diabetic diarrhoea in the absence of bacterial overgrowth), rotating antibiotics (for bacterial overgrowth) and stool softeners for constipation. Some patients with intractable diarrhoea may respond to octreotide.

Bladder dysfunction

Treatment of urinary retention initially consists of a strict voluntary urination schedule. Scheduled urinations may be coupled with bethanechol, which increases detrusor muscle contraction. More advanced cases require intermittent self–catheterization and, in extreme cases, resection of the internal sphincter at the bladder neck.

Sexual dysfunction

Oral sildenafil (a phosphodiesterase type 5 inhibitor) is an effective and well-tolerated treatment for erectile dysfunction in men with diabetes. Retrograde ejaculation has been treated with an antihistamine. Treatment for female sexual dysfunction involves vaginal lubricants and estrogen creams.

Key points:

- The development of diabetic neuropathy correlates with the duration of diabetes and with glycaemic control.
- Diabetic neuropathy may manifest as distal symmetrical polyneuropathy, polyradiculopathy, mononeuropathy and autonomic neuropathy.
- Distal symmetrical polyneuropathy is the most common form of diabetic neuropathy.
- With tighter glycaemic control, clinically detectable neuropathy is reduced in both type 1 and type 2 diabetes.
- Tricyclic antidepressants and duloxetine are usually the first-line treatments for pain control in diabetic neuropathy.
- Medical treatment of postural hypotension consists of increasing the plasma volume with the mineralocorticoid fludrocortisone, a high-salt diet and adequate hydration.

Chapter 40

Musculoskeletal and dermatological manifestations of diabetes

Diabetic foot ulcers and infections comprise the most common dermatological and musculoskeletal complications of diabetes. Neuropathic arthropathy (Charcot joint) and other musculoskeletal and dermatological manifestations of diabetes are covered in later sections of this chapter.

Diabetic foot ulcers

Foot ulcers are a major cause of hospitalization, morbidity and mortality in patients with diabetes. Diabetic foot ulcers account for a significant proportion of all non-traumatic amputations (e.g. about two-thirds in the USA). The lifetime risk of a foot ulcer for diabetic patients (type 1 or 2) may be as high as 25%.

Aetiology

Diabetic foot problems are often secondary to neuropathy and peripheral arterial disease.

Neuropathy is present in over 80% of patients with foot ulcers. Sensory neuropathy results in decreased sensation of temperature, pain and pressure and makes injuries and blisters less noticeable. Motor neuropathy and muscle imbalance can lead to foot deformities. Autonomic neuropathy can

cause reduced sweat and sebaceous gland secretion resulting in dry, cracked skin.

Peripheral arterial disease reduces the blood supply needed for the healing of ulcers and infections. Peripheral arterial disease in patients with diabetes is often both macrovascular and microvascular.

Trauma is the usual precipitating event for diabetic foot ulcers. After the tissues are injured, the above factors can prevent normal healing and increase the risk of infection. In addition, hyperglycaemia impairs neutrophil function and host defence mechanisms.

Clinical presentations

All patients with diabetes should have regular comprehensive foot evaluations. It is important to ascertain duration of diabetes, glycaemic control, presence of neuropathy, micro- or macrovascular disease, history of cigarette smoking, previous foot ulcers and lower limb bypasses or amputation.

Assessment of the diabetic foot should look for the clinical features summarized in Box 40.1.

Peripheral neuropathy

Sensory neuropathy can be detected by a *10g monofilament*. Monofilament testing detects patients who have lost the protective pressure sensation and are susceptible to ulceration.

Lecture Notes: Endocrinology and Diabetes. By A. Sam and K. Meeran. Published 2009 by Blackwell Publishing. ISBN 978-1-4051-5345-4.

Box 40.1 Clinical features in the assessment of the diabetic foot

Neuropathy
Ischaemia
Bony deformity
Callus
Swelling
Skin integrity/breakdown (especially between the toes and under the metatarsal heads)
Infection
Necrosis

The filament is pressed against the plantar aspects of the first and fifth toes, the first, third and fifth metatarsal heads and the plantar surface of the heel (Fig. 40.1a). The monofilament buckles at a given force of 10 g (Fig. 40.1b). The monofilament should not be applied at any site until callus has been removed.

Vibration sensation is assessed using a 128 Hz tuning fork. A neurothesiometer, if available, can also be used to detect sensory neuropathy. It is a device that delivers a vibratory stimulus to the foot that increases as the voltage is raised.

Peripheral arterial disease

Peripheral arterial disease should be suspected in patients with *intermittent claudication*, cool temperature, absence of hair and presence of foot ulcers.

An absence of *pedal pulses* (Fig. 40.2) and a prolongation of venous filling should prompt further investigation and referral to the vascular surgical team. To measure the venous filling time, a prominent pedal vein is identified with the patient in a supine position. The leg is then elevated to 45° for 1 minute to collapse the vein. The patient then sits up and hangs the leg over the examination table. If more than 20 seconds elapse before the vein bulges above the skin, important arterial disease is likely to be present.

The *ankle–brachial pressure index* (ABPI) is calculated by measuring the systolic blood pressure (using a small hand-held Doppler) in the brachial, posterior tibial and dorsalis pedis arteries. The

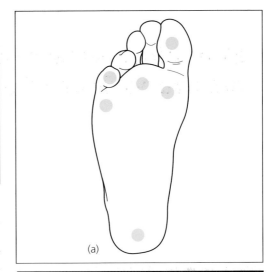

(a)

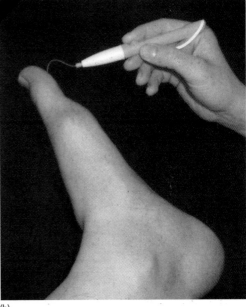

(b)

Figure 40.1 (a) Sites for 10 g monofilament testing. (b) 10 g monofilament testing.

highest of four measurements in the ankles and feet is divided by the highest of the brachial measurements. The normal ABPI is 1.0–1.3. An ABPI of 0.90 or less is diagnostic of peripheral arterial disease. An ABPI over 1.30 suggests the presence of calcified vessels, which is common in diabetes.

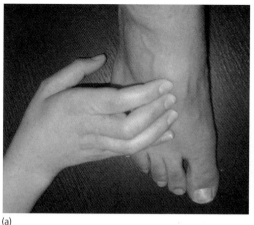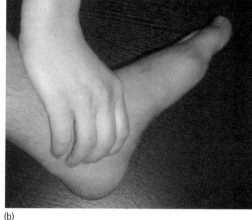

(a)   (b)

Figure 40.2 (a) Palpation of the dorsalis pedis pulse. (b) Palpation of the posterior tibial pulse.

Infected ulcers

Infections usually begin around cracks in the skin of the foot or around the toe nail bed (paronychia), or arise from ulcers. Diabetic foot infections are diagnosed clinically on the basis of:

- at least two of the following: erythema, warmth, swelling, tenderness
- pus coming out of an ulcer site or a nearby sinus tract.

Patients with cellulitis who have sensory neuropathy often do not experience pain. In necrotizing infections, purple/black discoloration of the skin, cutaneous bullae or soft tissue gas may occur.

Severity of ulcer infection

Diabetic foot infections may be mild, moderate or severe:

- *Mild infections (involvement of the skin or superficial subcutaneous tissues):* two or more markers of inflammation (erythema, warmth, swelling, tenderness), purulence and cellulitis extending for less than 2 cm around the ulcer.
- *Moderate infections (more extensive infection or involvement of deeper tissues):* cellulitis extending >2 cm around an ulcer, lymphangitic streaking, deep tissue abscess, gangrene (necrosis) or involvement of muscle, tendon, joint or bone.

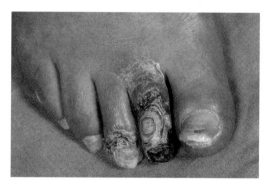

Figure 40.3 Diabetic foot with dry gangrene (caused by ischaemia), loss of hair and nail dystrophy.

- *Severe infections (signs of systemic toxicity or metabolic instability):* fever, chills, tachycardia, tachypnoea, hypotension, confusion, vomiting and blood tests showing severe hyperglycaemia, leukocytosis, metabolic acidosis and raised urea and creatinine (see 'Investigations' below).

Gangrene (necrosis) is caused by ischaemia and is classified as wet or dry. In wet gangrene, ischaemia is caused by septic vasculitis associated with soft tissue infection. The tissues are black, brown or grey, moist and often malodorous. In dry gangrene, ischaemia is caused by peripheral arterial disease. The tissues are black, hard and mummified (Fig. 40.3). There is a clean demarcation line between necrosis and viable tissue.

Up to two-thirds of patients with diabetic foot ulcers may have *osteomyelitis*. The following factors increase the likelihood of osteomyelitis in patients with diabetic foot ulcers:

- visible bone or the ability to probe to bone (using a sterile, blunt, stainless steel probe)
- ulcer size >2 cm × 2 cm
- ulcer depth >3 mm
- ulcer duration longer than 1–2 weeks
- erythrocyte sedimentation rate (ESR) >70 mm per hour (see 'Investigations' below).

Investigations

Blood tests

Blood tests should include full blood count, urea and electrolytes, ESR, C-reactive protein (CRP), blood glucose and glycated haemoglobin (HbA_{1c}).

Ulcer swabs and bone biopsy

Diabetic foot ulcers should be swabbed for *microscopy, culture and sensitivity*. Organisms isolated from superficial swabs may not reflect the organisms responsible for deeper infections. In the setting of deep tissue infections or osteomyelitis, cultures of deep tissue should be obtained at the time of debridement.

The correlation between superficial swab culture and bone biopsy culture is poor (up to 20%). Bone biopsy allows a histopathological diagnosis as well as microbiological culture and sensitivity. However, it is not always possible or practical to perform a bone biopsy as the incision made for a biopsy may not heal in those with peripheral arterial disease. Therefore patients may be treated empirically for the expected pathogens.

The microbiology of diabetic foot ulcers varies depending on the extent of involvement:

- *Superficial ulcers*: aerobic Gram-positive cocci including *Staphylococcus aureus, Streptococcus agalactiae, Streptococcus pyogenes* and coagulase-negative staphylococci. Methicillin-resistant *Staphylococcus aureus* should be presumed and treated empirically.

- *Deep, chronic ulcers*: Gram-negative bacilli such as *Pseudomonas aeruginosa* and *Proteus mirabilis*, in addition to the above pathogens.
- *Ulcers with extensive local inflammation and signs of systemic toxicity* should be presumed to have anaerobic organisms as well as the above pathogens.

In patients with chronic ulcers or those previously treated with antibiotics, infections are usually polymicrobial. When multiple organisms grow from a culture, it is difficult to determine which ones are true pathogens.

Imaging

In patients with diabetic foot infections, a *foot radiograph* must be performed to look for possible osteomyelitis.

If the foot radiograph is normal, the patient is treated for soft tissue infection for 2 weeks and the foot X-ray is repeated in 2–4 weeks. If the repeat radiograph remains normal, osteomyelitis is unlikely.

If either the initial or follow-up foot radiograph is characteristic of osteomyelitis, the person is treated for osteomyelitis after obtaining appropriate specimens for culture. Those with one or more of the risk factors for osteomyelitis (see above) whose radiographs are indeterminate for osteomyelitis should have a magnetic resonance imaging (MRI) scan (see below).

Radiographs are useful for demonstrating features of chronic osteomyelitis such as cortical erosion, periosteal reaction, mixed bony lucency, sclerosis and sequestra. Radiographs are of limited sensitivity and specificity in the detection of acute osteomyelitis. Osteolysis and periosteal new bone formation may not be evident until 2 weeks after onset of infection. However, MRI scanning demonstrates abnormal marrow oedema as early as 3–5 days after the onset of infection.

MRI identifies bone marrow oedema, soft tissue inflammation and cortical destruction. It cannot reliably differentiate between marrow oedema caused by osteomyelitis and that due to neuropathic (Charcot) arthropathy. MRI may also overestimate the extent of infection, since marrow oedema caused by osteomyelitis and surrounding reactive oedema cannot be distinguished. Furthermore, bone marrow changes may persist for weeks to months after osteomyelitis begins to respond to treatment. Gadolinium contrast-enhanced MRI is useful for demonstrating sinus tracts, fistulas and abscesses.

The *three-phase bone scan* uses a radionuclide tracer that accumulates in areas of increased osteoblast activity (e.g. ^{99m}technetium bound to a phosphorus-containing compound). Scans are performed immediately after tracer injection (blood flow phase), 15 minutes after injection (blood pool phase) and 4 hours after injection (osseous phase).

In patients with osteomyelitis, the uptake is increased in all three phases. In the setting of cellulitis, there is increased activity only in the first two phases. However, non-infectious disorders such as fracture or Charcot arthropathy are also associated with bone formation, and therefore increased radionuclide tracer uptake, leading to false-positive results. False-negative results are possible in the setting of chronic osteomyelitis with impaired blood flow or infarction or in early osteomyelitis.

Vascular investigations

Duplex ultrasonography allows anatomical localization of arterial stenoses and assessment of blood flow haemodynamics. The normal Doppler waveform is triphasic (a forward flow systolic peak, reversal of flow in early diastole and forward flow in late diastole). With progressive peripheral arterial disease, there is elimination of the reverse flow and a decrease in systolic peak.

Magnetic resonance angiography has shown promise to become a time-efficient and cost-effective tool for the complete assessment of peripheral arterial disease. It is usually performed if revascularization is being considered.

Angiography is considered the 'gold standard' of diagnostic evaluation for peripheral arterial disease. However, it is associated with the risks of iodinated contrast agents such as contrast nephropathy, and the risks inherent in percutaneous intervention.

Treatment

Advice for prophylactic foot care should be given to all patients with diabetes (see Chapter 35). Patients at high risk of developing foot ulcers must be referred to a podiatrist. Patients are at high risk of future plantar ulceration if they have neuropathy or neuropathic foot deformities, such as bunions or calluses, peripheral arterial disease or a previous history of foot ulceration or amputation.

The management of diabetic foot ulcers includes:
- attentive wound management and debridement
- antibiotic therapy
- relief of pressure on the ulcer
- revascularization
- glycaemic control.

Coordination of care among providers is important for keeping rates of amputation as low as possible.

Debridement

The management of patients with superficial ulcers includes debridement by a podiatrist, good local wound care and relief of pressure on the ulcer. Patients should avoid unnecessary ambulation. Open lesions are covered with a custom-fit piece of non-adherent dry dressing. Patients should be closely monitored. If the ulcer does not improve, hospitalization for bed rest and intravenous antibiotic therapy may be necessary.

Prompt surgical debridement and intervention is critical in the presence of:
- a large area of infected sloughy tissue
- infections complicated by abscess: localized fluctuance and expression of pus
- crepitus with gas in the soft tissues on X-ray (gas immediately adjacent to an ulcer may have entered the foot through the ulcer and is of less importance)
- purplish discoloration of the skin, indicating subcutaneous necrosis, or necrotizing fasciitis
- extensive bone or joint involvement.

Following surgical debridement, vacuum-assisted wound closure may be used in the treatment of open wounds to improve healing and closure. A sponge is secured under a clear dressing with tubing extending to a collection canister. A pump applies suction and causes fluid to flow out of the wound. Contraindications to vacuum-assisted closure include a visible vascular structure in the wound, incomplete debridement, malignancy in the wound, untreated osteomyelitis or an open fistula.

Antibiotics

Antibiotics used for the empirical treatment of mild, moderate and severe diabetic foot infections are summarized in Box 40.2.

The duration of antibiotic therapy should be tailored to individual clinical circumstances.

In patients with mild infection, oral antibiotics should be continued until the infection has resolved (usually about 1–2 weeks). It is not necessary to continue antibiotics for the entire duration that the wound remains open.

Box 40.2 Antibiotics for the empirical treatment of diabetic foot infections

Oral antibiotics for empirical treatment of mild diabetic foot infections
Regimens active against streptococci and MRSA
- Clindamycin
- Linezolid
- Penicillin + doxycycline

Regimens active against streptococci, MRSA, aerobic Gram-negative bacilli and anaerobes
- Amoxicillin–clavulanate + trimethoprim–sulfamethoxazole
- Clindamycin + ciprofloxacin (or levofloxacin)

Parenteral antibiotics for empirical treatment of moderate/severe diabetic foot infections
Vancomycin (active against MRSA) + one of the following (active against aerobic Gram-negative bacilli and anaerobes):
- Ampicillin–sulbactam
- Piperacillin–tazobactam
- Ticarcillin–clavulanate
- Imipenem
- Meropenem
- Metronidazole + one of the following: ceftazidime, ciprofloxacin or aztreonam

MRSA, methicillin-resistant *Staphylococcus aureus*.

In patients with infections requiring surgical debridement, intravenous antibiotics should be given perioperatively. In the absence of osteomyelitis, antibiotics should be continued until signs of infection appear to have resolved (usually 2–4 weeks). If there is a good response to intravenous antibiotics, oral agents can be used to complete the course of treatment. The optimal regimen and when to switch to oral antibiotics depends on the clinical features of each case.

Patients requiring amputation of the involved limb should receive intravenous antibiotics perioperatively. If the entire area of infection is fully resected, a brief course of oral antibiotics (for about a week) after surgery is usually sufficient.

If clinical evidence of infection persists beyond the expected duration, issues of compliance, antibiotic resistance, undiagnosed deep abscess and ischaemia should be considered.

The optimal duration of antibiotic therapy for osteomyelitis is not certain. Parenteral antibiotics should be continued at least until debrided bone has been covered by vascularized soft tissue. This usually takes at least 6 weeks from the last debridement. Long-term parenteral antibiotic administration may be accomplished on an outpatient basis via a long-term intravenous catheter with close monitoring. Monitoring may include weekly serum drug levels, renal function, liver function and/or haematological function, depending on the antibiotic used.

Relief of pressure: footwear and total contact casting

Devices used to relieve pressure on the ulcer ('mechanical off-loading') include removable cast walkers, half-shoes and total contact casts.

Total contact casting is an alternative to prolonged bed rest for the relief of pressure on the ulcer. This allows ambulation and is often preferred by patients. As many of the patients have markedly impaired sensation in their feet and legs, it is important to check regularly that pressure from the cast is not causing the formation of new ulcers. Total contact casting is contraindicated in patients with soft tissue infection or osteomyelitis.

Extra-depth and extra-width therapeutic shoes with special inserts are frequently prescribed for individuals with diabetes to prevent recurrence of foot ulcers.

Revascularization

In diabetic patients with peripheral arterial disease, revascularization and improvement of tissue perfusion help to control infection and promote healing of foot ulcers.

Angioplasty is indicated for single or multiple stenoses or short-segment occlusions of less than 10 cm. If angioplasty is not possible due to long arterial occlusions or widespread lesions, revascularization may be achieved by *arterial bypass surgery*. However, this is a major operation with its own inherent risks and should be reserved for patients who do not respond to conservative treatment and antibiotics, and require operative debridement with toe or ray amputation.

In arterial bypass surgery, an autologous vein is used to fashion a conduit from either the femoral or the popliteal artery down to a tibial artery in the lower leg, or the dorsalis pedis artery on the dorsum of the foot. After surgery, the leg has wounds at the sites of graft insertion and vein harvesting. Wounds overlying the arterial graft must be kept free from infection to avoid blockage of the graft. Postoperative oedema is common, and it is important to elevate the leg.

Novel therapies

Several novel therapies that may improve ulcer healing have been reported. These include custom-fit semi-permeable polymeric membrane dressings, cultured human dermis, platelet releasate, platelet-derived growth factor and human epidermal growth factor.

Charcot arthropathy

The following factors have been suggested to contribute to the pathogenesis of neuropathic (Charcot) arthropathy:

- Peripheral neuropathy and lack of proprioception may result in ligamentous laxity, increased range of joint movement, instability and damage by minor trauma.
- Autonomic neuropathy results in vasomotor changes, the formation of arteriovenous shunts and reduced effective skin and bone blood flow.
- There may be an exaggerated local inflammatory response to trauma (mediated by proinflammatory cytokines).

Neuropathic arthropathy in diabetic patients most commonly affects the joints of the foot and ankle: the tarsus and tarsometatarsal joints, metatarsophalangeal joints and ankle.

Neuroarthropathy affects about one in 700 diabetic patients with either type 1 or type 2 diabetes. These patients typically have longstanding diabetes and are in their sixth or seventh decade. However, younger patients may also be affected.

Clinical presentations

Patients with Charcot arthropathy may present with:

- a sudden onset of unilateral warmth, redness and oedema over the foot or ankle, usually with a history of minor trauma. About 30% of patients complain of pain or discomfort.
- slowly progressing arthropathy with insidious swelling over months or years, collapse of the arch of the mid-foot, and bony prominences and deformities.

The neuroarthropathy is bilateral in about 20% of cases.

Investigations

In acute Charcot arthropathy, the inflammatory markers may be increased. A plain radiograph of the foot may show mild or non-specific changes. Abnormalities that may be seen on a foot radiograph include:

- soft tissue swelling, loss of joint space and osteopenia

• forefoot: bone resorption, osteolysis of the phalanges, partial or complete disappearance of the metatarsal heads and 'pencil-pointing' of the phalangeal and metatarsal shafts

• midfoot and hindfoot: osseous fragmentation, sclerosis, new bone formation, subluxation and dislocation.

A *radioisotope bone scan* may show an increased uptake in neuropathic arthropathy. However, increased isotope uptake may be seen both in patients with diabetic neuroarthropathy and in those with peripheral neuropathy alone.

MRI scanning may facilitate the diagnosis of stress fractures and the visualization of torn ligaments and intra-articular fragmentation. However, the changes of acute neuropathic arthropathy may be indistinguishable from those of osteomyelitis.

Treatment

Acute-onset Charcot arthropathy is treated with *avoidance of weight-bearing* on the affected joint until oedema and erythema have resolved, and radiological signs have improved. A minimum of 8 weeks without weight-bearing is recommended for disease of the midfoot. Patients may progress through partial weight-bearing in a cast brace to full weight-bearing in approximately 4–5 months. Good chiropody and well-fitting shoes are essential.

Alternatively a *total contact cast* may be used from the time of diagnosis. This is a very efficient method of redistributing plantar pressure. The cast should be changed every 2 weeks. A transition to custom-made orthoses and commercial footwear accommodating the patient may be possible at about 9–10 weeks.

The swollen, uncomfortable, hot foot of active Charcot arthropathy may improve with an intravenous infusion of *pamidronate*. Oral bisphosphonates (alendronate) may also be useful. In patients with both Charcot arthropathy and renal insufficiency in whom bisphosphonates are contraindicated, intranasal calcitonin may potentially be useful.

Joint disorganization may be severe and irreversible in chronic cases of Charcot arthropathy. Common deformities such as the 'rocker-bottom foot' transfer weight-bearing to areas that may lack sensation and tolerate it poorly, leading to ulceration and infection. Surgical correction is best avoided in most patients. However, in carefully selected cases, acceptable alignment may be achieved by surgery, thereby preserving soft tissue viability and avoiding ulceration and amputation.

Other musculoskeletal manifestations of diabetes

A number of musculoskeletal conditions have been associated with diabetes mellitus (Box 40.3).

Limited joint mobility

Limited joint mobility is common in patients with diabetes mellitus. It is characterized by a limitation of joint movement, particularly in the small joints of the hands. Limited joint mobility is painless. It is commonly associated with thickening and waxiness of the skin on the dorsal surface of the fingers.

The risk increases with poor glycaemic control, duration of diabetes and cigarette smoking. It may be secondary to the deposition of abnormal collagen in connective tissue around the joints. Enzymatic and non-enzymatic glycosylation of collagen, abnormal crosslinking of collagen resulting in resistance to degradation, and increased

---

Box 40.3 Musculoskeletal conditions associated with diabetes

Diabetic foot infections
Neuropathic (Charcot) arthropathy
Limited joint mobility
Carpal tunnel syndrome
Dupuytren's contracture
Flexor tenosynovitis
Shoulder: adhesive capsulitis, calcific periarthritis
Diffuse idiopathic skeletal hyperostosis
Diabetic muscle infarction

collagen hydration may all play a role. Microangiopathy and neuropathy may contribute to contractures via fibrosis and disuse.

Stiffness and contractures result in decreased grip strength and difficulties with hand function. Examination of the hands may show contractures of the metacarpophalangeal, proximal and sometimes distal interphalangeal joints. Other joints may occasionally be involved. The 'prayer sign' test is performed by asking the patient to flatten the hands together as in prayer. This helps to identify contractures in the metacarpophalangeal, proximal and distal interphalangeal joints. Imaging studies are not typically used to diagnose limited joint mobility.

Limited joint mobility is difficult to treat. Glycaemic control should be optimized. Physiotherapy with passive palmar stretching and occupational therapy may improve hand function. Patients must be advised to stop smoking. Injection of the palmar tendon sheath with corticosteroids has been used.

Osteoporosis

The association between diabetes mellitus and osteoporosis remains controversial. Bone mineral density is lower in those with type 1 diabetes and normal or increased in those with type 2 diabetes. However, fracture risk appears to be increased in patients with both type 1 and type 2 diabetes. This is possibly related to factors in addition to bone mineral density, such as duration of diabetes, diabetic complications, treatment and risk of falling.

Diabetic muscle infarction

Diabetic muscle infarction is a rare condition characterized by an acute or subacute onset of muscle pain, swelling and tenderness, usually in the muscles of the thigh and calf. It affects patients with relatively longstanding diabetes. The pathogenesis is uncertain. The differential diagnosis includes infective myositis, intramuscular haematoma due to coagulopathy, venous thrombosis and neoplasm.

Investigations should include full blood count, creatine kinase, ESR, clotting screen, blood culture, plain radiograph, venous Doppler ultrasound and MRI of the affected and contralateral limb. MRI may show increased T2 signal in affected muscle, fascia and subcutaneous tissues.

The definitive diagnosis of diabetic muscle infarction requires biopsy of the affected area of muscle to demonstrate ischaemic necrosis and exclude infection. Surgical exploration and excisional biopsy is recommended in patients in whom a rapidly progressive infection of muscle or fascia cannot be excluded. Patients should also receive low-dose aspirin.

Dermatological manifestations of diabetes

Protracted wound healing and skin ulcerations are the most common dermatological manifestations of diabetes.

Diabetic dermopathy (or 'pigmented pretibial papules') begin as erythematous areas that evolve into areas of circular hyperpigmentation. The lesions are more common in elderly diabetic men and are caused by mechanical trauma in the pretibial region. Bullous diseases are also seen.

Necrobiosis lipodica diabeticorum is a rare skin manifestation of diabetes that predominantly affects young females with type 1 diabetes, retinopathy and neuropathy. These lesions start in the pretibial region as erythematous papules or plaque, gradually darken and develop irregular margins, with shiny atrophic centres.

Acanthosis nigricans (hyperpigmented velvety plaques on the neck or axillae) is a sign of insulin resistance.

Granuloma annulare (localized or generalized) are erythematous papules coalescing in rings especially on the backs of the hands and fingers.

Lipoatrophy and lipodystrophy can occur at insulin injection sites. Diabetic sclerodactyly is characterized by thickening and waxiness of the skin on the dorsa of the fingers and may be associated with limited joint mobility. Pruritus and dry skin are common in diabetic patients and are relieved by moisturizers.

Key points:

- Foot ulcers are a major cause of hospitalization, morbidity and mortality in patients with diabetes.
- Diabetic foot problems often occur secondary to neuropathy and peripheral arterial disease.
- Clinical evaluation of the diabetic foot should look for neuropathy, ischaemia, bony deformity, callus, swelling, skin integrity/breakdown, infection and necrosis.
- Investigations in a diabetic patient with foot problems include blood tests for full blood count, urea and electrolytes, ESR, CRP, blood glucose and HbA$_{1c}$, an ulcer swab for microscopy, culture and sensitivity, a foot radiograph, and duplex ultrasonography.
- The management of diabetic foot ulcers includes debridement, antibiotic therapy, relief of pressure, revascularization and glycaemic control.
- Neuropathic arthropathy in individuals with diabetes most commonly affects the joints of the foot and ankle.
- Acute-onset Charcot arthropathy is treated with avoidance of weight-bearing on the affected joint or total contact casts.

Index

269